D1272695

MENTAL AND ELEMENTAL NUTRIENTS

A Physician's Guide to Nutrition and Health Care

MENTAL AND ELEMENTAL NUTRIENTS

A Physician's Guide to Nutrition and Health Care

Carl C. Pfeiffer, Ph.D., M.D.
and the Publications Committee
of the Brain Bio Center

A Brain Bio Book

KEATS PUBLISHING, INC. New Canaan, Connecticut

Mental and Elemental Nutrients

Library of Congress Catalog Card Number 75-19543
ISBN: 0-87983-114-6
PRINTED IN THE UNITED STATES OF AMERICA

Keats Publishing, Inc., 36 Grove Street, New Canaan, Connecticut 06840

Contents

List of Tables

List of Figures

Preface

It is a pleasure and a privilege to welcome this sensible and much needed book, which draws together a great deal of information of value to the mentally ill and their families for planning appropriate nutrition. Yet this book should be equally useful to all of us.

It was self-evident to the older psychiatrists that a good diet was essential for their patients. Not only because of the nutrients which they ingested with their food, but because food was seen in the hospitals of the mid-nineteenth century as being a focus for the exercise of good behavior. To further this, the director of the hospital frequently sat down with his patients and ate with them, family style. This gave him an excellent opportunity to ensure that the hospital cooks were providing nutritious and tasty fare, while also allowing him to engage in conversation with patients and to observe their table manners.

The gigantification of the mental hospital made it impossible for the superintendent to do this. With that gigantification the quality of the food dropped so much that it would have required a cast-iron stomach and fortitude perhaps beyond the limit of human endurance for the superintendent to eat frequently with the patients. This omission tended to divert psychiatrists' attention from the importance of eating for patients, both as a nutritional and a social exercise.

I was walking through a mental hospital dining room the other day and was struck by its noisiness, smelliness and general bleakness. I am not sure how nutritionally sound the food was, but it was certainly not so inviting that I longed to seize a tray and join in the repast. Yet from almost a century before, we have descriptions of the excellent food in that same hospital, dainty ways in which it was served, the clean white napery, fine chinaware and glistening crystal. Food should not only be good, but it should be seen to be good and it should be served in a manner appropriate to its goodness.

Unluckily, those with grave mental illnesses are unlikely to be particularly well-fed in hospitals. In part at least because the hospital authorities often have the crudest ideas as to what the patients' requirements might be both nutritionally and psychosocially.

The psychiatric hospitals, instead of sticking to their own traditions for feeding patients well have tended to become more like the general hospital of fifty to a hundred years ago where patients might easily starve. Doctors Provost and Butterworth, of the University of Alabama School of Medicine, have shown that even today this lamentable event does occur due to a technical preoccupation with surgery and medicine rather than a general concern for the well-being of the patient.

The situation is certainly made worse in some mental hospitals and probably in general hospitals too, because vending machines carrying a variety of junk food snacks are frequently present on the hospital floors and provide temptations for patients who are not well enough fed in hospitals to be able to resist.

There are exceptions. I recall with gratitude the extremely good meals I had at Moorefield's Eye Hospital, London, England, following a cataract operation. These were made all the better because my greatly improved vision gave the food an almost psychedelic quality. I can still remember biting into the fried fish and how good it tasted. In the mid-nineteenth century cookery for the sick was considered a special aspect of the gastronomy and much thought and attention was given to it. I hope that *Mental and Elemental Nutrients* will be followed by a cookbook developed to accommodate the information provided here, which can be used in general and psychiatric hospitals. Its principles can be taught to patients and their families so that when they return home they can sustain themselves in the best possible nutritional state.

We live in a world where there is much malnutrition and in many areas a danger of starvation. In addition to malnutrition caused by poverty, there is probably almost as large and great an amount of malnutrition caused by what one might call perversity of taste. Anyone who watches T.V. advertisements soon notices that eating habits are encouraged in the very young, which are liable to do them much harm over the years.

What then can we do about this? Reading this book is certainly one step forward and carrying its message to hospitals of all kinds, schools and homes is clearly a citizenly duty which will repay those who undertake this labor manyfold in good health for their friends, children and themselves.

Humphry Osmond, MRCP., FRC Psych.
Tuscaloosa, Alabama

Commentary

Dr. Carl Pfeiffer and his clinical and research colleagues are pioneers and leaders in the field of orthomolecular psychiatric research. A research group may consider itself fortunate to make one new clinical finding. This group, one of the too few research groups in the world in this field, has made major contributions toward accurate diagnosis and toward improved treatment.

They have refined the schizophrenic syndrome by using biochemical assays for blood histamine levels, for urinary kryptopyrrole levels and for other substances which have proven very valuable in treatment of schizophrenic patients. They have shown that high kryptopyrrole levels produce a deficiency of zinc and pyridoxine and they have demonstrated the immense importance of trace elements in the prevention and treatment of mental illnesses.

Since this group is only beginning an epoch marked by enormous creativity and productivity one can only wonder at the discoveries which will pour from their laboratory over the next ten years. This book will be a preview of the future.

I advise every family which has any history of severe neuroses or psychoses to read it with care and to apply the principles to themselves for only in this way will there be any significant reduction from the human waste and ravages of mental illness. Standard psychiatry (tranquilizers and talk) has proven itself bankrupt. This book represents the wave of the future.

Abram Hoffer, Ph.D., M.D.

MENTAL AND ELEMENTAL NUTRIENTS

A Physician's Guide to Nutrition and Health Care

Introduction

"Wastebasket diagnoses" abound in medicine and psychology. The excuse often given by the medical and psychological fraternities is that a label on the patient saves the patient's (or his parents') money in that they don't go shopping around among doctors for a cure that doesn't exist! However, the search for more effective treatment should never be relaxed by patient, parent or doctor. Biological science is at best only a progress report, so the "wastebasket" of today may be the goldmine of tomorrow.

We have had an older patient come to us with a diagnosis of mental retardation when actually the other wastebasket diagnosis "schizophrenia" would have gotten her help as early as the late 1950s. Now after twenty years this mentally retarded patient is found to respond to standard antischizophrenic medication. This is indeed sad, because the patient wasted many years with her mind imprisoned and her body rocking back and forth while she squawked like a chicken.

Clinical diagnoses such as minimal brain damage, learning disability, neurological deficit, mental retardation, schizophrenia, neurosis, psychosis, maladjustment reaction, autism, emotional disorder, alcoholism, drug addiction, hypoglycemia, schizoid, juvenile delinquency and senility can all be wastebaskets. Even if the label is a valid diagnosis when given, the progress of medical knowledge is such that many patients can be better diagnosed and treated if their illness is reviewed at five-year intervals. Rather than mental retardation, the term "mental dormancy" might be used, with the result that scientists would continue looking for the actual causes. The pediatrician has a simple label for some cases, namely "failure to thrive." This "without prejudice" labeling highlights the fact that it is the doctor's job to find out *why* the patient doesn't thrive!

Psychiatric diagnoses are only diagnoses of elimination. In the well-studied mental patient, the internist and radiologist and neurologist apply all the tests they know as of the present time. If all are negative they may suggest psychiatric help. If the patient were to see these same diagnosticians in 1985, a factual diagnosis would be more likely, and differential diagnosis probably would be more complete because of our ever increasing wealth of medical knowledge.

One must always ask the individual who makes a "psychogenic" diagnosis (diagnosis by elimination) this question: What, in your handling of a thousand such cases, would make you state positively that one case was *not* of psychogenic origin? This positive yardstick is applied constantly by the inquiring scientist and should be used more often in medicine. At present there probably isn't a Freudian psychiatrist (or psychologist) who could give a valid and scientifically acceptable answer to this simple question.

Patients and lay authors sometimes use the word "cure," but medically trained persons soon learn to be more circumspect. The disease is "arrested" or the "effect of the disease process is stabilized." Workers treating patients with nervous and mental disorders soon learn to assess the "social rehabilitation" of their patients. Similarly, workers in cancer cite "five- and ten-year survival" as goals in therapy of these difficult-to-treat disorders.

I learned as a medical student to avoid "cure" (as well as "incurable") from walking Ellis Avenue in Chicago each day on my way to medical school past a building where the words "Chicago Home for Incurables" were engraved in stone over the doorway. This was in 1936. I hope the building, with its negative words, has become outmoded and demolished by now. How much better it would have been to have a temporary sign, whose date would be changed each year, stating "Untreatable by methods available in 1936." After all, sulfa drugs were introduced in 1937 and so much more happened after that—the TB sanatorium, for example, has been completely eliminated.

We shall attempt in this book to provide a progress report

on nutrients for the interested and educated reader. After many unscientific diet books, any book on nutrition written in part by a medical doctor might be suspect. We have, however, used a committee of scientifically trained individuals to consult the original and current literature in order to provide the reader with the basic information.

Carl C. Pfeiffer, Ph.D., M.D.
Princeton, New Jersey, 1975

PART ONE

Nutritional Background

INTRODUCTION

Good nutrition, we believe, is the key to the large task of preventing disease states. But what is good nutrition? Unfortunately, nutrition has been overlooked by medical schools and by physicians—almost none of whom have clinical nutrition as their specialty. Other groups such as osteopaths, dentists and chiropractors are more interested in nutrition and frequently give better advice on this subject than physicians.

In this first section, we introduce the elements of nutrition—proteins, fats, carbohydrates—and discuss their relation with vegetarianism, the maligned egg, and the almost forgotten nut. Next, we analyze the American diet and present alternatives. Special diets for different types of patients are discussed. Specific nutrient-rich food sources and recipes are detailed. Then the various weight-watching regimes are assessed and hints for making dieting easier are given. Finally, we warn the consumer about food additives, artificial sweeteners and some of the hazards of the marketplace.

CHAPTER 1

Nutrition as Preventive Medicine

The well nourished American is a myth. Despite the high level of education and the abundance of available food, many people make poor food choices and are badly nourished. Advanced stages of vitamin deficiency diseases still occur in America. Scurvy, beriberi, pellagra, rickets and other deficiency diseases are found in large city hospitals. Recent evidence has shown that these classic syndromes constitute only a small segment of the total results of malnutrition. Undiagnosed subclinical malnutrition of trace elements and protein may exist and subtly cause such significant physiological damage to body and brain as stunted growth, premature aging and early death. Using nutrition as preventive medicine, we can check the destructive course of malnutrition.

Malnutrition—a Present-Day Problem

Malnutrition (or bad nutrition) may afflict up to 80 percent of the nation's population, according to Drs. Cheraskin and Ringsdorf. National nutritional surveys have indicated that most people have low levels of one or more essential nutrients, relative to the traditionally recommended levels. A study at Jersey City Medical Center showed that 83 percent of patients admitted to the hospital have at least one vitamin deficiency and 68 percent have two or more deficiencies. Malnutrition is not new, yet many were shocked by the CBS documentary called "Hunger in America" and by "Hunger USA" published by the Citizens Board of Inquiry.

What exactly is malnutrition? In the report "Malnutrition and Hunger in the United States" by the AMA Council on Foods and Nutrition, malnutrition was defined as:

> A state of impaired functional ability or deficient structural integrity or development brought about by a discrepancy between the supply to the body tissues of essential nutrients and calories, and the biologic demand for them.

The etiology of malnutrition may be divided into two categories, primary and secondary. Primary malnutrition results from the faulty or inadequate intake of nutrients caused by faulty food selection, lack of money, poisoned and contaminated foods, insufficient soil nutrients, or by food shortages. Secondary malnutrition is due to factors interfering with the ingestion, absorption, or utilization of essential nutrients, or to stress factors that increase their requirement, destruction, or excretion. (See Table 1.1 for causes of malnutrition.) Primary and secondary malnutrition may exist together, and great care must be taken to separate and correct the interrelated factors for each individual.

TABLE 1.1

Basic causes of malnutrition

Food crop failure

Lack of water	**Inadequate sun**
Poisoned soil	**Floods**
Inadequate soil	

Manure failure

Only nitrogen, potassium and phosphate	**Too much copper, phosphate, nitrate, selenium, acid, or alkali**
No trace elements	

Poverty

Overpopulation with inadequate arable land
Farming ignorance
Wage-earner illness
Unemployment
Inadequate protein
Neglect of children

Medical factors

Diarrhea
Nausea
Operations
Parasites
Food allergy
Prematurity
Vitamin dependence
Chronic infection
Pregnancy
Lactation
Malabsorption
Crash diets
Bad eating habits
Medications
Individual variation
Infirmities
Vitamins *plus minerals*
Loss of taste
Cancer
Anorexia nervosa

Improper food storage

Potato carcinogen
Wheat and peanut fungus
Bacterial growth

Contaminated food

Swordfish with mercury
Seed grain with organic mercury
Pigs with methyl mercury
Rice with cadmium
Wheat with selenium
Oils with antiknock
Ginger Jake paralysis
Milk with Tremitol

Food processing

Milling of grain that removes vitamins and trace elements
Boric acid
Technical mistakes
Flame-retardant chemical
Freezing (with chelators) that reduces trace elements in commercial green vegetables
Sterilization in cans may remove vitamin C and pyridoxine (B-6)
Canning adds tin and may add lead and cadmium to foods
Aluminum added to food in cooking needs investigation by modern methods

Poisoned water

Excess copper, cadmium or lead with acid well water
Bacterial contaminated water
Inadequate calcium and magnesium to lime the pipes
Nitrates from surface drainage

Both primary and secondary malnutrition contribute to the disorders already discussed. Our nutritional section will deal mainly with correcting primary malnutrition.

Malnutrition is a very real and insidious problem, and the effects may be severe and lasting. Adequate nutrition is essential for proper and optimal growth. David Kallen, Ph.D., asserts that malnutrition during development leads to high infant mortality and smaller physical size. Severe malnutrition may lead to intellectual impairment. However, the relationship between moderate malnutrition and intelligence is still unclear. Winick had illustrated a critical period of the first six months of development in animals and in man, during which time cell division takes place and malnutrition will produce irreversible damage. The late Professor B.S. Platt of London's School of Tropical Medicine, found that protein-calorie deficiency during pregnancy in dogs caused neurological dysfunction simulating that of central nervous system (CNS) damage in human infants. The negative effects of malnutrition on intellectual capacity and on physiological development result in reduction in growth rate, delayed physical maturation, and decreased learning ability.

Furthermore, a synergistic interrelationship exists between malnutrition and infectious disease, the two largest world health problems. Malnutrition results in loss of productivity, disease creates metabolic demands, and this cycle is further complicated by parasitic infestations. Infections may be associated with pregnancy and the post-partum (after birth) state and diabetes. Perinatal mortality is high: over 45 per 1,000 in 1972 for "staff" deliveries at Wayne State University School of Medicine in Detroit; over 40 per 1,000 for nonwhites in the entire state of North Carolina in 1972. Obviously little help stems from monitoring mother and fetus during the last few days of pregnancy when both have suffered months of malnutrition. Pregnancy is a severe nutritional stress. Good nutrition should begin many years before pregnancy.

Malnutrition and Preventive Medicine

These statistics show the need for preventive nutrition. A lifetime of better nutrition can contribute significantly to modifying the development of many diseases. According to Dr. Edith Weir, assistant director of USDA's human nutrition research division, diet has played an important role in recent decades in reducing the number of infant and maternal deaths and deaths from infectious diseases, especially among children, and in extending the productive life span and life expectancy. A team of scientists at the University of Alabama Medical Center believes that Americans suffer from varied ailments, insomnia to cancer, largely because of improper diet. Overweight is linked to heart disease, hypertension, rheumatic disease, and other conditions. Some specialists are of the opinion that better diet would result in reduced incidence of respiratory, infectious and heart diseases. They project a 25 percent reduction of heart disease in people under 65 as a result of improved nutrition.

Because of human biochemical individuality, each person must find out which nutrients are individually needed; that is, some may need minimum attention to some vitamins or trace elements while others may need much attention to stay well. Many scientists, such as Dr. Roger Williams and his colleagues of the University of Texas, argue that because of individual variability in nutritional requirements, essentially no one can be fed adequately on an average American diet. Although this is far from proven, many people—some schizophrenics, drug addicts, alcoholics, and others on the upper end of the spectrum of biochemical need—have shown particular deficiencies in some nutrients.

Emphasis should be placed on a preventive approach to disease rather than on the role of diet in treating health problems after they develop. Most doctors and hospitals are not nutritionally oriented and rarely advise patients about dietary needs. Many physicians still state that three square meals a day is all anyone needs. Among them are the surgeons who believe their post-operative patient can live for five days on intravenous saline alone, and the obstetricians who tell the zinc and B-6 deficient mother with nausea of early pregnancy to "eat later in the day but don't gain weight." Or the doctor who doesn't believe in vitamins or trace elements at all!

Nutrition receives little attention in the medical school

curriculum and most American physicians have not yet recognized that nutrition is an essential part of good medicine. Nutrition is a young science and our present knowledge about human nutritional needs is limited, especially for conditions such as pregnancy and old age. The gaps in human nutritional knowledge aren't being filled fast enough. Some doctors now feel that nutrition should properly be a specialty within medicine, emphasizing biochemistry and clinical nutrition. (And we agree!)

Malnutrition may be prevalent among hospitalized patients. Despite sophisticated diagnostic procedures and drugs in hospitals, patients' nutritional status does not necessarily receive adequate attention. Basic principles of nutrition are being ignored in the care of hospitalized patients. Dr. Elizabeth Prevost of the University of Alabama School of Medicine has emphasized this point. Dr. Prevost conducted a study surveying the nutritional status of 100 medical surgical patients hospitalized for two weeks or more.

Very few test data or other basic information relating to general nutritional health (such as weight and height) were normally collected at the hospital. Dr. Prevost found that almost one-third of the patients had histories of nausea, decreased appetite, and weight loss, which are potential indicators of nutritional problems. Two-thirds of the patients who actually had been weighed lost weight while in the hospital. About half had low serum albumin levels (blood protein) but high protein diets were prescribed for only about two-thirds of the patients with this condition. About one-third were anemic when admitted, and about one-fifth became anemic while staying at the hospital. Few tests were done to determine vitamin status, despite the known association of various conditions and drug therapies with vitamin depletion. Evidence of vitamin depletion was found in about one-quarter of the patients but no vitamin therapy had been prescribed. Dr. Prevost found further hospital procedures potentially detrimental to patient nutrition: withholding of meals, failure to observe food intake, and prolonged use of glucose infusions.

Further evidence for the slighting of nutritional needs by hospitals and doctors was offered by Dr. Charles E. Butterworth, Jr., director of the nutrition program at the University of Alabama, Birmingham, and chairman of the AMA's Council on Foods and Nutrition. He has charged that hospital diets are often inadequate to maintain health or, at times, so bad as to worsen health. From visits to several hospitals and an intensive study at one, he found surgery performed without first preparing the patient's internal environment for the stress, followed by oversight of adequate post-operative nutrition. Unfortunately, post-operative neglect led in some cases to advanced states of malnutrition and occasional death.

Furthermore, as the patient knows, hospital diets (as in other large institutions) are usually overcooked, stored in steam tables, unappetizing, flavorless, and not well varied. One patient is reported to have pushed back the dinner tray and asked for seconds on the intravenous drip! Obviously, the nutritional status and supervision of patients should be of utmost importance in hospital care. Unfortunately, most of our hospitals emphasize corrective, rather than preventive, medicine. Yet, many doctors are becoming aware of the essential importance of nutrition in medicine, as is indicated by the recent book, *New Breed of Doctor: Nutrition For a Healthy Mind,* by Alan Nittler.

Diet is important to virtually every facet of your life. Good nutrition is more than just avoiding bad health and disease, says Nicholas Johnson of the Federal Communications Commission; it is one of the basic essentials to attain the more abundant life. As he said before the graduating class of the College of Arts and Sciences, American University, "Diet affects your physical appearance, your energy levels, your intellectual and creative abilities, your mental health and general feeling of well-being, even your ability to enjoy love and sexuality." Anthelme Brillat-Savarin, renowned writer on foods, said, "Tell me what you eat, and I will tell you what you are."

Learning and practicing intelligent nutritional habits and correct food combinations should be of primary concern, essential to physical, mental, and emotional health. We believe that nutritional education should begin early in schools to equip youngsters with some knowledge of what they eat and why they eat it. The brain is composed, as is the rest of the body, of cells which must be nourished by nutrient biochemicals to function properly. Malnutrition may result in impaired brain function.

Logically, mental illness may be best prevented by vitamins, minerals, and other nutrients. George Watson, author of *Nutrition and Your Mind,* says that in most cases there is no motivation for abnormal behavior (as psychotherapy would have it), that this behavior is a result of an undernourished brain, an exhausted nervous system or any of a number of other physical problems directly related to imperfect mind function. Strong psychological stress or sudden shock can exhaust tissues of certain chemicals necessary for normal functioning. If your senses play tricks on you, if you hear or see things you know aren't there, you are probably suffering from a vitamin deficiency, a block in utilization in your body, or an increased need for some nutrient. Simple insomnia can precipitate these symptoms and biochemical imbalance. This somatic base of mental disease has traditionally been neglected. The importance of malnutrition as a major cause of mental illness is now being more widely recognized and accepted.

Poor dietary habits often stem from emotional disturbances and follow back to them. Poor nutrition can be at the root of behavior which perfectly imitates that of the neurotic or psychotic, sometimes with no overt physical evidence of nutritional deficiency. An example is pellagra or subclinical pellagra, the disease resulting from a deficiency of niacin, whose mental symptoms mimic those of schizophrenia. Pellagra is a vitamin *deficiency* condition, while some mental illnesses are vitamin *dependency* conditions. Pellagrins can relieve their disease promptly by small quantities of niacin, while those with certain types of mental disorders, notably schizophrenics, must remain on higher quantities of nutrients due to a greater need for those nutrients.

A study conducted by Irene Payne, Ph.D., and Mildred M. Hudson on the dietary histories and actual three-day eating habits of forty-nine first admission mental hospital patients revealed nutrient deficiencies similar to those of other groups in the U.S. Why did these people become mentally ill and not others? The RDR of nutrients used to judge the adequacy of intake may not apply to mental patients, who may have increased needs. The individual's requirements vary greatly, much more so than is traditionally believed. Individual differences must be taken into account in the treatment of emotional and mental disorders.

We know that by altering man's physical state in very slight ways, emotional and mental responses are altered. This can be seen in everyday life. This is also evident in the working of drugs. Nutrients work to correct a biochemical imbalance usually more slowly than drugs, although some vitamins, such as inositol, have drug-like action. Drugs can have unpleasant and sometimes damaging side effects, whereas nutrients are safer and cheaper. Wherever possible in medicine, nutrients should be used as the first choice; however, this does not obviate the use of drugs when needed.

Proper nutrition and nutrient therapy have helped many schizophrenics, some of whom had been given up as hopeless after both drug and psychotherapy treatments. Learning problems, senility, alcoholism, and suicidal tendencies have been affected. The psychological state of healthy individuals has also been improved on nutritional therapy. Some nervous and physical disorders do require more than proper nutrition, but the regenerative powers of the body, mind, and emotions are greatly enhanced by proper nutrition. However, nutrient therapy does not work for everyone; for some it may be unnecessary. Self-treatment could be dangerous or even fatal. Some nutrients become toxic at high levels; and what is needed by one person may be too much for another. We stress that the patient should not attempt self-diagnosis; proper clinical biochemical testing may be needed.

Biochemical treatment, or orthomolecular medicine, is the correction of faulty biochemistry. Linus Pauling coined the term "Orthomolecular Medicine" which involves the provision of the proper quantities of nutrients for the individual, not huge mega or pharmacologic doses. Pauling defines Orthomolecular Medicine as:

> the preservation of good health and the prevention and treatment of disease by varying the concentrations in the human body of the molecules of substances that are normally present, many of them required for life, such as the vitamins, essential amino acids, essential fats, and minerals.

He states that in two years of experience with more than 1,000 schizophrenics, 60 percent treated with megavitamins either improved considerably or had complete relief of symptoms. Now, after further experience and research, higher recovery rates are obtained. The Canadian Schizophrenia Foundation found an 85 percent recovery rate using the original megavitamin therapy. Here at the Brain Bio Center in Princeton, New Jersey, the estimated improvement rate is 90 percent using the biochemical approach. These figures are relative to a 35 percent complete spontaneous recovery rate, and an approximate 50 percent recovery rate for other more traditional therapies such as psychotherapy (however, this 50 percent may include the masked 35 percent of spontaneous recovery.)

The North Nassau Mental Health Center compared its five years of experience using the orthomolecular approach with its previous five years using traditional psychiatric approaches. They found the orthomolecular approach to be more effective, shorter in duration, and cheaper. Also, the orthomolecular approach required less professional manpower, and allowed the treatment of more patients with greater efficiency.

Dr. John Blass, physician and biochemist at the Neuropsychiatric Institute at UCLA, believes that megavitamins are a useful treatment which will eventually benefit 20 million Americans. The combination of good natural foods plus the correct nutritional supplements could eliminate most of the mental health problems (as well as physical illness) and is inexpensive when compared to drugs and doctor bills. Pauling pointedly states that:

> A psychiatrist who refuses to try the methods of Orthomolecular Psychiatry (nutrition as related to mental health) in addition to his usual therapy in the treatment of his patients is failing in his duty as a physician.

References

American nutrition: ignorance in abundance. *Med. World News* p. 6, 5 January 1973.

Brewer, T. Total blackout on role of malnutrition. *Medicine,* 24 October 1973.

Deadly hospital food? *Time,* 22 July 1974.

Kallen, D. J. Nutrition and society. *JAMA* 215:1:94, 1971.

Moser, R. Mango malnutrition déjà vu. *Med. Opin.* p. 72, November 1971.

National nutrition. *Science* 183: 1062, 1974.

Nittler, A. *A new breed of doctor.* New York: Pyramid Publications, 1974.

Nutrition held overlooked in care of patients in hospitals. *Intern. Med. News,* 1 July 1974.

Payne, I., and Hudson, M. Dietary intakes of mental patients. *AJPH* 62:9:120, 1972.

Sackler, A., One man . . . and medicine: is nothing known? *Med. Trib.* 10 July 1974.

CHAPTER 2

Nutrients vs. Drugs for the Good Life

What constitutes the good life? This obviously depends on the age and maturation of the individual questioned! If we consider only the young adult and adult, however, there are various facets to the good life, some of which may diminish with advancing age. Table 2.1 attempts a summary of these numerous complexities.

Many facets of life can be regulated by good nutrition and work habits to allow each individual steady maximal performance limited only by the abilities with which he has been endowed. Yet, some are night owls and like night life, and others are morning larks who follow the old American Indian motto, "Sleep when the birds no longer fly; rise when the first faint dawn appears."

Bertrand Russell (1872-1970) was one of the first to emphasize man's love of excitement and, conversely, man's discontent with boredom. Russell pointed out that in Australia, where rabbits are many and people are few, boredom can be relieved by the excitement of an annual rabbit hunt. In London, where people are many and rabbits are few, some other means of excitement to relieve boredom must be found. Russell further suggested that artificial waterfalls should be erected in

TABLE 2.1

The "good life" has various facets

	Young Adult	*Adult*	*Senior Adult*
Good physical health	+	+	+
Good mental health	+	+	+
Financial security	+	+	+
Intellectual challenge	+	+	+
Intellectual productivity	+	+	+
Sex relations	+	+	?
Peer esteem	+	+	+
Freedom from fears	+	+	**Fear of death**
Freedom from prejudice	+	+	+
Steady maximal performance limited only by natural abilities	+	+	+
Need for excitement	+	—	—

each large city so that bored young people could shoot the rapids daily in exceedingly fragile canoes. He emphasized exercise, saying that a man would be less likely to cheer the onset of war if he had walked twenty-five miles that day. Russell also said that boredom can be prevented by the pursuit of scholarly knowledge. Scientific discovery leaves no room for boredom even when initial hypotheses are disproven.

Dr. A. Hatch has found that isolated rats placed in an empty environment become caricatures of the lonely housewife. They gained weight, were jumpy and nervous, and even showed signs of nervous disorders. Bored humans thus can place an extra burden on our medical care systems. Boredom allows many trivial aches and pains to surface as seemingly life-threatening symptoms.

If good nutrition does not provide steady maximal performance, then the disappointed individual may seek out drugs for this purpose. Easily available drugs are caffeine as in coffee, tea, and cola drinks; alcohol, as in beer, wine and hard drinks; amphetamines, as in diet pills and some nose drops. Tobacco, betel nut, marijuana and other drugs may also be tried.

The urge to try psychedelic drugs may have a firmer basis than youth's usual fling with those accepted agents which alter man's moods—namely, alcohol, tobacco and betel nut. The open rebellion of youth in this respect may be a repudiation of "talking therapy" in favor of the more potent drug therapy which has evolved in the past ten years. The modern drugs will lift depressions, control schizophrenia, produce sleep and elevate moods. "Talking therapy," if expertly directed, will help solve the problems of everyday life. If inexpertly directed, "talking therapy" may cause destructive emotional upheaval and increase stress and mental disorders.

Modern youth is assailed with so-called healing talk from the cradle to driver's license age. Much of this talk is necessary, particularly the occasional sharp "No!" followed by a slap, and more often the approving "good boy" or "good girl" followed by a hug. However, a modern youth may start at cradle age with talk instead of discipline, at preschool age receive talk instead of training, and be referred for one reason or another to the talking specialists annually until he is able to grow a beard. By this time, he is adequately toilet trained (mainly for his own comfort), but not otherwise disciplined. He knows that insofar as he is concerned "talking therapy" is water off a duck's back, so he goes in for the more potent street drugs to provide excitement and to change his unhappy and disillusioned mood and to try to solve his problems.

Young people are not against "talking therapy;" they engage in it constantly among themselves. But some have learned all of the reasons, blessings and maledictions—to such an extent that they may be disillusioned with "talking therapy" as elaborated by our best behavioral theorists both modern and ancient. In their disillusion, they may believe that only drugs are left. These seem good because "They are *real,* man"—as positive in their action as a karate chop.

Many adults remember, from their early youth, the reported effects of "ammonia cokes," aspirin cokes, or the effect of a beer spiked with a leaf from a Benny inhaler. (The first two were not effective, and the last is fortunately not available because Benny inhalers are no longer marketed.) If man can achieve the good life through the judicious use of nutrients, then the need for street drugs and "talking therapy" will be eliminated!

What Constitutes Good Nutrition for the Good Life?

A good balanced diet should provide the normal individual with the following nutrients:

1. adequate protein intake
2. adequate vitamin intake
3. adequate mineral and trace metal intake
4. adequate fluid balance
5. sufficient starch to supply energy needs
6. adequate fats

Coffee and doughnuts make very little contribution to good nutrition. The cake flour customarily used in doughnuts is devoid of minerals and trace elements, while the coffee provides liquid and caffeine, a stimulant to which an individual can quickly develop a tolerance. It is wise to reserve coffee, tea and cola drinks to those periods in life when an added stimulation may be sorely needed. Coffee or tea will then be effective as a stimulant.

What Constitutes the Normal Person?

Ever since the Greeks divided man's personality into four basic humors, man has been reclassifying the personalities displayed by his fellow man. The study of personality is called typology, and the subdivisions vary according to the discipline of the worker who makes the classification.

Thus, psychologists and sociologists have attempted subdivisions and correlations of the personality according to behavior, while physiologists and biochemists have tried to do the same thing with physiological and biochemical tests. (Some of the most recent of these tests show promise for the objective classification of personality.)

From the standpoint of good nutrition and the good life,

the individual's basic personality is important. The "morning lark" should not be placed as a roommate in college with the "night owl," and yet colleges seldom bother to classify freshmen in accordance with such basic characteristics. Marriage counselors and dating bureaus might also make better matches if this simple aspect of personality were considered. (Table 2.2 summarizes some of the characteristics and the ways in which they have been classified.)

TABLE 2.2

Progress in the science of typology according to disciplines

Typology	*Types*			*Source*
Historical	Choleric "Night owl."	Sanguine	Phlegmatic melancholic "Morning lark"	Greek body humors Layman's interpretation
Psychological	Extrovert Hypomanic Outer directed Aggrandizer Extratensive	Normal " or bimodal " " "	Introvert Depressive Inner directed Minimizer Intratensive	Jung
Physiological-psychological	Field independent	Normal	Field dependent	
Educational-sociological	Overachiever Expressive	Normal "	Under- achiever Instrumental	
Anatomical	Endomorph	Mesomorph	Ectomorph	Sheldon
Physiological	Ergotonic Slow oxidizer Low energy EEG Blocked alpha waves	Normal " " "	Vagotonic Fast oxidizer High energy EEG Normal alpha waves	 Watson Goldstein
Biochemical	Hyperthyroid	Euthyroid	Myxodematous madness (hypothyroid)	Asher

Typology	*Types*			*Source*
Biochemical cont.	**Histapenic**	**Normal histamine**	**Histadelic**	**Pfeiffer**
	High copper	"	**Normal copper**	**Pfeiffer**
	Over-abundant catechol amines	**Normal**	**Inadequate catechol amines**	**Murphy, Bunney and Brodie Davis**
	Dopamine	**Normal**	**Dopamine**	**Soloman**
	Under-methylation of biogenic amines	**Normal**	**Over-methylation of biogenic amines**	**Pfeiffer**

Karl Jung is generally credited with coining the terms "extrovert" and "introvert." Since then many terms have been used to describe various degrees of high and low mood swings. Much is now being made of dopamine as a neurotransmitter while histamine is still underrated because of lack of interest on the part of granting agencies. Biogenic amines are compounds which are involved in the transmission of nerve impulses. There is a widely accepted hypothesis, the overmethylation hypothesis, that addition of methyl groups to these compounds is responsible for such schizophrenic behavior as mania, hallucinations and paranoia. Indeed, administration of such methylated amines as bufotenine, dimethyltryptamine, and mescaline will evoke such symptoms in normal people. Rhoda Papaioannou of the Brain Bio Center believes, however, that small amounts of such methylated biogenic amines are essential to normal functioning. If there is such an abnormality as overmethylation, there must be an opposite side to the coin, that of undermethylation and this inability to produce normal amounts of methylated biogenic amines might well lead to depression. Undermethylation would also allow for the accumulation of such amines as histamine as in our high-histamine, depressed patients.

CHAPTER 3

We Shall Overcome—Inadequate Diet!

Adelle Davis, the famous nutritionist, noted that entire civilizations rise and fall on their diets. Food should contribute in a positive way to building up and maintaining the health of our bodies. Proper eating habits promote productivity and longevity, while poor eating habits deprive body cells and tissues of substances necessary for vital functions, causing weakness and increased susceptibility to disease.

Today, more than 50 percent of Americans eat poorly, displaying a decided preference for those foods which are least nutritious. Many are unaware that general health suffers as a result.

What's Wrong with the Way I Eat?

For career-oriented and other active people, meal preparation often seems a troublesome routine which interrupts more interesting and important projects. TV dinners and fast-food chain restaurants offer convenient alternatives to laboring in the kitchen. Mothers find that children with fussy eating habits, who pick indifferently at meat and vegetables, will readily devour French fries and greasy hamburgers served in attractive cardboard containers. Many busy people and irrational dieters forego breakfast and lunch, relying on sugar-laden confections to revive waning energy in mid-afternoon. Schoolchildren, enticed by colorful packaged products in glittering machines, often invest lunch money in potato chips and candy bars rather than in more nutritious foods.

Within the past fifty years, consumption of fats and refined carbohydrates has increased tremendously. Saturated fats are a factor conventionally associated with high cholesterol levels and heart disease. Fats account for approximately 40 percent of the calories in an average daily diet. Hydrogenated oils and shortening, lard, butter and bacon provide the most concentrated sources of saturated fats. Animal feeding practices in the United States result in saturated fat marbled into lean meat, especially beef, providing an additional, invisible source of fat. Although a limited amount of fat (preferably unsaturated) is needed in the diet for the absorption of fat-soluble vitamins A, D, E and K and for several other functions, the body cannot handle the large quantities of fats now consumed.

Refined carbohydrates, which supply 45 percent of the calories in an average daily diet, but only 10 percent of the essential nutrients, deserve worse than the term "empty calories" since their contribution is largely negative. An English cancer specialist, Dr. Dennis Burkitt, contends that a diet high in refined carbohydrates leads to a high bacterial count and slow bowel movements, increasing the probability of developing cancer of the colon. Candy, ice cream, doughnuts, soft drinks and other such confections also contribute to the development of heart disease, alcoholism, diabetes, hypoglycemia, tooth decay and other disorders. Dr. John Yudkin, sugar researcher, states that "if only a fraction of what is already known about the effects of sugar were to be revealed in relation to any other material used as a food additive, that material would promptly be banned."

Both fats and refined carbohydrates are "fattening." Carbohydrates contain four calories per gram while fats contain nine. High consumption of these foods has fostered the myth of well-fed America when, in reality, such consumption promotes numerous health problems. Should Americans continue to pursue their current eating patterns, their general health will progressively deteriorate and American civilization could indeed enter upon the path of historical decline.

It's Not My Fault— Look What They're Doing to My Food!

For years, representatives of numerous public health groups have promoted that familiar adage, "To enjoy good health, eat a balanced diet," certain that the average individual will receive all the nutrients his body needs provided he consumes adequate amounts of food from the four traditional groups: dairy products; meat, fish and eggs; fruits and vegetables; and grains. They have worked on the assumption that an appropriate combination of these foods should supply the Recommended Daily Allowances (RDAs) of vitamins and trace elements necessary for the maintenance of sound muscles and organs. Despite these proclamations, recent nutritional surveys reveal a general ignorance regarding what constitutes a properly balanced diet and, worse still, the fact that even a well-balanced diet can produce borderline or outright deficiencies in one or more of the essential nutrients.

RDAs specify the nutrient requirements necessary for the prevention of severe deficiency diseases, not for optimal health. Individual need for nutrients varies. Genetic abnormalities, pregnancy, illness, great occupational stress or drug use often create a greater need for certain vitamins and trace elements in the body than the sparse quantities specified as RDAs.

Human Diet Must Be Supplemented for Rats

A study conducted by Dr. Donald Davis, assistant professor of chemistry at the University of California at Irvine, revealed striking deficits in a diet composed of accepted staple foods. In his three-month study, rats were placed on the following diets:

(1) an approximation of the American diet, consisting of white bread, sugar, eggs, milk, ground beef, cabbage, potatoes, tomatoes, oranges, apples, bananas and coffee; (2) the same diet as (1) supplemented with twelve vitamins and thirteen trace elements; (3) Purina Rat Chow (which is commercially balanced specifically for laboratory rats and contains unrefined grains and fish meal fortified with vitamins and minerals, plus a small amount of molasses as the only sugar); and (4) Purina Rat Chow diluted with enough glucose to provide 70 percent of the total calories.

Results showed the undiluted rat chow to be the best diet! The *supplemented* human diet followed, as a close second to the rat chow, in fulfilling the animals' nutritional needs, while rats maintained on the remaining diets trailed behind those of the first two groups in size, physical maturity and general health. Since humans certainly do not have *less* exacting nutritional requirements than rats, the average human diet, nutritionally unfit for rats, must be equally unsatisfactory or even more so in meeting human needs.

What is wrong with the type of "well-balanced" diet eaten today? An answer to this perplexing problem lies in the inadequacy of foods available to today's consumer.

Beginning as tiny seeds imbedded in the soil, every farmer's crops travel a long and deleterious route to the table. Tiny calves, suckling pigs, little lambs and baby chicks follow a similar path to the meat platter. Nutrient-deficient soils, chemical fertilizers, time required for shipping and storage, and finally, processing and treatment with chemical additives, successively deprive plants and animals of vital nutrients as they journey from the farm to the consumer.

Deficient Soils and Chemical Fertilizers

Soil today differs greatly from the fertile earth the American Indians relied upon for survival. Centuries of continuous planting, failure to rotate crops or allow fields to lie fallow for a season, and natural weathering agents have depleted the once-rich earth of many essential trace elements. In thirty-two states of the United States alone, the zinc content of soils falls below the adequate level. Plants will continue to grow despite suboptimal nutrient conditions, but suboptimal health will be noted in animals and humans consuming plants raised in deficient soils. Zinc deficiency in animals and man results in retarded growth, delayed sexual maturity, loss of taste and prolonged wound healing. Other deficiency syndromes ensue from a lack of other trace elements in the soil.

Chemical fertilizers often exacerbate the deficiencies. Plants absorb nitrates from nitrogen fertilizers and the nitrates, in turn, destroy vitamin A, one of the essential vitamins found in plants. Even the "organically grown" label on a food does not necessarily guarantee nutritional superiority since the manure or compost used as fertilizer may vary greatly in nutrient content. Fertilizers should have trace elements added when deficiency is indicated by soil or crop analysis.

Storage

Foods continue to lose nutrients during the time required for harvesting and shipping crops. Even under the best storage conditions, vegetables kept too long decrease significantly in nutritive value. For example, spinach, potatoes and lettuce can lose up to 50 percent of their vitamin C content during warehouse storage.

Processing of Foods

As the next step in bringing food to the consumer, farmers and distributors deliver their raw goods to processors who then manufacture a variety of packaged products for the supermarket. Processing retards food spoilage. Canned and frozen meats and vegetables, prepared breads and cereals, refined flour and sugar, which remain attractive and succulent on supermarket shelves for considerable periods, represent a modern convenience. But the price paid for this convenience amounts to a drastic reduction in available nutrients.

Processing=Loss of Vitamins and Trace Elements

Processing yields greener vegetables and "purer" oils—the kinds of products the consumer has come to classify as being of high quality. In reality, such processing decreases the quality of foods by removing vital nutrients.

At the commercial freezing plant, during the freezing process, green vegetables may be scalded with the chelating agent EDTA, partially removing trace metals such as zinc, manganese and calcium. Because the surface metals are removed, the vegetables will remain a bright green rather than turn gray when cooked. Processing with EDTA reduces the zinc and manganese content of green peas to 20 percent of the expected normal range. Due to widespread use of EDTA in food processing, man may consume as much as 100 mg of this chemical per day, further affecting the body's intake of trace metals.

Metals are also removed during processing of such foods as peanut butter and oils. Oils are naturally a dark color, due to what processors consider to be "impurities." These "impurities," which contribute odor and flavor, are actually nutrients! Other nutrients destroyed during this type of oil processing are vitamins E and A and phosphorous compounds such as lecithin. Vitamin E and lecithin are natural antioxidants which prevent rancidity. Processing companies remove them only to replace them with synthetic antioxidants called preservatives. Today there is no such thing as an unrefined vegetable oil on the market except in health food stores.

Wheat and Sugar Are "Purified"

Similar to the process of refining oil are processes used to refine whole wheat and whole sugar. Each of these foods contains a natural abundance of vitamins, minerals, enzymes, lipids, and protein. In processing, both become stripped down to devitalized, tasteless products which are nutritionally inferior to the whole foods.

When whole wheat is milled into white flour, the bran,

middlings and wheat germ are extracted from the kernel. Since these wheat byproducts furnish a rich source of trace elements and vitamins, refined white flour loses most of the chromium, zinc, iron, manganese, B vitamins and vitamin E originally present in the whole wheat kernel. Stripped of these vital nutrients, what remains of the wheat kernel is then bleached white as snow.

Why is wheat processed to such an extent? Whole-grain flour just doesn't keep as well as refined flour. If the oil and protein in the wheat germ and all the B vitamins were not extracted, flour would have to be treated as a product, like nuts, that goes rancid—a commercial inconvenience.

Sugar cane suffers an equally tragic fate. At the sugar mill the juice is pressed out of the cane, removing the iron- and calcium-rich molasses. The remaining raw sugar, still rich in minerals and vitamins, is then refined and whitened. In the process, thiamine, riboflavin, niacin, calcium, phosphorus and most of the iron and potassium are stripped away until only the naked carbohydrate sucrose remains. Sugar companies correctly label their white-sugar products "pure sugar"! (Even "unrefined sugar" and brown sugar are largely sucrose with a small amount of impurities either not extracted or added back.)

After processing, the nutrient-rich wheat and sugar residues serve as ingredients in animal feed. Ironically, then, man selectively receives carbohydrates, but how well fed indeed are the animals!

Several major deficits result from the removal of vital nutrients from whole wheat and sugar. White flour and sugar supply plenty of calories, but lack the nutrients necessary for the proper utilization of those calories. Vitamin B-6, vitamin E, chromium, manganese, zinc and magnesium, all contained in the "refuse" left after processing, play a significant role in the body's use of starches and sugars.

Chromium, for example, occurs in the glucose tolerance factor needed to burn sugar. Chromium levels rise in response to sugar ingestion. With each rise, some chromium is lost in the urine. Refined white flour retains only 13 percent of the chromium found in whole wheat and refined sugar only a trace of the chromium found in sugar cane. Consequently, the refined foods do not have enough chromium to utilize the sugar, so that the body must rely on the chromium content of other foods in order to metabolize carbohydrates. Often these other foods do not form part of the daily diet.

Processing results in the removal of a greater percentage of some vitamins and minerals than others, thus upsetting the natural balance among the nutrients present in whole foods. An example is cadmium's relationship to zinc. Whole wheat contains cadmium and zinc in a ratio of 1 to 120, but after processing the ratio in white flour becomes 1 to 20. Cadmium competes with and displaces the vitally important zinc in man. An excess of cadmium interferes with zinc metabolism and can produce high blood pressure.

Dietary Fiber Is Important

Deficiencies and imbalances resulting from the refining of foods can be correlated with some diseases. During World War II Denmark stopped refining flour, an action which was not accompanied by any other marked changes in living habits. Later it was found that the death rate had dropped and that there had been a marked decline in cancer, heart disease, diabetes, kidney trouble and high blood pressure. Some of these diseases are related to the loss, during refinement, of roughage, or fiber, in the form of the bran and cellulose of plants.

Inadequate dietary fiber can, furthermore, lead to constipation. Constipation, an ailment of civilization, is largely due to the consumption of food that leaves little or no residue, one that is completely digested, such as refined carbohydrates. The body receives an abundance of worthless calories through refined sugar consumption rather than valuable calories through fiber foods such as fruits, vegetables and whole-grain bread. For example, the white bread eater receives 87.5 percent less fiber than the whole-wheat bread eater. Chronic constipation can cause diverticular disease of the colon and other bowel problems, especially in the aged.

Through the years, doctors have recommended relaxation, laxatives, prunes and enemas to relieve constipation. However, constipation can be easily prevented and cured by returning fiber to the diet. Unrefined bran, a rich source of food fiber, absorbs large amounts of water, has almost no calories and allays hunger. The amount of fiber required varies with the individual.

White Bread Is Not the Staff of Life

Although so obviously devoid of nutritive value, refined flour and sugar supply nearly half the total daily calories in an average American diet. White bread, for example, which is composed primarily of refined white flour, serves as a major staple food, though it provides almost none of the essential nutrients. Dr. Jean Mayer, Harvard nutritionist, believes that American white bleached dough products would not even receive the label "bread" in his native France, where flour is coarser and contains more vitamins and trace elements. At one time bread (made from whole wheat) merited the distinction "the staff of life," but today's white bread is about as life-sustaining as tissue paper!

Are Cereals Really Snacks?

Most packaged breakfast cereals provide other notorious examples of processed and nutritionally worthless foods. These cereals are composed mostly of refined grains, shortening and additives, and are loaded with refined sugar; some cereals contain as much as 50 percent sugar!

Michael Jacobson, consumer advocate, suggests that cereal products be categorized as snacks, rather than cereals—a term which implies a valid food. In most breakfast cereals, the natural nutrients have been processed out and some vitamins and minerals (but not important trace metals) added so that the food can be advertised as "vitamin-enriched," thereby increasing the advertising appeal. The consumer is fooled into believing that a nutritious food is offered. "Natural" breakfast cereals now on the market are certainly better; however, the manufacturers still insist on adding an excess of sugar.

In this generation, people raised on white bread, sugary breakfast cereals, commercial ice cream and other prepared foods have no concept of the truly wholesome foods from which these products originated. Food industries have convinced the public that a whiter, purer, longer-lasting, easier-to-prepare product is as nutritionally good, if not better, than the original food.

Clearly, tinkered foods at present available to the consumer simply do not provide all the nutrients essential to optimal physical and mental health. Despite Dr. Davis's and other researchers' evidence that even the best diet today is inadequate, the U.S. Food and Drug Administration (FDA) has slapped controls on the sale of nutrient supplements because they fear "health faddists" will receive overdoses. Yet, as Dr. Davis states, "No normal daily amount of a vitamin supplement gives 10 percent of a lethal dose." Moreover, the individual concerned with the quality of his or her food is not usually a faddist, but merely someone who recognizes the need for more than the manufacturers can offer.

A Do-it-yourself Score Card

In fairness to the food industry, we have listed some real improvements which have resulted from food processing. You may have items that you will want to add. Keep in mind that coconut oil is the most saturated oil and that soybeans are high in copper and low in zinc. Also, most aerosol propellants are air pollutants.

1. Sliced bread	11.
2. Widespread refrigeration	12.
3. A standard fresh egg	13.
4. Some frozen foods	14.
5.	15.
6.	16.
7.	17.
8.	18.
9.	19.
10.	20.

The list is short. Perhaps you can add other items.

Restoration, Enrichment and Fortification

In response to appeals from concerned nutritionists, notably the Food and Nutrition Board of the National Academy of Sciences, efforts have been made to increase the nutritive value of processed foods through restoration, enrichment and fortification. Restoration replaces in foods those nutrients which were present naturally but have been lost in processing (from 110 to 150 percent of the original value). Enrichment supplies foods with specific nutrients in conformity with a standard developed by the government. Fortification enhances foods by adding one or more nutrients which were not present or were present in small amounts before processing.

Federally endorsed in the United States, these practices have resulted in the enrichment of flour, bread, rice, cornmeal and other grain products with thiamine, riboflavin, niacin and iron; the fortification of whole, skim and nonfat dry milk with vitamins A and D; the addition of vitamin A to margarine; and the fortification of table salt with iodine. In some areas of the country, water is fluoridated to protect against dental caries.

While such modifications have improved the nutritional value of widely used processed foods to some extent, allowing most people to adhere to their preferred eating habits without suffering severe deficiency diseases, nutritional deficits persist. Ironically, the enrichment, restoration and fortification program itself has engendered new problems.

Rats Die on Enriched White Bread

At present, four nutrients (iron, thiamine, riboflavin and niacin) are used to enrich most commercial grain products. In his now well-known study, Dr. Roger Williams, former Director of the Clayton Foundation Biochemical Institute at the University of Texas (who discovered the B vitamin pantothenic acid), fed rats on standard enriched white bread. Within ninety days, two-thirds of the rats died while the others suffered severe malnutrition, resulting in stunted growth. An improved enriched bread to which Dr. Williams added the essential minerals magnesium, manganese, sulfur, copper, phosphorus and calcium plus the vitamins A, E, folic acid, pyridoxine (B-6), pantothenic acid and the amino acid lysine, maintained healthy rats indefinitely. A key supplement was lysine, an amino acid in wheat and rice, which enhanced the protein quality of the bread. Nutritional experts have urged the addition of lysine to wheat flour for years. On the basis of his findings Dr. Williams, too, advocates further enrichment of grain products.

In complete accord with Dr. Williams, the National Academy of Sciences' National Research Council now recommends the addition of six more (for a total of ten) vitamins and minerals (vitamin A, pyridoxine, folic acid, calcium, magnesium and zinc) to foods made from wheat, corn and rice. Since junk foods and snacks made from these grains are replacing wholesome foods as dietary staples, contributing 26 percent of the average daily caloric intake, the Food and Nutrition Board recognizes the compelling need to augment the nutritional value of these popular products.

Enriching a refined, sugar-laden food will indeed provide the consumer with a few more vitamins and minerals, but it will not alter a product's fundamental inadequacy. Advertising fosters the mirage that a nutritious product is offered because several nutrients providing some percentage of the RDAs have been added back when, in reality, it remains grossly inferior to the original natural food. The four nutrients currently used to enrich most flour and grain products, plus the six suggested additions, together comprise far fewer nutrients than those that were crushed, ground and squeezed out of the grain during processing. Vital metals such as molybdenum are lost from them forever. Moreover, food factors always work as a team, producing a synergistic (cooperative) effect, and a balanced intake is essential.

Royal Lee, D.D.S., recognized that the synergistic principle (the whole is greater than the sum of the effects of its individual parts) applies to nutrition when he stated, "Single synthetic fractions of foods used to imitate the whole substance cannot equal Nature's own concentration of nutritional factors." Natural foods (before processing) contain important functional nutrients, not yet recognized scientifically as essential, which enhance the action of vital nutrients. Present practices of food supplementation are not at all scientific, but rather amount to tinkering.

Hazards of Tinkering

Due to present enrichment procedures, many people may receive excessive amounts of certain trace metals. For example, commercial enriched white bread contains more iron than whole-wheat bread, and government officials advocate a still greater increase in the iron content of bread. The stated reason is that a specific portion of the American population may be anemic because their diets lack sufficient iron, a view fostered by the results of a ten-state nutritional survey in 1967 which showed that 27 percent of the women and girls studied had anemia.

Not *all* anemias are caused by lack of iron, so perhaps we would be better off treating the anemia individually with vitamin B-6 *or* iron supplements. A sweeping increase in the iron content of bread is not only shortsighted but potentially lethal. Iron can seriously intensify (possibly cause) Parkinson's disease, thalassemia, sickle cell disease, siderosis, hemochromatosis, Laennec's cirrhosis and porphyria cutanea tarda. These are disorders in which iron is improperly used in the body so that the victims must restrict their iron intake. (High iron levels have also been implicated in depression and in some forms of schizophrenia.) These people will either be forced to forego bread and cereals because of an artificially raised iron content, or suffer the consequences.

Moreover, the iron added to white bread is of questionable value as it is the ferric form, which the body does not absorb well, rather than the ferrous form which is better suited to human chemistry. The inorganic iron (ferric form) tends to combine with and inactivate vitamin E in the body, thus interfering with the antioxidant and therapeutic effects of this vitamin. Therefore, the true value of any iron-enriched bread is debatable.

Lactose Intolerance

Another important problem with the present enrichment program concerns the foods treated. Milk, for example, is an excellent food for many people. However, the majority of the world's population does not have the enzyme, lactase, needed to digest lactose, the sugar contained in cow's and goat's milk. In this country alone, lactose intolerance affects about forty million people. The net effect is that the fortification of milk with vitamins A and D provides no benefit to 20 percent of our population because they cannot drink milk. Although fortification of milk with A and D has benefited the millions who can drink milk, a way must be found to supply the rest of the population with these two vitamins.

Conserve Rather Than Restore

In contrast with the present practices of overrefining with subsequent enrichment, processing practices that conserve the nutrients natural to foods should be mandatory. The Food and Nutrition Board of the National Academy of Sciences urges industry to improve processing techniques aimed at conservation of nutritional quality, rather than to depend on restorative addition. A still more fundamental approach would be extensive nutritional education, restriction of the refinement processes and elimination of the multitude of nonfoods now so widely consumed. The practices of restoration, enrichment and fortification can be beneficial, but not when used as compensation or justification for extensive refinement and processing.

Food Additives

During the nineteenth century, unscrupulous and concealed adulteration of foods with chemical substances to maintain and enhance color, flavor and texture gave rise to public attempts to establish a consumer protection agency. Harvey W. Wiley's poison squad and Upton Sinclair's book *The Jungle* played major roles in securing the Pure Food and Drug Act of 1906. Wily manufacturers, however, could easily circumvent this law since any prosecutor had to prove "intent to defraud the public."

In 1958, the U.S. government authorized a Food Additive Amendment stipulating that any substance added to a food must be proven safe by the manufacturer before being offered for sale. On the basis of this amendment, FDA officials compiled a list of additives "generally recognized as safe" (GRAS). Safety criteria include probable consumption and safety factors set by animal testing, but the GRAS list continually fluctuates as some additives prove dangerous *subsequent* to their approval and sale. Cumulative effects of these chemicals in man remain largely unknown, and the possible interaction of some food additives has seldom been considered since toxicity studies usually deal with individual additives.

Commonly defined as "those substances the use of which results or may be reasonably expected to result, directly or indirectly, in their becoming a component or otherwise affecting the characteristics of any food," some 2,500 to 3,000 food additives are currently in use. Among those most often employed are: preservatives (to keep food fresh during storage, shipping and shelving); antioxidants (to retard oxidative breakdown of fats and oils which causes rancidity at room temperature); antibiotics (to extend the fresh life of food and cause animals to grow more rapidly); hormones (to fatten animals with less feed); stabilizers and emulsifiers (to keep food a uniform, smooth texture); sequestrants (to separate trace elements that might otherwise interfere with food processing); buffers and neutralizers (to make foods more or less acid); and colors and flavors. Also used in foods are solvents (to keep other additives properly distributed); coating agents (to make such foods as chocolates and oranges shine); propellants or aerating agents (to add carbonation to beverages or allow foods with creamy textures to be ejected from aerosol cans); and bleaches, moisteners, drying agents, extenders, thickeners, conditioners, curing agents (in meat), hydrolizers, hydrogenators, fortifiers, sweeteners and compounds with particular purposes too numerous to mention.

Few of these additives have any nutritional value and many are unnecessary; they are added simply at the discretion of the processors. On an average, the consumer swallows five pounds of additives per year, suffering the possible risk of toxicity. To illustrate the potential and real hazards of food additives, the following pages offer detailed information concerning a variety of these substances.

Preservatives

Preservatives, which include antimicrobials, antioxidants and antibiotics, serve as merchandising aids which are commonly used in processed foods to prolong shelf life. "Antimicrobial" preservatives are used to inhibit, not prevent, bacteria or mold growth. One such antimicrobial agent, diphenyl, is used in the wrapping material on citrus fruits to inhibit mold growth and disguise true age. The antioxidants commonly used to combat rancidity in fatty foods include butylated hydroxyanisole (BHA), butylated hydroxytoluene (BHT), propyl gallate, lecithin and alpha tocopherol (vitamin E). The necessity for antioxidants is questionable, as oils (especially natural unprocessed oils) will keep perfectly well if refrigerated.

BHT and BHA provide good examples of the unnecessary use of synthetic food additives. They are used by some manufacturers of breakfast cereals, chewing gum, vegetable oil, shortening, potato chips, candy and other oil-containing products. Some manufacturers produce these same foods without using BHT or BHA, which illustrates the superfluous nature of these chemicals. Despite the fact that they accumulate in body fat, BHA and BHT have not been adequately tested for possible toxic effects such as the production of cancer. Both BHA and BHT are maintained on the GRAS list, though they do not benefit the consumer and are unnecessary.

Two preservatives which have received much publicity are sodium nitrate and sodium nitrite. Sodium nitrite is used in meats to prevent the growth of bacteria which cause botulism. Nitrite also imparts the characteristic pink color to cured foods and contributes slightly to the taste. Sodium nitrite appears in luncheon meats, ham, hot dogs, many other processed meats, and smoked fish; Americans cannot purchase bacon that has not been processed with this additive.

Both sodium nitrate and sodium nitrite are toxic at levels only moderately higher than the levels used in food. We know that sodium nitrate is potentially dangerous to small children, can deform the fetus in pregnant women and can cause serious damage in anemic persons. Infants have died from nitrite poisoning and many others have been incapacitated.

Nitrite's toxicity is due to its affinity for hemoglobin, which is converted to methemoglobin. At high levels, death results from failure of oxygen transport. Despite the fact that infants are much more susceptible to methemoglobinemia than adults, nitrite and/or nitrate are added to some meat-containing baby foods. Furthermore, nitrites are potentially dangerous, in that they can be transformed into nitrosamines, which are carcinogens (cancer-causing chemicals) either by heating or by the action of stomach acids.

Dr. Michael Jacobson, codirector of the Center for Science in the Public Interest, has stated that he considers bacon a most dangerous food because of the carcinogen formed by heating. Maximum tolerance levels should be set for the use of sodium nitrite and sodium nitrate, and a substitute sought.

Antibiotics and Hormones

Antibiotics such as chlortetracycline or oxytetracycline act as preservatives and are used to promote rapid animal growth. Penicillin and other antibiotics are used to treat mastitis, an udder infection of cows, and residues may be found in milk brought to market by farmers.

Antibiotic residues are sometimes left in meat, possibly producing undesirable effects. Some experiments indicate that antibiotics alter the intestinal flora, lowering ability to synthesize vitamins while allowing the development of antibiotic-resistant bacteria. One poisonous and meat-transmitted bacterium is *salmonella*, the most common kind of food poisoning in America. In addition, antibiotics administered to combat infections may be rendered ineffective by prolonged ingestion.

At one time hormones, such as phenylarsonic acid and diethylstilbestrol (DES) were generally used to increase animal growth. DES is a synthetic estrogen, or artificial female sex hormone, which increases the rate of weight gain per pound of feed in male animals. DES was first used in chickens, then in cattle. It was found to have carcinogenic and possibly sterilizing effects, and repeated small doses are more destructive than a single large dose. Although the use of DES in animal feed has been banned, it is currently allowed in the form of animal implants to encourage growth, and may be used until tests are concluded to prove that they are harmful. This is characteristic of the legal turmoil engendered by this apparently profitable substance. Despite the known hazard, enough people work to keep DES in use so that its status has been in a state of flux since its effects have been discovered.

Stabilizers

Brominated vegetable oil (BVO) is a stabilizer. Flavoring oils in soft drinks would float to the surface without BVO, which has the same density as water and helps to disperse the lighter-than-water oils throughout the drink. Studies indicate that BVO accumulates in animal tissue and is harmful to certain body organs of the rat, but possible long-term toxic effects, such as cancer or birth defects, remain unknown. BVO was banned in Sweden in 1968 and in Britain in 1969, but Americans still add BVO to soft drinks and other snack-type foods that are devoid of nutritional value. Again, safe alternatives are available.

Emulsifiers

Synthetic emulsifiers, used by manufacturers to make water mix with the fats in a product, replace a product's natural emulsifiers destroyed by processing.

An excess of emulsifiers in the body poses a serious threat, since they disturb the biochemical action of the linings of the stomach and intestine, thereby enabling ingested poisons to pass more easily into our systems. For example, in test animals emulsifiers increased the intake of iron from foods; the concentration of the excess iron in the animals' spleens and livers resulted in cirrhosis and cancer. In man, some emulsifiers can cause a tremendous increase in the absorption of fat-soluble vitamin A, which is toxic at high levels. Emulsifiers may also accelerate the absorption of carcinogenic food additives; but, though many have voiced concern, the emulsifiers have not been tested with other additives.

Food Colorings

Among the additives which may be rapidly and excessively absorbed by the body due to the presence of emulsifiers are the coloring agents. Since coloring greatly enhances food appeal, the coloring agents form the most prevalent group of food additives. Although substances derived from plants, insects and minerals color some foods, more than 90 percent of the coloring agents used in America are synthetic chemicals known as "certified" food dyes because the FDA must certify their use. Uncertified colors are generally not considered dangerous, but the certified colors are almost universally suspect as carcinogens.

Every year, four million pounds of certified dyes are added to foods manufactured in the United States. Despite regulation by the FDA, the history of their use is replete with surprises.

In 1919, the famous "butter yellow" was found to produce cancer of the liver and was removed from the market. In 1960, the certified colors FD&C Orange Nos. 1 and 2 and Red No. 1 were banned from the market because they were found to damage internal organs. Yellow Nos. 1, 2, 3 and 4 were discovered to induce intestinal lesions, heart damage and other harmful effects in animals. FD&C Red No. 32 was used in a dyebath for more than half the Florida orange crop before being banned. Violet No. 1, used to stamp the Department of Agriculture's inspection seal on meat and to color candy, beverages and pet food, was banned in April 1973 due to evidence of cancer and skin lesions. Note the irony: the dye used to indicate safe meat was itself dangerous!

At present, eight certified food dyes may be used in any food: Blues 1 and 2; Green 3; Reds 2, 3 and 40; and Yellows 5 and 6. Three others are restricted in use: Red 4, Citrus Red 2 and Orange B. Red 4 is restricted to use in maraschino cherries on the basis that no one would eat *that many* candied cherries.

Red 4 had wide use in foods until the discovery that high doses harmed the adrenal glands and urinary bladders of dogs. In 1965, Red 4 use was about to be banned entirely in food, but the maraschino cherry lobbyists convinced the FDA that one only eats a few cherries at a time, which would not provide enough Red 4 to cause harm.

Citrus Red 2, used only to color the skin of oranges (the FDA doubts that anyone would want to eat the peel) may be a weak carcinogen. (Many people make marmalade using orange peel.) At least eleven states and Canada have now banned the sale of artificially colored oranges.

Orange B, which has been used since 1966 to color frankfurters, is chemically related to Red No. 2. Red No. 2 is widely used to impart the striking cherry tinge to certain soft drinks, candies, ice cream, baked goods, cherries and even sausages. Red 2 was banned in the Soviet Union on the grounds that in laboratory rats it caused birth defects, impaired reproduction and induced cancer. To date, this has been the only dye that has been tested for birth defects. Russian experts claim that only two of our certified food dyes are harmless.

Other dyes used today have engendered some concern. The International Union Against Cancer rates Green No. 3 and Blue No. 1 as unsuitable or potentially dangerous for man or animals. When injected in animals, both have been reported to produce cancer, yet we have been consuming Green No. 3 since 1927 and Blue No. 1 since 1929. Studies of Yellow No. 6, widely used to color butter, margarine and chicken skin, indicate it is safe. However, one study shows that it affects the eye, sometimes causing blindness. The leading British authority, Dr. Bicknell, believes the azo dyes (Yellows 5 and 6 and Reds 2 and 4) to be particularly dangerous.

Such dyes, believed by many to be hazardous due to

their carcinogenic and other damaging effects, may pose a still greater threat when combined with emulsifiers in the same product (i.e., ice creams, margarines, some breads and candy).

Although the 1960 Food Coloring Law established more severe safety regulations for food dyes, many doubtful colorings continue to enjoy widespread use.

Artificial Flavorings

Flavorings comprise one of the largest and most important categories of additives. Artificial flavorings mask the absence of more expensive natural flavors, sometimes improving flavor or even providing new flavors. Approximately 70 percent of the currently marketed flavorings are completely synthetic. (This figure does not include the laboratory duplications of natural flavoring substances.) Despite the enormous daily consumption of flavorings, most of the thousands of flavorings, natural or synthetic, have not been tested for their ability to produce cancer, birth defects or mutations.

Monosodium Glutamate

One flavoring additive which has, however, received much attention is monosodium glutamate (MSG) which was developed in Japan. Millions of pounds are used in Japan as in the United States to enhance the flavor of protein foods by exciting the taste buds. But MSG's ability to overexcite nerve endings may cause brain damage, especially in infants, who do not have a well-developed blood-brain barrier to inhibit MSG from travelling freely to the brain. Baby food manufacturers recently agreed to omit MSG from their infant products since MSG was only placed in the food to make it taste better to the mother!

Dr. Ho Man Kwok, in 1968, found MSG to be responsible for what he called "the Chinese restaurant syndrome." Susceptible individuals complained, shortly after ingesting food at a Chinese restaurant, of a burning sensation in the back of the neck, headaches and chest tightness. Today, monosodium glutamate remains a controversial item because many authorities consider it harmless, if not salutary. MSG, as a flavor enhancer, remains on the FDA's GRAS list.

"All-American" Products

The usual supermarket probably contains about eight thousand food items, more than two-thirds of which were never seen in a store before World War II. Nearly all of these new items are processed foods or formula foods, items which are partially or totally artificial. Sourpuss, for example, is a sour synthetic lemon juice that is sometimes used instead of real lemon juice in mixed drinks. Other synthetics are sold in the shape of a lime or a lemon and bear the label "imitation lime juice" or "imitation lemon juice." Tang is synthetic orange juice and contains no vital trace elements. White vinegar is pure 5 percent acetic acid. Many "fruit punches" are highly synthetic with artificial flavors and colors.

Hot dogs, America's favorite "meat" product, may actually contain little meat, but may instead be comprised largely of water, spices, additives (including sodium nitrate, sodium ascorbate and glucona delta lactose) and fillers. Fatty parts of the animal (which the consumer would ordinarily avoid) may supply the meat in hot dogs. To increase the protein content of hot dogs, dry milk and soy flour are added. Other binders may include cereal or starchy vegetable flour. For a time, FD&C Red No. 4 was used on hot-dog casings, but eventually it was found that this dye damaged the bladders of test animals; vegetable dyes are currently used.

The mustard that is applied to hot dogs may contain even more chemical additives than the hot dog. The bun wrapped around the hot dog typically is made with hydrogenated vegetable oils (the process of hydrogenation destroys essential fatty acids by saturating them); BHT or BHA to keep the shortening from oxidizing; emulsifiers; chlorine dioxide to bleach the refined flour; and potassium bromate and iodate to make the dough elastic and stable. Some hot-dog buns are even dyed yellow, apparently to convince the consumer that eggs and/or butter have been added.

And consider that great American invention called ice cream. The FDA does not require ice cream packagers to list the additives in their products, but many chemical additives, being cheaper than natural factors, are often used. As a result, most inexpensive, prepacked ice creams may be almost totally artificial. Laboratory analyses from Drs. Francis J. Waickman and Joseph L. Kloss of Cuyahoga Falls, Ohio, disclosed that the following were found to be constituents of synthetic ice cream:

> Diethyl glucol—a cheap chemical used as an emulsifier to substitute for the lecithin in eggs.
>
> Piperonal—extensively used as a substitute for vanilla. This is also used to kill lice.
>
> Aldehyde C17—used to flavor cherry ice cream. This liquid is used in aniline dyes, plastic and rubber.
>
> Ethyl acetate—used to achieve pineapple flavor. This also serves as a cleaner for leather and textiles and as a solvent for lacquer.
>
> Butyraldehyde—gives ice cream various nut-like flavors and is commonly an ingredient of rubber cement.
>
> Amyl acetate—gives banana ice cream its flavor and is used commercially as an oil paint solvent.
>
> Benzyl acetate—provides strawberry flavor to ice cream and is used as a solvent for plastics.

Of course, not all ice creams contain these artificial additions. (There are natural ice creams, but they are more expensive. Cheaper products with artificial additives are often used for this reason.)

Dietetic products generally are not better and are sometimes worse. The following is taken from the label of a well-known dietary frozen dessert:

> concentrated skim milk, water, sugar, microcrystalline cellulose, polyglycerol esters of fatty acids [emulsifier], fructose, artificial flavor, cellulose gum, guar gum, carrageenan, artificial color, ascorbic acid [C], ferrous sulfate [iron], niacinamide [B-3], vitamin A palmitate, pyridoxine hydrochloride [B-6], thiamine hydrochloride [B-1], riboflavin [B-2] and folic

acid [B-vitamin]. (Our inserts are in brackets.)

We all know how great Mom's old-fashioned apple pie tastes; we shouldn't be fooled by some of the convenient premade pies available at the grocery store. We offer a sample of an ingredient label from one such concoction:

> water, sugar, shortening, corn syrup, coconut, whey solids, dextrose, food starch-modified, sodium caseinate (a milk protein), whole milk solids, mono- and diglycerides, salt, artificial flavor, vanilla, polysorbate 60 and stearyl-2-lactylate [emulsifiers], hydroxpropyl cellulose, monosodium phosphate, guar gum, lecithin, and artificial color in a crust of wheat flour, shortening, sugar, corn syrup, rye flour, water, salt, invert syrup, molasses, leavening, and artificial flavor.

An important point to remember when reading the ingredients of a product is that they are listed in decreasing order of concentration (note that sugar and water are at or near the beginning of the above lists).

Learning What to Eat

Faced with an appalling abundance of adulterated foods and the frightening fact that most "All-American" convenience foods represent thoroughly debased products, the consumer may indeed wonder, "Well, what *should* I eat?" Short of the radical decision to "live off the land," one cannot avoid all processed and chemically treated foods, since relatively few economical substitutes are currently available.

To obtain an adequate balance of essential nutrients, one must reject the spurious notions of food quality fostered by manufacturers and advertisers. Fortunately, a careful selection of foods from the supermarket, plus several natural items from health food stores, and more enlightened methods of food preparation afford the rudimentary basis for a healthier way of life.

Become an avid label reader; avoid those products loaded with synthetic chemical additives. Push that shopping cart past the refined carbohydrates, and avoid canned foods immersed in sugary syrups. Shun bakery products. As a sweetener, use honey as a substitute for sugar in baking and in tea and coffee, or use artificial sweeteners in restricted amounts. Experiment: try carob molasses, carob syrup, unrefined molasses and date sugar. If possible, resist the clarion call of a sweet tooth and omit sugar completely. Within a few weeks, the desire for sweets will begin to disappear.

Linger at the fresh fruit and vegetable counters. Fruits and vegetables provide a wealth of vitamins and minerals, aid in the reduction of blood cholesterol and promote regularity.

Nuts, the dried fruits and seeds of many plants, are another nutritious and delicious food. Nuts are high in unsaturated fats and incomplete protein, and are rich sources of important nutrients, especially the trace minerals. Because nuts are high in fat, they are digested slowly, thus allaying hunger.

If concerned about the fat (especially the saturated fat) content of foods, remember that animal fat is 100 percent saturated. Use more lean meats, poultry and fish. Avoid the high-fat, sausage-type meats and filled luncheon meats. Turn to alternative sources of protein such as eggs, dairy products (especially cheese—low in fat, if preferred), soybeans, nuts, legumes, lentils, whole grains, wheat germ and wheat bran and maize. Limit use of lard, butter, margarine, hydrogenated shortening and processed peanut butter and bacon. Use more liquid vegetable oils.

The Hunzas, who subsist primarily on grains (wheat, barley, maize), fruits (fresh and dried) and goat's milk and butter, enjoy robust health, phenomenal energy and endurance. American consumers can benefit similarly from a combination of these foods; and, as consumers selectively avoid inadequate adulterated foods, the magic wand of supply and demand will eventually banish them from the market.

Take supplements of those nutrients most difficult to obtain in foods. At the very minimum, purchase a multivitamin formula which contains no copper or iron but does contain zinc.

Improved methods of preparing and cooking foods will prevent loss of nutrients. Since iron knives oxidize vitamin C, a stainless steel or plastic knife should be used when slicing fruits and vegetables high in C such as oranges, lemons, grapefruit and cabbage.

Man is the only species who overheats his food, and many

people will stoutly defend the assumed value of hot foods. Arhenius proved many years ago that most chemical reactions double in rate with every 10°C rise in temperature. The vitamins in food obey this law and some disintegrate rapidly on steam tables, in boiling water, and with the time added for the rituals involved in preparing hot foods. However well intentioned it may be, the whole "hot lunch program" frequently amounts only to an endeavor that keeps a maximum number of people employed in a glittering stainless steel empire.

Vegetables should be steamed in minimal water to the point of palatability. Only one meat (pork) and some kinds of fish need to be well done. Other meats can be cooked to taste. A few plants and legumes must be well cooked. A pressure cooker prepares food rapidly, retains nutrients and requires little water. A wok (a Chinese cooking vessel) steam fries vegetables in a tasty manner. All pot liquors and juices should be saved to make a delicious soup.

Overall health will be immensely benefited as we employ better methods of preparing foods and begin to reeducate our taste buds.

Suggestions for Making Nutritious Natural Cereal

Now that big food processors have jumped on the profitable bandwagon of "natural" cereal breakfast foods, the time has come to set guidelines for such foods if they are to be termed "natural."

1. Cooking must be avoided or minimized. (Too much cooking destroys vitamins.)
2. Sugar should not be added.
3. Wheat germ should not be "toasted."
4. Extra vitamins or minerals should not be added.
5. The product may contain a mixture of dried natural fruits which can be easily hydrated with milk. Fresh fruit should always be added if available.

Since none of the "natural" products meet all these simple standards, it is cheaper and better to make your own. A week's supply can be made and stored in the refrigerator.

Base: Wheat bran, rolled oats, or freshly puffed maize (popcorn). (Popcorn and milk is an old New England Sunday-night-supper dish.)

Sea kelp powder, if desired.

Dried fruits (chopped or cut in a blender): pitted dates, dried apples, peaches, apricots, prunes, raisins.

Chopped nuts: pecans, peanuts, almonds, cashews, filberts, etc.

Seeds: sesame, sunflower, pumpkin.

Wheat germ (not the toasted variety).

Brewer's yeast (numerous powders available).

Sweetener (from plastic squeeze bottle): cane molasses, sugar beet molasses, citrus molasses or honey (possibly aspartame).

Homemade Granola

3 pounds rolled oats
1½ pounds rolled wheat
½ to 1 pound sunflower seeds
½ to 1 pound sesame seeds
½ to 1 pound wheat germ (raw)
¼ pound dry milk
1 pound or more nuts (almonds, cashews, peanuts)
½ pound shredded coconut (optional)
vegetable oil, approx. 1 quart
1 to 1½ pounds honey
1 pound raisins or dates

Combine and mix all ingredients except oil, honey and raisins. Add enough oil to just slightly wet the ingredients and mix thoroughly. Add honey to taste and mix again. Place thin layer on baking sheets in a 300 degree oven and watch carefully. (The first batch takes a while to start cooking, but after the pans heat up, the granola can easily burn.) Once the granola starts to roast, stir every few minutes (especially around the edges of the pans) to prevent burning; take out when light golden brown. Spread on paper to dry and cool; add raisins and store in closed containers.

This is a basic recipe which can be varied to suit your taste. It yields about 10 pounds of granola; one can cut down all ingredients for a smaller quantity.

Snack Mix

Mix together any of the following:
sesame seeds
sunflower seeds
pumpkin seeds
raisins
dates, figs
cashews
walnuts
almonds
peanuts

Dietary Soup

To bouillon cubes (beef or chicken) add puffed maize instead of croutons.

Puffed Maize as a Breakfast Cereal

The convenience of a ready-to-eat cereal may be great compared to other breakfast foods. With these guidelines a week's supply of good-to-chew natural food can be quickly and easily made in your own kitchen.

Start with 1 cup chopped nuts or seeds. Add 1 cup wheat germ, ¼ cup brewer's yeast, 4 cups wheat bran, puffed and slightly blended maize, rolled oats or any combination of the three; 2 cups chopped dried fruit; and ½ teaspoon dried kelp. Mix well and store in refrigerator. Use honey or molasses from a plastic squeeze bottle when serving with milk.

The puffed maize can easily be made in a deep kettle with lid. Two tablespoons of polyunsaturated oil is placed in the bottom of the pan and heated at the three-quarter speed on an electric burner. Initially one kernel of maize can be placed in the kettle to test the temperature. When the single kernel starts to sizzle, or puff, enough of the rest to cover the bottom in a single layer can then be added. No shaking is necessary. When all popping noise stops, the product is ready for serving. Salt to taste.

Puffed maize can be used instead of croutons in all soups. It can be used instead of white bread as a base for stuffing for poultry and meatloaf. Puffed maize can be the basis for home-made granola, since the slow speed of any blender will cut the puffed maize into a tasty cereal.

Rather than permit a child to go off without breakfast, one can hand him a bag of puffed maize as he runs for the school bus.

Puffed maize is unique as a cereal food. The outer shell of the maize is strong, to resist attacks by insects. The nutritional value is that of all corn. (It is low only in protein—and the specific protein it does contain is low in tryptophan and lysine. This, however, is true of all grains.) Many people find puffed maize, with its content of natural husk or bran, to be laxative. Better bowel movements are the great advantage of eating the whole natural grain.

Shelf life is certainly two to three years, and the method of preparation is simple—namely, the application of heat. In dry climates maize is less likely to puff fully. However, it will puff if the moisture is restored to the kernel.

The price of maize is lower than or competitive with that of other cereal grains. The yield per acre is less than that for wheat or field corn, but maize needs less extensive processing. As of 1975, maize costs 30 cents a pound, barley 19 cents and some less nutritious ready-made breakfast foods about $1.00 a pound.

References

An apple a day—does it really keep the doctor away? *Seed, U.C.I. Monthly,* April 1974.

Bauman, H. E. What does the consumer know about nutrition? *JAMA* 225:61, 1973.

Bricklin, M. Bathroom death and how to prevent it. *Prevention* p.71, July 1974.

Food and your family. Bulletin, Ada, Michigan: Amway Corp., 1972.

General policies in regard to improvement of nutritive quality of foods. *Nutr. Rev.* 31:324, 1973.

Hawken, P. and Rohe, F. *The oil story.* Boston: Organic Merchants.

Henkin, H., Merta, M. and Staples, J. *The environment, the establishment and the law.* Boston: Houghton Mifflin, 1971.

Improvement of the nutritive quality of foods. *JAMA* 225:116, 1973.

Jacobson, M. F. *Eater's digest: The consumer's factbook of food additives.* Garden City, New York: Doubleday, 1972.

Kirschman, J. D., director, Nutrition Search. *Nutrition Almanac,* U.S.A. Minneapolis, Minn.: Associated Litho. 1973.

Lear, J. The flimsy staff of life. *SR* p. 53, October 1970.

Lederman, L. The acid in the sweetness. *The Sciences* p. 6, July/August 1974.

Marine, G. and Van Allen, J. *Food pollution: The violation of our inner ecology.* New York: Holt, Rinehart and Winston, 1972.

Poppy, J. *Adelle Davis and the new nutrition religion.* New York: Schizophrenics Anonymous of White Plains, N.Y.

Wickenden, L. *Our daily poison.* Old Greenwich, Connecticut: Devin-Adair, 1956.

Williams, R. Should the science-based food industry be expected to advance? Presented to Nat. Acad. Sci., 21 October 1970.

CHAPTER 4

Those Publicized Weight-reducing Regimes

People are never at a loss to find new ways to wither away unwanted poundage. The Ice Cream diet, the Drinking Man's diet, the Sweet-tooth diet, the Grapefruit diet, the Operant Conditioning diet, Dr. Atkins' Diet Revolution, Dr. Stillman's Quick Weight Loss diet and countless others have all appeared in the past decade or so. Some who say they "have no willpower" rely instead on appetite suppressants, even though there has been considerable concern about the risk of psychological and sometimes physical dependence on amphetamines and similar drugs.

The continuing plethora of new weight-reduction regimens testifies both to the ingenuity of the human mind and to the average dieter's lack of perseverance. Since Americans continue to try one after another, it might be prudent to ask: are reducing diets helpful or harmful in effecting weight reduction while maintaining body nutrition and sanity?

One currently popular diet is the "Cider Vinegar, Lecithin, Kelp and B-6" diet. This consists of 1,000 calories a day accompanied by the use of these four adjuvants. The creator of this diet states that she lost 12 pounds in two weeks. In our opinion, the effectiveness of the cider vinegar, the kelp and even the lecithin for weight reduction is questionable. Vitamin B-6, however, is known to aid fluid and weight loss. (The diet's originator, Mary Ann Crenshaw, was careful to supplement her B-6 intake with a source of all the B-complex vitamins. This, in our view, is an important guideline for anyone trying the diet.)

Two other popular and much-publicized diets are Dr. Stillman's Quick Weight Loss Diet and Dr. Atkins' Diet Revolution, both of which advocate a high-protein, low-carbohydrate regimen designed to induce ketosis—the presence in the body of excessive amounts of ketone (acetone) bodies, an indication that unwanted fat is being burned off as fuel. (The presence of ketone bodies in the urine indicates that ketosis has been established.)

The basic Stillman diet allows only lean meats and poultry, lean seafood, eggs and low-fat cheeses plus vitamin supplements and eight glasses of water a day. In a study by Bonnie Worthington and Linda Taylor, matched subjects were put on this diet or on a balanced low-calorie diet for two weeks and were then tested for any changes in body state. The only positive result was an initial rapid weight loss for the Quick Weight Loss dieters. Tests also revealed a definite increase in the frequency and amount of urinary ketones and a resultant depression of appetite. This sounds appealing, but one must remember that some carbohydrates are needed by the body to regulate protein and fat metabolism and to maintain adequate functioning of brain and nerve cells. To eliminate carbohydrates from the diet is to induce an abnormal metabolic state which may cause complications leading to permanent cellular damage.

Recently Rickman et al. reported a rise in serum cholesterol levels averaging 33 mg percent in subjects kept on the Stillman diet from three to seventeen days. (By way of contrast, Svacha et al. studied serum cholesterol levels of men ingesting three eggs a day for three weeks and found that their levels increased by only 13 mg percent.) Thus, not only is necessary carbohydrate intake severely restricted on the Stillman diet, but increases in serum cholesterol occur which may foster or enhance cardiovascular difficulties.

Dr. Atkins' diet in some respects parallels the Stillman diet but allows the individual to eat any and all the protein and fat he wants, with a zero-carbohydrate intake at first, thus utilizing stored fat as fuel rather than available carbohydrates. (Another difference is that Dr. Atkins does not stress the use of great quantities of water. He says not to limit fluids but that there is no need to "force" them.)

But again, ketosis indicates an abnormal metabolic state due to lack of carbohydrates, which is very dangerous for some people. Such a diet, while successful in inducing rapid weight loss, may have serious long-term effects. This diet is extremely high in cholesterol and saturated fats, and when the body weight stabilizes, such a diet tends to increase serum cholesterol and B-lipoprotein levels, which may possibly promote atherosclerosis and cardiovascular complications in later life. Although the immediate result of this diet is rewarding, nausea can occur with rapid weight loss. Also, it would seem likely that individuals, seldom able to withstand dietary restrictions for more than a month, would revert to their previous higher carbohydrate intake.

Other diets somewhat similar in that they restrict the *kinds* of food eaten are the so-called Mayo Diet (which did *not* originate at the famous Mayo Clinic), and the Drinking Man's diet. The so-called Mayo Diet advocates grapefruit for its supposed fat-dissolving qualities (not true!). Other foods such as eggs, meat, fish and some vegetables are also allowed. The Drinking Man's diet substitutes high-calorie alcohol for some of the dietary carbohydrate allowance.

All of these diets do cause weight loss, as any low-calorie diet would in most individuals, but at what price? Usually, the cost of the book, plus the mental anguish caused by severely imbalanced dietary intake and a desire to eat those foods prohibited by the diet.

The "Zen" macrobiotic diet is not a reducing diet in its intention, but because of its restrictions it can cause weight loss and irreversible damage to health. It has even been found to constitute a threat to life. This diet, which really has little connection with Zen Buddhism, was invented by and named by George Ohsawa and is claimed to be a means of creating a spiritual awakening or rebirth.

The seven stages of the diet serve to reduce the variety of food ingested while purportedly helping the individual to achieve well-being. In the first stage of the diet such foods as chicken, fruit, vegetables, seafood and cereals are allowed. Brown rice is emphasized. Successive stages call for a gradual reduction of foods until, in the last stage, all that one ingests is brown rice and tea. Fortunately, most individuals following this diet never reach the last stages, but with persistence in following some of the preceding diets one stands in great danger of incurring severe nutritional deficiencies.

Several people have suffered advanced malnutrition in the seventh stage of the macrobiotic diet. One patient lost her teeth, became severely anemic, stopped menstruating and finally died. Cases of scurvy, hypoproteinemia, hypocalcemia, emaciation due to starvation, loss of kidney function due to restrictive fluid intake and, finally, death have all been reported following continuous macrobiotic dieting. (How can one hope to reach a state of well-being when the body is deprived of nutrients essential to proper brain and body function?)

People who decide to undertake a crash diet may fail to realize that the most important aspect of weight reduction and weight control is keeping weight off by learning proper eating habits. An ideal reducing diet must satisfy nutritional needs in order to maintain mental health (which, in turn, can make it easier to muster the necessary determination).

By omitting or severely restricting the kinds of foods which contain any of the body's basic requirements (carbohydrates, proteins and fats) we deprive it of the essential vitamins and minerals needed to maintain optimal mental function. Dizziness, fatigue, and even psychotic or neurotic behavior patterns may result from lack of vital nutrients.

References

Atkins, R. C. *Dr. Atkins' diet revolution.* Philadelphia: David McKay, 1972.

Crenshaw, M. A. My amazing cider vinegar, lecithin, kelp, B-6 diet. *Family Circle,* January 1974.

Rickman, F.; Mitchell, N.; Dingman, J. and Dalen, J. Changes in serum cholesterol during the Stillman diet. *JAMA* 228:54, 1974.

Stare, F. The diet that's killing our kids. *JAMA* 218:394.

Worthington, B. and Taylor, L. Balanced low-calorie vs. high-protein-low-carbohydrate reducing diets. *J. Amer. Dietetic Assoc.* 64:52, 1974.

CHAPTER 5

Eat to Live— Don't Live to Eat

Whether for health reasons or merely aesthetic ones, many of us seek to alter our body weight or shape. There are a few trim persons unnecessarily obsessed with body fat, but most of the weight imbalances people worry about are very real and can pose a threat to health. However, not all persons with weight problems are responsible for their condition. About 5 percent of all weight problems, both overweight and underweight, in our country are attributable to physical malfunctions, such as glandular disorders. Therefore, any weight control program should be preceded by a physical checkup. Once the possibility of a physical complication has been eliminated, a rational dieting plan can be put together to suit one's needs. In this chapter, we offer some tips on how to lose weight, followed by a discussion of the few cases in which weight gain is needed.

Tips on Weight Reduction

In this "land of plenty," it happens that many of us have underdeveloped arm muscles and are unable to push ourselves away from the dinner table until long after our bodies' physiological needs have been satisfied. However, for many overweight and obese persons, it is more a matter of quality than quantity. They don't merely eat too much; rather, they eat the wrong foods and take little physical exercise. Ironically, they are overweight yet malnourished.

The terms overweight and obesity are defined relative to desirable weight. Between 10 and 20 percent over desirable weight is considered overweight; 20 percent or more above desirable weight is defined as obese. Obesity is one of the major nutritional problems of our country. A comprehensive study representing the experience of twenty-six life insurance companies between the years 1935 and 1954 indicated that average weights for men and women of most ages are 15 to 25 pounds over desirable weights, and that an estimated 30 percent of our men and 40 percent of our women above age forty are obese. The prevalence of "overweight" was even found to range from 15 to 30 percent among children and adolescents. This increasing problem is serious because overweight and obese persons are more prone to hypoglycemia, diabetes, heart disease and early death.

In the quest to lose weight, many dieters embrace bizarre and often physically dangerous measures. Some undergo gut operations, others wire their jaws together, and still others spend hours on exercise machines or follow severely unbalanced diets. A professional wrestler may think he knows a good way to get down to his match weight, which may be 15 pounds below his usual weight. His routine procedure is to eat nothing but vitamins, work out, run a mile or two, sit in a sweat bath for two hours, and finally spit out saliva into a mason jar until he has lost the last pound! He thinks he knows all about vitamins, but he may not know about the trace elements lost in sweat and saliva. Important trace elements found in sweat are zinc, manganese, and nickel. In saliva one finds zinc, potassium, magnesium, and calcium. The wrestler may therefore get to the desired weight but be so depleted of trace elements that his muscles will not perform maximally and the strategy of the match may be lost in his befuddled brain. Such crash dieting can produce a feeling of unreality, depression, disperceptions, and even hallucinations.

It is not worth losing pounds or inches if the price paid

is your physical and/or mental health. Therefore, any weight-reducing regime must include a nutritionally sound diet. Rational diet construction must also consider energy expenditure. Exercise is fundamental for obesity control and physical fitness. Psychological and behavioral considerations are the third essential factor. Dieting demands motivation, determination and a burning desire to lose weight. The worth of any dieting program is negated if the dieter cannot follow it regularly.

A nutritionally adequate diet is one which provides sufficient amounts of all the essential nutrients. This must satisfy vitamin and mineral as well as protein, fat and carbohydrate needs. Because the dieter must economize on calories, foods must be chosen wisely. All foods eaten should contribute nutritional value to the diet; no empty calories should be consumed. Wholesome foods for daily selection vary widely: fish, poultry, lean meat and eggs; milk and dairy products; vegetables, mainly green, yellow and orange; citrus and other fruits and fruit juices; and whole-grain cereals and breads. The dieter should select foods from each of these groupings daily and follow the nutritional guidelines set in previous chapters. Nutritious foods can be chosen carefully to fit within the boundaries of a low-calorie diet.

Lose Two Pounds a Week

Be realistic about the amount of weight that can be lost in a week's time. The average weight loss should not exceed 2 pounds per week. The dieter needs sufficient calories to maintain physical vigor; an allowance of about 1,000 calories should be adequate for most but at the same time low enough to permit weight loss. About 300 calories per meal should permit reasonably sized servings, but no second helpings. The following hints may make your dieting easier.

Make Those 1,000 Calories Count

Remember, you are allowed only 1,000 calories, so make those calories nutritious. An egg is 75 calories, as is a slice of bread, but the egg is so nutritious that a whole baby chick can grow from one egg in twenty-one days while rats fed on a white-bread-and-water diet will die from malnutrition in about ninety days. So it would be nutritionally economical to have at least one egg per day, and the bread which you allow yourself should be as unrefined and wholesome as possible. In your search for nutritional calories, avoid junk foods made up mostly of fat and refined carbohydrate; they provide too many empty calories. Bakery confections and most commercially prepared breakfast cereals are good examples of junk foods; "frosted" cereals are 45 percent sugar.

Frequent Snacks

If you suffer from hypoglycemia, try six small meals a day rather than your accustomed two or three large ones. This may reduce hunger and can be helpful in relieving hypoglycemia. Carry your nutritious foods around as snacks (vegetables, seeds, nuts, fruits, hard-boiled eggs, cottage cheese, etc.). When food is available at your fingertips for snacking, hunger is reduced and the desire for those high-calorie, low-nutrient foods is curtailed. You may even find your total food consumption to be lowered as a result of more frequent feedings.

If you are *not* hypoglycemic and you are not bothered by hunger pains, then the best meal plan for weight loss may be an adequate breakfast, a light lunch or nutritional low-calorie snack, and a modest dinner which is high in protein and low in fat. These two alternate courses are merely suggestions. Each individual has his own ideal time interval between meals or snacks, and this must be individually determined.

Instant Broths and Bouillon Cubes

Instant chicken and beef broths can be made into delicious soups which have many nutrients and only 12 calories per cup. The coffee break need not be tea or coffee but can be a cup of broth. This can be repeated many times each day. Various brands of instant broth and cubes are available at only 2 to 10 cents per serving. Hot water is, of course, needed to reconstitute the broth, but a thermos bottle can be loaded with broth before leaving for work.

Use Fats Sparingly

In planning your diet, the fat, carbohydrate and calorie content must be considered. Fats are required by the body, but because they are so calorific (more than twice as many calories per unit of weight as proteins or carbohydrates), fat should be limited. This can be accomplished by avoiding the use of fats in cooking, as in frying or in gravies, and by using some low-fat products, such as low-fat dairy foods and lean meats. Refined carbohydrate foods should be avoided, as these are the most nutritionally empty foods. The body needs some carbohydrate, but choose carefully—a piece of fruit (for dessert instead of pastries), salad, vegetables and perhaps a slice of bread (whole grain) with the meal. Alcoholic beverages should be avoided.

Avoid Sweeteners

Table sugar is the most "empty" of all the refined carbohydrates. Try to avoid refined sugar of all kinds both in cooking and eating. However, don't rely on dietetic candy, cookies or soft drinks to stay your appetite either. None of the available artificial sweeteners is intended for daily consumption in large amounts. Certainly saccharin, cyclamates and others are safe if used only to sweeten tea or coffee once or twice a day, but when used in large doses in calorie- and nutrient-restricted diets, the total effect is not predictable. Sensitization may occur and undernourished organs may be harmed. Remember, these are artificial chemicals, to be used prudently.

Honey Yogurt

You might try the various types of molasses and honey which, when used sparingly, can sweeten acid fruits, rhubarb or sour apple sauce. Any of these dishes is "fit for a king." Honey used in tea enhances its flavor, and a small amount of honey in plain yogurt has fewer calories and is more nutritious than the inch of sugary jam often found at the bottom of flavored yogurts. If you like fruit-flavored yogurt, try adding fresh fruits rather than settling for preserves found at the bottom. Honey and molasses can be placed in plastic squeeze bottles such as are used to dispense catsup or mustard. The trace element content of honey or molasses (see Table 5.1) is appreciable and needed by the body.

TABLE 5.1

Analysis by atomic absorption spectograph of trace elements in honey and molasses, ppm

	Element				
	Zn	**Cu**	**Fe**	**Mn**	**Cr**
Orange-blossom honey	**0.98**	**0.05**	**0.59**	**0.17**	**0.02**
Clover honey	**0.82**	**0.08**	**1.81**	**0.29**	**0.05**
Cane molasses	**1.08**	**0.55**	**20.4**	**4.14**	**0.08**
Beet molasses*	**3.02**	**1.75**	**30.2**	**5.83**	**0.30**

Data of The Brain Bio Center

*Beet molasses is highest in all of the trace metals measured. This molasses is usually not available in health food stores because of a more bitter taste than cane molasses. Beet molasses would be ideal for baking and cooking. At present it is used as cattle food.

Try Cold Water

Quenching one's thirst has always been a problem for dieters in this soda-pop-oriented country. Club soda is a good thirst quencher and can provide the bubbles without the non-nutritional syrup and calories. A small amount of unsweetened fruit juice added to your club soda makes for a great-tasting and nutritional carbonated drink! Furthermore, remember that a glass of cold water is God's gift to man. Imagine yourself in those countries of the world where water must be boiled before drinking and ice cubes, if available, may often contain bacterial impurities. Knowing the value of a glass of cold water will allow you to have this regal drink, with or without ice, four to five times a day. It is cheap and contains no calories. It washes the acid from your stomach and decreases hunger pains, and adequate water intake promotes the elimination of excess salt which tends to swell the body tissues.

Weight Loss by Edict

The word of the doctor takes precedence over that of friends or relatives. The doctor should advise every overweight patient to lose weight, and every obese patient should be given dietary instructions. Otherwise, the patient will conclude that the doctor condones his excess weight and poor dietary habits. This advice should be kindly at the first visit, at which time studies undertaken by the doctor may elicit some deficiencies or hidden hungers. With each succeeding visit, however, the doctor should become more stern and dictatorial, even to the point of edict. "Lose weight or else your health will suffer!" This firm stance will help to fortify drug and nutrient therapy of obesity. If the patient is lazy, the doctor should ask him to park far from his office to get the exercise, and far from the supermarket and, in addition, to walk to the library each day.

Set Your Mind on Nutrition

Your new-found nutrition-conscious frame of mind should enable you to dispel preconceived notions of what a meal should involve. Enjoy your green salad before the regular meal, but skip the rolls or bread. Lemon juice or cider vinegar can season your salad, and a hard-boiled egg may be sliced over the top. If no salad is available, eat celery, carrot sticks, green peppers, pickles or radishes. Cabbage or lettuce can be eaten as a wedge out of the hand and can be wrapped in plastic for the lunch box.

A lunch need not be a sandwich with bread and mayonnaise. Be inventive! A lunch can be a chicken drumstick, a hard-boiled egg, a slab of cheese, the above vegetables, and carefully counted out nuts or fresh fruits. Allow five calories for each nut you eat. If restaurant foods tempt you beyond your calorie budget, start a lunch club and let the members vie with one another in creating nutritious, low-calorie lunches. When dinner time rolls around, cook enough food for you and one other, then invite two additional dieting friends. Each of you will consume only two-thirds as many calories.

Keep a Food Diary

At the risk of being called eccentric, buy a small diary-type notebook to itemize all that you eat and drink each day. Write down the items after each meal, and in the evening go over the list to see if you have exceeded your 1,000-calorie diet. If the total is high, resolve to do better the next day.

Set up a Shining Example

Ambitious dieters have attached pictures of huge, obese or slim, trim persons to the refrigerator door with the idea that these will remind them of what they want to get away from or what they strive to become. Willpower-maintaining devices are helpful; after the first couple of refusals to give in to your appetite, you'll find that it is easier to say "No," as your desire for those fattening foods fades.

Repeat Your Diet Slogan

Diet and exercise are inherent in any sound reducing plan, but no regimen can be complete without including a method of maintaining motivation and willpower—in other words, placing mind over matter. You might create a motto or slogan or even a Transcendental Meditation *mantra* that reflects your reasons for needing weight reduction. Psychologically, this can be effective as a means of allaying hunger when it strikes.

The usual reasons for weight reduction are (1) to achieve a better body figure—to redistribute body weight from hips, buttocks or breasts, or to fit back into clothes worn when one was thinner; (2) to have better energy and less weight to carry around; (3) to meet an absolute job requirement, as for modeling, acting or being a stewardess, policeman, military man or athlete; and (4) to prepare for surgery or to prevent or minimize the effects of medical problems such as hypertension, cardiac ailments, diabetes, gout, varicose veins or joint pain. One example of a *mantra* for a better body figure might be BET-BO-FIG. You may want to recall an old slogan or make up a new one that is especially helpful to your willpower; an example is "a minute on the lips, forever on the hips." A slogan or *mantra* can be repeated to yourself at weak moments.

Shop after Eating

The worst time to shop for food is when hunger is striking hard, for that is when the candy bar and cookie shelves look most tempting. Plan your shopping trip after a meal so that appetite does not rule reason. The nutritionally conscious shopper can cut costs if she or he learns that sugar*less* does *not* mean tasteless.

Win a Bet

If you are the gambling type, bet a friend that you can lose more weight in three months than he or she can. The money saved by dieting can be appreciable so that the bet can be sizeable, perhaps five dollars a week to be deposited weekly. At the end of twelve weeks the winner takes all, namely sixty dollars. You'll be able to buy a new swim suit and perhaps go to the seashore on that money. If you work hard enough and raise the bet, the trip may not cost you a cent. So line up your gullible friend and have a reliable third party accumulate the stakes.

Keep Occupied

Many a woeful dieter exclaims, "I'm fine until after dinner and then I go berserk." Have you considered that those frequently interrupted television programs may have you running to the refrigerator to avoid the commercials? Try reading an interesting book; you will find that reaching for the potato chips and concentrating just don't mix. If you must watch television, perhaps uninterrupted shows might prevent you from walking away as easily. Do you have a hobby? If not, get one. Needlework, auto mechanics, plant care, photography, refinishing furniture and playing the piano or guitar are only a few of the thousands you might try. Complete attention tends to make the time pass quickly; before you realize it, you will have spent the evening without once having had the urge to eat.

Exercise Away Your Frustrations

Don't soothe your frustrations, jealousies, anger or boredom with overeating; exercise away your emotions. Exercise is the second essential constituent of your weight-reducing program, and its importance cannot be overemphasized. Everyone should spend half an hour daily working on an individual program of exercise. Active exercise will make you sweat, burn fat and build muscles. Jogging, cycling, swimming and tennis are a few suggestions. Stretching exercises done on the floor can also offer some assistance in mobilizing fat. Sitting in a steam bath will induce sweat, but it leaves you with too much time to think about food. Hard physical exercise may be so exhausting as to allow you to go to bed hungry and sleep until breakfast. A hot bath at night is relaxing and may enable you to sleep on an empty stomach.

Sex Is Exercise Too

A great form of exercise which also has the added benefit of enabling you to relax into sleep is sex. Yes, sex is estimated to burn off a few hundred calories! This may be one-third of the allotted daily calories. Adequate sexual foreplay is, of course, part of the calorie-consuming value of sexual activity.

Sexual performance is enhanced by beer or pleasant wine at dinner, but it is inhibited by strong empty-calorie beverages such as liquors and mixed drinks. You may want to plan an intimate dinner for two; serve wine, and in place of dessert approach your companion and say, "I'm on a strict diet and need to burn off 400 calories tonight!"

The Group Efforts

Motivation is half the battle. Group efforts instill motivation in many dieters. Special organizations designed for the purpose (for a fee) will give you some motivation and companionship in your quest. The encouragement received from the group is similar to that in other groups with a specific purpose; in this instance, the purpose is to keep losing weight. When dieters have lost weight during the week, they receive unanimous approval. When they haven't lost or they've gained, they experience negative reinforcement and embarrassment.

Some dieters turn to a type of group effort which employs more extensive behavior modification techniques. Professionally organized group therapy with active behavior modification is based on the premise that while diet and exercise are fundamental for obesity control, behavioral modification or environmental factors such as cues, stimuli and people provide the underlying motivation essential for long-term regulation. A program of this sort seeks to alter the reinforcements received by the dieter from these environmental factors in order to discourage overeating and the overweight state.

Anyone can mimic a behavioral program (without the fee) by maintaining a daily chart of weight, foods eaten and exercise time, and by having others give verbal or other rewards when weight is lost. When a group agrees to adhere to this program, for collective reinforcement, each achieves the desired result while saving the fee for membership in a commercial enterprise.

The hints and suggestions we have proposed for diet, exercise, and motivation may be adequate for most. But for some persons, a more rigid, supervised program is needed to produce greater weight loss or to enhance and maintain psychological incentive. The severely obese person may even require careful psychiatric evaluation and appropriate psychiatric treatment.

Nutrients and Medications for a Weight-loss Program

Maintaining the body's supply of essential nutrients is of the utmost importance during weight reduction, when food intake is limited. A few nutrients even assist you in your efforts.

A multipurpose vitamin tablet should be taken daily. This tablet must be mineral-free because copper is not needed in a supplemental dose by adult man and can produce harmful effect. Five brewer's yeast tablets should be taken three times a day, since brewer's yeast is the best source of the B-complex vitamins and of the "glucose tolerance factor" which will help burn sugar.

In addition, a source of zinc such as 20 mg zinc gluconate should be taken twice a day since the entire world population is probably deficient in zinc. This gets rid of one prominent hidden hunger. Fasting of any kind exaggerates this zinc deficiency and is apt to deposit white marks in the finger nails. Vitamin B-6 should be taken twice a day, since zinc given without adequate vitamin B-6 (pyridoxine) may increase any feeling of unreality and pyridoxine also aids in weight reduction. Depending on individual requirements, a large dose such as 200 mg of B-6, morning and night, may be needed.

Don'ts

Swallowing baking soda to allay hunger pains can cause water retention. The dieter also should not use calcium or magnesium salts to deaden hunger because excess calcium may cause kidney stones and magnesium salts can cause diarrhea. A supplemental dose of calcium and magnesium, if desired, may be taken in dolomite tablets or, as they occur naturally, in bone meal. Don't use pep pills! Don't use patent or highly advertised boob-pills! Don't arrange to get injections of chorionic gonadotropin (CGT) or injections of anything else such as hormones or estrogens! If your doctor wants to give you vitamin B-12 injections to relieve tiredness, that is acceptable. However, only sensible diet and the exercise of your less-tired body will result in a healthful weight loss. Beware of the interest of a clinic that specializes only in weight loss! Often, greedy professionals give daily injections of worthless claptrap!

Medical Supervision

Most doctors will be happy to supervise a weight-reduction program. Some may let you attend a club, with monthly medical supervision. The doctor can decide if you need additional thyroid to help you lose weight. He or she will probably, if necessary, prescribe the judicious use of diuretics (water pills) to prevent that annoying weight gain before the menstrual period. This hormone-induced swelling and water retention has been responsible for many a fat woman's saying, "I took only water for three days and yet I gained 3 pounds." There is an up-and-down flow in a woman's weight which must always be considered in the personal weight-reduction program. If it is not considered, discouragement may set in. The water pill counteracts this tissue swelling and frequently will allow weight loss to continue when a plateau or stalemate is reached. Maintaining a low-salt diet also helps to prevent tissue swelling.

Obesity and Schizophrenia

When schizophrenia begins at or before adolescence and is of the histapenic (low histamine) type, then a disproportionate fat deposition, termed "stalagmitic" obesity, may occur in the lower legs and buttocks. The obesity only occurs in histapenic and never in histadelic (high histamine) patients. The disorder may be more prevalent in the female, but the male adolescent schizophrenic with paranoia and stalagmitic obesity is frequently encountered. Remission or effective therapy of the schizophrenia results in weight reduction with a more normal distribution of the fat. Lack of exercise is probably not a factor since some of these patients get adequate exercise; some are even professional athletes.

Some people, not ordinarily classifiable as schizophrenic, have learned for themselves, while attempting crash diets, that the thin state is not the best for them insofar as normal perception and mood are concerned. In these individuals it is obvious that the fatty tissues act as a buffer to pick up abnormal stimulants and thus give them more productive lives and personalities they can more easily live with. The productivity and originality of some overweight and eccentric people may be positively amazing to their friends, but the secret may really be that a mild schizophrenic process plus body fat makes them highly productive and loaded with nervous drive.

Tips on Weight Gain

It sounds like a fairy tale to many, but there are at least two instances in which gain of weight and muscle are desired. The economics of professional football provide us with an example. A good lineman may be turned down by a professional coach because he weighs a mere 220 pounds and the opponents have "lines" who average 260 pounds. He may be six-feet-three and be all muscles, but the coach says, "Gain 40 pounds."

Doctors who advise these athletes in body building produce such weight gains with diets of 9,000 calories per day given in five meals. These are combined with weight lifting and other muscle-building exercises so that the extra weight is added as usable muscle. The traditional Japanese Sumo wrestlers eat tremendous amounts of food, especially rice and bananas, to maintain their great girth. It is possible to take a person whose weight is perfect for his height and have him reach a superperfect weight for a specific purpose.

There are others besides athletes who require weight gain. Persons who have difficulty maintaining a normal weight may have overactive thyroids, intestinal worms or mechanical obstructions, or they may be fast oxidizers or even poor converters of food into muscle. When tests for all these possibilities are exhausted and the weight loss threatens their lives, their condition is termed "anorexia nervosa," meaning lack of appetite because of nerves.

Anorexia nervosa, the relentless pursuit of thinness

through starvation, has recently been classified as a psychotic illness. The onset may begin between the ages of ten to fifteen and is usually precipitated by a stressful event such as time spent away from home or a chance remark about baby fat. The first signs are toying with food; later there is a preoccupation with losing weight and an avoidance of all foods which may possibly take the form of a phobia. If allowed to progress too far, this illness may cause damage which can not be remedied by any diet. It affects teen-age girls predominantly and may become so severe as to cause death.

Many symptoms accompany anorexia nervosa. The individual's perception of her body becomes dangerously distorted; she may deny any interest in sex; most importantly, she feels a need for excess energy expenditure so that she continuously walks the hospital corridor. Although her body is in need of food, she sullenly maintains, "I do not need to eat." One young lady, aged sixteen, entered a hospital weighing 61 pounds, had protruding ribs and shrivelled breasts, and had to be tube-fed to be kept alive, yet she denied that her skeletal appearance was in any way extraordinary.

Therapy has consisted mainly of restoration of body weight through tube-feeding, high-calorie diets, bed rest and close observation. If treatment is successful, the anorexic individual usually realizes the bodily damage her pathological preoccupation has caused.

Psychotherapists have claimed that anorexia nervosa patients subconsciously reject pubertal development and by starving themselves hope that secondary sex characteristics will subside or go away. In other words, they hope to retain their infantile dependency. One such psychotherapist, Dr. S. A. Finch, says, "Anorexia nervosa is a non-classic psychophysiological disorder in which it is difficult to postulate the existence of a biological factor."

Recent data, however, may be more revealing of biological factors in anorexia when all implications and ramifications have been adequately explored. Robboy et al. of the Department of Obstetrics at the University of California at Los Angeles studied several groups of patients including those with anorexia, normal age-matched controls and patients with malnutrition due to other causes. They studied the vitamers with vitamin A activity in the blood of all three groups. The beta-carotene and other vitamers were extremely high in patients with anorexia; the actual levels of beta-carotene (a substance which can be converted into vitamin A) for the three groups were 90, 20 and 8, respectively. The investigators postulated an acquired inability to use vitamin A. This suggestion needs further study. A. A. Crisp et al. working in London, have found that anorexia nervosa patients have the typical early-morning insomnia of depressed patients, although the anorexia patient rarely complains of insomnia. The sleep disturbance may be related to simple malnutrition.

The findings of Robboy et al. and other investigators may be a significant biological keystone which will allow us to understand the biochemistry of anorexia patients more fully. With understanding, the proper therapy may be indicated.

We hope we have advised, even inspired you to commence a nutritious diet regime. If you want to gain weight, focus on a widely varied calorie diet; and if you want to lose those extra pounds, don't delay—start today! The hints offered in this chapter supply you with a foundation for your future eating habits. Good luck!

References

Crisp, A. H., Stonehill, E. and Fenton, G. W. The relationship between sleep, nutrition and mood: a study of patients with anorexia nervosa. *Postgraduate Medical Journal* 47:207-213, April 1971.

Halmi, K. and Fry, M. Serum lipids in anorexia nervosa. *Biological Psychiatry* vol. 8, no. 2, 1974.

Hussey, H. H. Anorexia nervosa: treatment by behavior modification. *JAMA* vol. 228, no. 3, 15 April 1974.

Maxmen, J. S., Siberfarb, P. M. and Ferrell, R. B. Anorexia nervosa. *JAMA* vol. 229, no. 7, 12 August 1974.

Robboy, M. S., Sato, A. S. and Schwabe, A. D. The hypercarotenemia in anorexia nervosa: a comparison of vitamin A and carotene levels in various forms of menstrual dysfunction and cachexia. *Amer. J. Clin. Nutr.* 27, April 1974.

CHAPTER 6

Cholesterol, Sugar, Fats and the Frequently Maligned Egg

A strong case has been made against the consumption of eggs in an effort to reduce cholesterol intake. Doctors, voluntary health-oriented associations and even some nutritionists have convinced the public that eating eggs, with their appreciable cholesterol, will increase serum cholesterol and increase the risk of coronary heart disease. Probably as a consequence of this advice, the average American consumption of eggs per person in 1973 was estimated at 292, a 5 percent drop from the previous year. As recently as 1945, the average American was eating 403 eggs a year. We recommend 2 eggs per day or 700 per year!

Cholesterol

Cholesterol enters the body as food, but it is also manufactured within the body. It is one of the several important lipids that normally circulate in the blood. Cholesterol is present in small amounts in almost all body tissues, but its concentration is highest in the liver, nerve fiber sheaths, white matter of the brain, and adrenal glands. From cholesterol the body synthesizes provitamin D, bile salts and the steroid hormones of the adrenal cortex. Cholesterol is also, however, a major component of the plaques that build up in the blood vessels to produce atherosclerosis or hardening of the arteries.

Cholesterol is an important source of the natural adrenal steroid hormones. These include hydrocortisone, the glucosteroids, and DOCA—the salt- and water-balancing steroid. Without these hormones, patients may develop Addison's disease or adrenal insufficiency. The adrenal gland is normally filled with cholesterol waiting to be transformed into useful steroid hormones, so that a reduction in cholesterol consumption could possibly result in low blood pressure and swelling of the tissues with salt and water due to the body's inability to synthesize DOCA.

Cholesterol is synthesized by the liver to meet body needs, and the liver regulates the quantity and activity of cholesterol in the body. The liver thus controls the amount of cholesterol circulating in the blood, the removal of cholesterol from the circulation, the production of bile acids from cholesterol and the excretion of cholesterol and bile acids in the form of bile into the intestine. The liver uses mostly saturated fats and refined carbohydrates for cholesterol synthesis, but whatever a person eats beyond his energy requirements (excess carbohydrates, fats and proteins) can be used by the liver as raw material for cholesterol. (See Figure 6.1.)

The liver and the intestine are the major locations of cholesterol synthesis; however, nearly all cells, if properly nourished, can produce some cholesterol. This endogenous, or internal, production of cholesterol is estimated at 1,000 to 2,000 mg (1 to 2 gm) daily. This is three to four times as much as the usual diet supplies. Dietary cholesterol and fasting both inhibit cholesterol bio-synthesis, but high-fat diets speed up the manufacture of cholesterol. Once in the blood, saturated fats transport more cholesterol than unsaturated fats.

Cholesterol and Saturated Fat

Now that we have presented some of the background data on

Figure 6.1

The Biosynthesis of Cholesterol

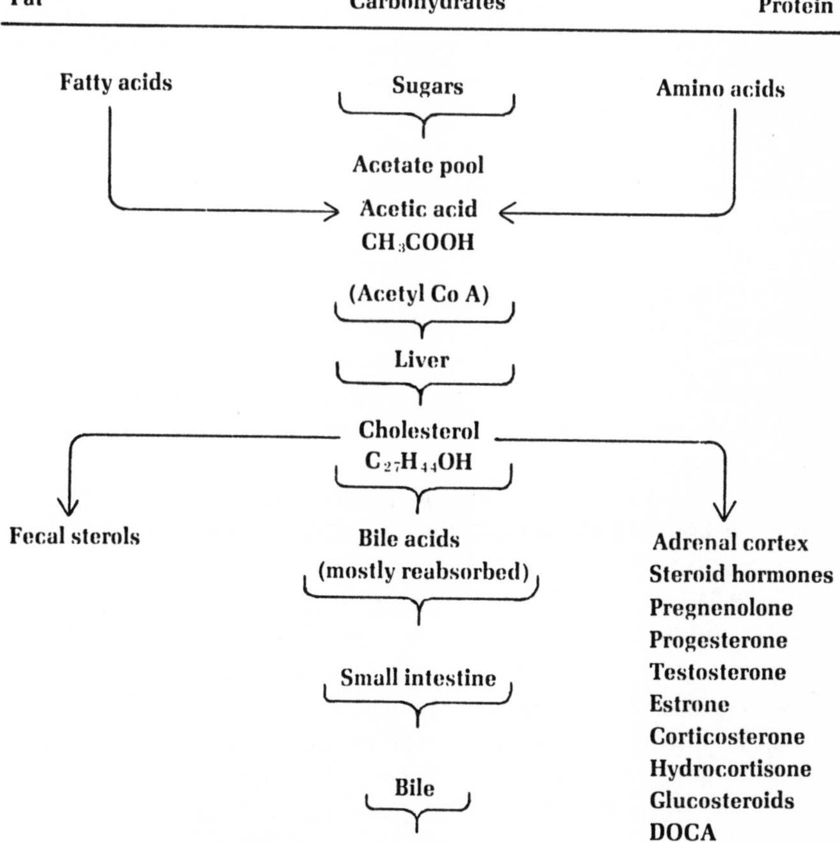

cholesterol, let's examine the relationship to heart disease of cholesterol and saturated fats.

Cholesterol has been associated with atherosclerosis since 1913 when Nikolai Anichkov, a Russian pathologist, showed that rabbits fed large amounts of cholesterol and animal fats rapidly developed hardening of the arteries. Since then, further studies have confirmed this. For instance, it is true that the chicken and rabbit (herbivores), when forced to eat food containing 5 percent of cholesterol, will develop atherosclerosis. Man (an omnivore eating 500 gm of food per day) seldom gets more than 1 gm of cholesterol (0.2 percent). Omnivores handle cholesterol better than herbivores, yet these two herbivores have been the most frequently used animal models.

A correlation nevertheless exists between the incidence of atherosclerosis and high consumption of saturated fats and cholesterol. In Western diets, most fats are saturated. Forty percent of the calories in the average American diet are from fats, and about 17 percent of those dietary fats are saturated. The well-known long-term Framingham study, starting in 1949 and using more than 5,000 subjects, (one-fifth of the town of Framingham, Massachusetts) indicated a relationship between coronary heart disease and the typical American diet, high in saturated fats.

In Western and other countries where diets are typically high in saturated fats, more people have atherosclerosis than in those regions where diets are low in saturated fats. However, there are several exceptions to this relationship, going both ways. Vegetarians (eating a diet low in saturated fats) often develop atherosclerosis. Eskimos (eating a diet high in saturated fats) rarely have it. This indicates that other factors are involved. Although the risk of heart attack has increased in the United States in the last sixty years, saturated fat consumption has not. Furthermore, correlations exist between atherosclerosis and almost any aspect of the affluent society—for example, number of automobiles, income, lack of exercise and high sugar consumption.

Scientists never claim a cause-and-effect relationship

—and not something else—is a cause of atherosclerosis. Neither is it proven that eating eggs increases the risk of heart attack.

In the meantime, elevated serum cholesterol is indeed an important prognostic factor. Blood pressure, serum cholesterol and the cold pressor test are three measures which collectively are good predictors of susceptibility to coronary heart disease. Statistically, a man's risk of coronary artery disease rises exponentially with his cholesterol level. The cholesterol level is the easiest of the lipid levels to measure and is indicative of some patients' degree of atherosclerosis. Our population, relative to that of other countries, has high serum cholesterol. The usual cutoff point is 240 mg percent. There is no increase of risk at levels below 240, but above 250 the risk rises very sharply.

Saturated fats are not always the sole aggravating factor. Five types of blood-fat abnormalities are involved in atherosclerosis. These are determined by triglyceride, free fatty acid, and cholesterol levels; in each of the five types one or more of these may be elevated to varying degrees. Type II and Type IV are the most common. The Type II individual may have trouble metabolizing saturated fats and therefore should probably abstain from eating these. The Type IV individual has his cholesterol level elevated by carbohydrates, particularly refined sugar and alcohol. For these people, the carbohydrates are a greater problem than saturated fats or cholesterol. They must avoid starches and sugars.

In some other classifications, emphasis is placed on free fatty acids and beta lipoprotein. Free fatty acids are mobilized by adrenalin, and beta lipoproteins are elevated by testosterone therapy. Both adrenalin and testosterone, the male sex hormone, are implicated in atherosclerosis. Niacin blocks the transport of free fatty acids released by adrenalin.

No one can prove beyond a doubt that atherosclerosis is caused entirely, or even primarily, by factors of diet. Most people tend to forget all the other factors associated with heart disease risk, which may be equally important or more important than the simple cholesterol level: high blood pressure, cigarette smoking, high consumption of carbohydrates, lack of exercise, overweight, diabetes, gout, individual reaction to stress, and genetic differences in people's ability to metabolize cholesterol and fatty acids.

Stress and Other Factors

Many factors regulate cholesterol level. Diet alone cannot control the cholesterol level in your blood.

How you feel can raise the level without any change in food intake. Stress (releasing adrenalin) causes an acute rise in cholesterol level. Nerve-induced high cholesterol may result from anxiety when the doctor prescribes a heart-disease-oriented diet. Yet much of the publicity related to heart disease still uses the fear-oriented approach.

Smoking also raises the serum cholesterol; the heavy smoker increases his risk at least six-fold.

Eating too much in relation to expended energy also raises the cholesterol level.

Of extreme importance is exercise, which has been shown to lower cholesterol levels in animals and man. Human studies have indicated that regular exercise offers some protection against heart disease and improves the chances of surviving a heart attack.

The risk appears to be highly related to lifestyle and personal stress, as exemplified in our affluent society. Low-income people generally, irrespective of race or diet, are less vulnerable to heart attack than people who must deal with the pressures imposed by social status. Interestingly, wild baboons who live in regimented troops but whose diets are not high in saturated fats get atherosclerosis, whereas more easygoing primates with the same diet do not.

Sugar and Cholesterol

Recently, attention has been drawn to high consumption of refined carbohydrates as a possible cause of the pandemic incidence of atherosclerosis. (You will recall that cholesterol is manufactured in the liver from refined carbohydrates as well as saturated fats.) Dr. John Yudkin has associated coronary heart disease with refined sugar intake rather than with saturated fats or cholesterol. He draws support from correlational and experimental evidence.

In the past century, sugar consumption in America has increased by a much higher percentage than the consumption of fats. Yudkin has calculated that Britons now eat as much refined sugar in two weeks as eighteenth century Britons ate in a year. Just in the past hundred years, the average sugar intake has increased nearly fivefold in Britain, America and other "developed" countries. As a result of feeding rats amounts of sugar similar to those consumed by people, Yudkin found enlarged and fatty livers, enlarged kidneys and shortened life spans (premature aging).

Diets low in fats and high in natural polysaccharides, such as the complex sugars or carbohydrates found in legumes, cereal grains and vegetables, are usually associated with lower cholesterol levels. Consumption of natural carbohydrates has decreased in American diets, while the consumption of refined carbohydrates has increased. Americans, as we have seen, get 45 percent of their calories ("empty calories") from refined carbohydrates, especially sugar.

Total Lifestyle

Likely no one factor (dietary or otherwise) is responsible for heart disease. As we have seen, many factors have been found to be important, and some of these are probably synergists in atherosclerosis. A variety of factors may be important for some people, while others may be affected by a single dominant factor. In this light, it is probably not worthwhile for everyone to modify his diet drastically so as to consume less cholesterol. Some studies are being done along these lines, but no conclusion is yet available.

Good dietary and health habits must begin early in life. *The preventive approach to all disease is by far more effective than later corrective procedures.* For instance, it is useless for a man with a sedentary office job, without proper exercise and diet, to start late in life by eliminating eggs. Egg-restricted diets might be prescribed for high-risk patients, mainly middle-aged men with high serum cholesterol levels or Type II patients. This does not imply that others should forego the nutritional benefits of eggs.

Butter vs. Margarine: the Polyunsaturated Issue

Another food which some people now avoid because of its high saturated fat content is butter. Many Americans have switched to margarine in their quest for a healthier food. Polyunsaturated fats (liquid at room temperature and most commonly found in vegetable oils) are supposed to lower cholesterol levels but some evidence says *No!* Linoleic acid, a polyunsaturated fat found in large amounts in corn oil, safflower oil and other liquid fats, is an essential fatty acid and should comprise about 2 percent of the daily calories.

The fallacy with regard to some margarines is that the unsaturated oils are artificially hydrogenated to become saturated fats. Polyunsaturated fats turn rancid easily, and hydrogenation gives them not only a more solid consistency at room temperature but also a longer shelf life, by saturating the carbon-to-carbon double bonds. (The double bonds are responsible for the unsaturated nature of fats.) Hydrogenation can make the oils even more saturated than some fats commonly called saturated! For instance, hydrogenated soybean oil produces a higher level of cholesterol in rats than corn oil.

The unsaturated oils are chemically reactive. They not only go rancid on standing, but on heating (or hydrogenation) may change their geometric design from left to right and front to back. While this may be one hazard of hydrogenation, this process also occurs when oils are heated, as in cooking. The housewife may already have noted that French-frying oil becomes more solid when used repeatedly for cooking. The oil then is less polyunsaturated and is more hydrogenated.

When margarines contain hydrogenated oil, this is indicated on the label. The rule for labeling margarine is that the first item listed must represent at least 50 percent of the product. If the first item is hydrogenated (hardened) oil, you know that at least half of that margarine is hydrogenated oil. If the first item listed is liquid vegetable oil, you know that product is at least half polyunsaturated oil, which is desirable in margarine.

Another source of confusion is coconut oil, which is about 99 percent saturated and thus contains a much higher percentage of saturated fat even than meat or butter fat. Nondairy creamers, which are used extensively as an alternative to cream or milk, are made with coconut oil. They are carefully not labeled cream, but the stewardess on the airline says, "Cream with your coffee?" as she hands you the emulsified coconut oil. Crackers, aerosol whipped creams, many puddings and the vegetable shortening in pastries from most commercial bakeries are made from coconut oil, which is used to prevent rancidity.

Nutrients Involved in Cholesterol Regulation

It seems logical that, since cholesterol naturally circulates in the blood, some nutritional deficiency may be what allows plaques to form and build up in the arteries. This may result either from an imbalance or a deficiency of vital nutrients. Choline, vitamin B-12, biotin, lecithin, pangamic acid and possibly inositol are lipotropic substances—substances which must be present to prevent accumulation of fat in the liver. Since the liver regulates cholesterol, these vitamins may be very essential.

Deficiencies of magnesium, potassium, manganese, zinc, vanadium, chromium or selenium, or of vitamins C, E, niacin (B-3), folic acid or pyridoxine (B-6) may be significant. Adelle Davis reminded us that magnesium is essential to keep the blood cholesterol down and to prevent heart attacks. Magnesium has protected against atherosclerosis in experimental animals on atherogenic diets. A deficiency of chromium (glucose tolerance factor) in experimental animals allows the appearance of fatty deposits in blood vessels, which is similar to the clogging of arteries in man. We believe that stretch marks in the skin and white spots in the fingernails are signs of zinc deficiency. Perhaps atherosclerosis is a similar break in the arteries caused by lack of zinc in our diets.

Zinc supplements have greatly improved the condition of patients suffering from hardened arteries. Dr. Harold G. Petering and his associates at the University of Cincinnati Medical Center have found that blood fat levels decreased when blood zinc levels increased. A Scottish researcher has found more cholesterol in the adrenal glands of laboratory rats on diets deficient in zinc than in those of rats kept on diets plentiful in zinc. At the University of Rochester, more than half of the patients treated with zinc for atherosclerosis showed improved tolerance to exercise and increased warmth in hands and feet.

It is known that niacin (B-3) reduces blood serum cholesterol. It has also been shown that vitamin C can lower cholesterol. Various theories have been proposed to account for these actions. Vitamin C may produce its effect by complexing the calcium and thus dissolving the plaques in blood vessels; by lowering serum surface tension (and thus increasing solubility of cholesterol in the serum); by regulating the rate of the formation of cholesterol in the body; by aiding in the synthesis of steroid hormones from cholesterol in the adrenal cortex and competing with free fatty acid release; and finally by assisting in the conversion of cholesterol to bile acids for removal from the body. As adrenocortical activity increases, the concentration of ascorbic acid (vitamin C) and of cholesterol in the adrenal gland decreases. A significant direct correlation exists between the vitamin C concentration in the liver and the rate of cholesterol transformation to bile acids. Whatever the active role of vitamin C, a deficiency speeds the formation and deposition of cholesterol, and adding C to the diet helps clear blood vessels. One scientist believes atherosclerosis to be due to a long-term deficiency of vitamin C. (Refer to page 131 for further detail.)

Many fats are naturally protected by the presence of antioxidants such as vitamin E and lecithin. Lecithin is found naturally in eggs, soybeans and vegetable oils. This phospholipid is manufactured in the body and is also an emulsifier which is used by some firms in the food industry to prevent rancidity.

The phospholipids, as emulsifiers, have an affinity for water and break up fat into tiny particles so that it can be dissolved in water. Their vital role in metabolism stems from the fact that they are essential to the digestion and absorption of fats by the cells. Some say lecithin is the natural antagonist of cholesterol, and animal studies have shown that lecithin can dissolve atheromatous plaques in blood vessels. However, the evidence is far from conclusive. Lecithin's effect may be due to the choline molecule which is part of the structure.

The Maligned Egg

There has been much publicity concerning the bad effect of eggs on blood cholesterol, but let's look at the accurate assay of the effects of eggs (or egg yolks) on the cholesterol levels of normal people. (All 275 mg of cholesterol in the egg is contained in the yolk.)

Svacha et al. at Auburn, Alabama fed three eggs per day to fourteen normal men, several of whom smoked tobacco habitually. Only the smokers had a significant total rise of 27 mg percent in serum cholesterol (9 mg per egg). Nonsmokers had a nonsignificant rise of only 2 mg percent (0.7 mg per egg). It should also be noted that smokers inhale poisonous cadmium, which antagonizes zinc, one of the useful trace metals contained in egg yolk.

In yet another study, Takeuchi and Yamamura of Osaka, Japan compared the responses of thirty-one young men with ten middle-aged men when each group was given nine egg yolks per person per day. The young men had an average rise in cholesterol of 17 mg percent (2 mg per egg) while the middle-aged men had a rise of 35 mg percent (4 mg per egg). The mean cholesterol levels at the start were 185 mg percent for the young and 195 mg percent for the middle-aged men.

These scientific studies in man contrast with the statement of Dr. Castelli, director of the laboratory in the Framingham study: "I have lowered my cholesterol from 250 to 200 mg percent partly by eliminating eggs and other measures, such as diet and exercise." Trager, in *The Bellybook*, says, without presenting a scientific basis for the statement: "If a man eliminates 2 eggs per day he can lower his cholesterol by something like 25 mg percent," and "Every 100 mg of cholesterol a man eats per day raises his serum cholesterol by 5 mg percent." If this last statement were true, then the men eating three eggs in Auburn, Alabama, should have had a rise in their cholesterol of 275 X 3 eggs X 5 mg%÷100 mg percent or a 41 mg percent rise! Actually the result was 2 mg percent for nonsmokers and 27 mg percent for smokers! What a difference!

The Japanese men cited above as eating nine yolks a day should have had a rise of 275 X 9 yolks X 5 mg%÷100=124 mg%. Actually, the rise was only 17 mg percent for young men and 35 mg percent for the middle-aged men. An easy answer lies in the fact that the egg yolk is a balanced nutritional delight which contains not only cholesterol but lecithin, zinc, iron, sulfur and other trace elements which provide the biochemical cement to build the native cholesterol into steroid hormones and other useful body bastions against disease.

The egg is an ideal natural food supplied in a hard (calcium and magnesium) disposable (for your compost pile) shell. If the shell were made of tough protein (as is the turtle's) the present-day consumer would get only frozen yolks and whites, and the shell would be snatched away by processors for use as animal food. At present, feeding the hens limestone (which is cheaper than egg shell) supplies the needed calcium. The brittle egg shell has almost completely prevented commercial adulteration of the egg. Only healthy hens will lay eggs, so the egg farmer goes to great pains to see that his hens are healthy. The only trace of adulteration is that American hens are fed additional B carotene and vitamin A in order to produce an egg with a deep orange yolk. Of some interest is the fact that the bones of the baby chick get their calcium, phosphorus, magnesium, sulfur, selenium, fluoride and iron from the yolk of the egg.

At six months of age the human infant's first dose of iron and sulfur ordinarily comes from the feeding of cooked egg yolk. This is needed since milk is deficient in iron. The egg also has a built-in warning device in that, when old or stored in heat, the sulfur compounds start to decompose, become noticeable, and the smell of "rotten eggs" warns the consumer.

Believe it or not, this smell of rotten eggs is one of the reasons that we recommend two eggs per person daily. The odor means that sulfur is present. Man needs sulfur and its natural contaminant, selenium, for skin, hair, fingernails and toenails, to build the amino acid taurine in the cells and brain and to make sulfonated compounds for the joints. The essential amino acids containing sulfur (cysteine and methionine) are not enough. Grandma, when she gave sulfur and molasses each springtime, was correct in believing that the body needs sulfur.

A Whole Chicken Develops from One Egg

Chicken eggs provide excellent food, since the protein balance is of the best biological value possible. The egg has the amino acid pattern in the proportion closest to the needs of your body. The egg is low in fat, rich in protein and vitamin A, low in calories and economical (much cheaper and higher quality protein than meat). It is, furthermore, a good source of vitamin B-12 if you are a vegetarian. (B-12 is found only in animal products.) It also contains (some in larger amounts than others) choline, tryptophan (precursor of niacin), pyridoxine (B-6), biotin, folic acid (a B vitamin), riboflavin (B-2), thiamin (B-1) pantothenic acid (a B vitamin), selenium, zinc, phosphorous, calcium and sulfur.

The yolk of an egg is almost the only food that will blacken a silver spoon because of its high sulfur content. (One other is hot red pepper.) So if you need sulfur for your skin and fingernails, you have little choice but to eat two eggs a day. As the old professor of nutrition said as the clincher to his lecture, "What other food product will grow a whole chicken or even an ostrich?"

Two eggs per day eaten somehow and anytime, at breakfast, in an eggnog, hard-boiled, sliced over salad, or even "deviled" are one way to assure added energy and maximal mental functioning for the day. One sometimes wonders if the effective nervous drive of some active and capable members in our society is not in part owing to their ability to maintain a high blood cholesterol. In clinical experience we have found that patients with rheumatoid arthritis or hypoglycemia or mental disease need these two eggs, and usually do not like eggs. In the case of the hypoglycemic, more hard-boiled eggs may be eaten as between-meal snacks.

An average egg yolk contains 0.165 percent elemental sulfur, which means 165 mg of sulfur per 100 gm of yolk. The sulfur amino acids, methionine and cystine, account for 91 percent of the sulfur in the yolk. There are approximately equal amounts of methionine and cystine. The body needs 850 mg of all kinds of sulfur per day. The whole egg contains 67 mg of sulfur or 8 percent of our daily needs. This cannot easily be found in other foods. In addition, one whole egg contains 0.7 mg zinc, 1.2 mg iron, 5.5 mg magnesium, 16 mg inositol, 27 mg calcium, 76 mg potassium, 253 mg choline and 590 units of vitamin A. The egg can thus be considered the ideal model of the exact nutrients to take with you to a desert island! The protein is complete, with all the essential amino acids, and the ratio of minerals is perfect for the purpose of growth.

Note again that the egg contains 27 mg of calcium and nearly 6 mg of magnesium—a ratio of four to one, whereas dolomitic calcium-magnesium contains these two elements in a ratio of six to four. But phosphorus is higher (100 mg) than either sodium (66 mg) or potassium (76 mg). Perhaps the ideal calcium-magnesium supplement might also include some bone meal for its phosphorus content.

Sea salt is 1.9 percent chlorine, 1.0 percent sodium, 0.135 percent magnesium, 0.08 percent sulfur, 0.04 percent calcium and 0.038 percent potassium, with much less phosphorus. Most of the sulfur is as the sulfate, which is easily used by ruminants but not by man. The main extra mineral to be obtained from the use of sea salt on your egg is magnesium.

It is true that the egg is high in cholesterol, averaging 275 mg. Since the average daily consumption of cholesterol is about 800 mg, you can see that eggs are a major contribution. The individual who eats no eggs or organ meats probably takes in about 200 mg of cholesterol a day. If he or she uses skim milk and vegetable margarine, the intake may be as low as 100 to 150 mg per day.

Our recommendation may exceed the generally advised upper limit; however, this amount of balanced egg cholesterol has not been proven to be harmful. Furthermore, it is substantially less than the 1 to 2 gm the body manufactures every day. Dr. Roger Williams says that it is a fundamental nutritional error to exclude eggs from the diet. He believes that the cholesterol will be utilized if the other foods eaten contain the needed trace metals. Doctors and others worried about heart disease have unduly placed the blame on the egg.

Egg eating does not explain or cause heart disease. Instead of blaming eggs, it would seem wiser to concentrate on correcting an otherwise poor diet. As we have seen, nutrients such as vitamin C, niacin, magnesium, zinc and chromium, possibly lecithin, and other factors such as natural carbohydrates and regular exercise produce and maintain lowered cholesterol levels, which are negatively associated with atherosclerosis. High cholesterol levels are promoted when the diet is mainly refined junk foods without trace elements.

The high-risk cholesterol patient should be tested for adequate zinc, excess copper levels and his spectrum of serum lipids. He can then be advised as to whether his total nutritional status will allow the addition of eggs to his diet. The person who eliminates eggs will still have the basic problem which allowed the initial build-up of cholesterol in the arteries in the first place! So, by all means, unless you are a high-risk coronary patient, have your one or two eggs a day for good economical nutrition.

The cholesterol war between the American Heart Association (AHA) and the egg industry continues, with the public trying to guess how it will all turn out. Both sides appear to be short on science and long on hot air. Perhaps some quotes will illustrate.

Dr. Jean Mayer: "Both sides are fighting over your heart." He advocates only two eggs per week and calls the egg industry "the heart-disease Mafia."

The egg industry: ". . . absolutely no scientific evidence that eating eggs, even in quantity, will increase the risk of a heart attack. . . . Eggs do not contain food additives."

Dr. Henry Blackburn of the University of Minnesota: "We have simply gone too far in consumption of egg fat, dairy fat and meat fat."

Dr. Roger Williams: "I think the egg advertising tends to

counteract the anti-egg promotion of the AHA which is not justified. They're such good food. I believe the cholesterol in eggs will take care of itself if the other foods you eat are good."

Dr. Theo. Cooper, National Heart and Lung Institute (NHLI) Director: "We're trying to determine whether reducing blood lipids including cholesterol will prevent coronary heart disease."

Dr. Ray Reiser, Professor of Biochemistry at Texas A & M: "First recognize individual differences. There's no increase in risk at cholesterol levels below 240, and such people are in no danger from eating eggs. The advice is: See your doctor, find out your cholesterol level and be treated as an individual."

Even as we eat our delicious morning eggs, the news media tell us that scientists have found a way to remove cholesterol from eggs just as they removed wheat germ from wheat. One method is simple. The stirred-up yolk is centrifuged so that the fatty esters and cholesterol are whipped off the top along with the fat-soluble vitamins. The product is then sold in the frozen state, probably with a stabilizer and preservative to prolong shelf life.

A Standard Brands subsidiary has a cholesterol-free egg substitute called Egg Beaters which is sold in the frozen state. When thawed, this product has the appearance of beaten eggs but is mostly egg whites with selected vitamins, minerals, fat and even protein added. The 1-pound package is said to be the equivalent of eight large eggs and without detectable cholesterol. A prominent label says, "Cholesterol-free Egg Substitute." In fine print, we find "egg white, corn oil, non-fat dry milk, emulsifiers (vegetable lecithin, mono- and diglycerides and propylene glycol monostearate) cellulose and Xanthan gums, trisodium and triethyl citrate, artificial flavor, aluminum sulfate, iron phosphate, artificial color, thiamin, riboflavin and vitamin D." The tinkered product has lost almost all zinc, all usable sulfur, all B-6, all vitamin A and all niacin, not to mention the trace metals and nutrients which allow a whole baby chick to develop from the yolk.

What happens to all those yolks from the tinkered eggs? A company public relations man says that various things such as cosmetics, bakery products and pet food absorb the yolks.

Dr. Roger Williams says, "The dogs are again better fed than man." We say, "Let them eat their tinkered eggs. Whole fresh eggs or fight is our motto!"

The little red hen says, "I spend my nights using 10 percent of my very bones to properly enclose the egg and keep meddlers from tinkering."

Humpty Dumpty says, "All the king's horses and all the king's men are needed to protect me."

References

Adams, R. and Murray, F. *Minerals: Kill or cure?* New York: Larchmont Books, 1974.

Ginter, E. Cholesterol: vitamin C controls its transformation to bile acids. *Science* 179:702, 1973.

Lewin, S. Evaluation of potential effects of high intake of ascorbic acid. *Comp. Biochem. Physiol.* 46 B:427, 1973.

Medical World News, pp. 22-24, 15 March 1974.

Robinson, C. H. *Fundamentals of normal nutrition.* New York: Macmillan, 1973.

Rickman, F.; Mitchell, N.; Dingman, J. and Dalen, J. E. Changes in serum cholesterol during the Stillman diet. *JAMA.* 228:54, 1974; *Nutritional Reviews Supplement*, p. 24, 1974.

Spittle, C. Atherosclerosis and vitamin C. *Lancet* p. 1280, 11 December 1971.

Svacha, A. J., Wesson, N. C. and Waslein, C. I. Effect of egg intake and tobacco smoking on serum cholesterol. *Fed. Proc.*, 33:690, 1974.

Takeuchi, N. and Yamamura, Y. Effects of egg yolk and moctamide on serum lipids in man. *Clin. Pharm. and Ther.* 16:368, 1974.

Trager, J. *The big, fertile, rumbling, cast-iron, growling, aching, unbuttoned bellybook.* New York: Grossman, 1972.

CHAPTER 7

Artificial Sweeteners

As an alternative to sugar, many have turned to artificial sweeteners. Originally used as sugar substitutes for diabetics, artificial sweeteners are now being consumed in large quantities by dieters and the general populace. They thus ignore labeling stating that the sweetener "should be used only by persons who must restrict their intake of ordinary sweets." Concern has frequently been expressed as to the safety of the widespread use of nonnutritive food additives.

Saccharin (Ortho-sulfamido-benzoic acid) $C_6H_4SO_2NHCOOH$

Saccharin was discovered in 1879 when Constantin Lahlberg tasted bread which had been accidentally contaminated by a coal tar derivative he had synthesized. This sweet-tasting coal tar derivative has been sold commercially since 1900, and for the first half of the century was used to sweeten foods consumed almost exclusively by persons with diabetes. Saccharin is not converted by the body to glucose and thus can be utilized by the diabetic as an alternative to sugar. Early work showed that it was absorbed by the body and almost totally excreted in the urine. Since the early 1960s, however, the general public has been encouraged by manufacturers to buy artificially sweetened "diet products."

Saccharin is about four hundred times sweeter than sugar and ten times sweeter than cyclamate. It is without caloric value and may have helped obese persons to lose weight. Four million pounds (2,000,000 kilos or 2,000 tons) were produced in the year 1967. It is used in many products, including carbonated beverages, dry beverage bases, dietetic foods, home sweetener preparations, and a few nonfood substances. Popular soft drinks may contain up to 150 mg of saccharin, the individual tablets 15 mg, and packets such as Sweet and Low 15 to 50 mg, which is the equivalent of one to three teaspoons of sugar. Saccharin is not used in canned foods or drinks that are sterilized by heat because the decomposition products are less sweet.

Saccharin is currently the synthetic sweetener most commonly used in the United States. Its safety has recently been, and continues to be, investigated. Experiments have been designed to examine possible harmful effects in the body. Some of the experiments are reviewed here.

Safety of Saccharin

Saccharin, in doses several times greater than the amount to which humans would be exposed, was fed to pregnant mice, rabbits and rats during the sensitive period of their pregnancy, and detectable birth defects were not found in the fetuses. In a 1951 study by the FDA saccharin concentrations of above 0.1 percent of the diet caused kidney damage, but not cancer, in rats. In 1970, another feeding study in female mice did not indicate cancer, but the urinary bladders were not examined.

In 1957, a controversial experimental method was introduced in saccharin studies in which a pellet composed of the sweetener mixed with cholesterol was implanted in the urinary bladders of mice. Several mice developed bladder cancer. (In this same study, however, tumors did not result from large and continued injections of saccharin in the mice.) The experimenters did not conclude that saccharin was cancer-producing. Some scientists believed that the saccharin simply served to intensify the known ability of cholesterol pellets to cause tumors. Just after the long cyclamate fight, however, in March 1970, biologists at the University of Wisconsin, using the bladder-cholesterol implantation technique, found that saccharin quadrupled the incidence of malignant bladder tumors.

Implantation methods do not conclusively prove the cancer-producing potential of saccharin. However, as a result of the possibility of carcinogenicity, the FDA moved to review the safety of saccharin. In July 1970, the FDA assigned to the Food Protection Committee of the National Academy of Sciences, National Research Council, the task of reviewing all scientific studies on saccharin. Their report concluded that the present and projected usage of saccharin in the United States did not represent a dangerous risk.

The testing continued. Several lifetime rodent-feeding studies have been conducted. Preliminary analysis in March 1972 of one such study at the Wisconsin A.R.F. Institute found malignant bladder tumors in several of the male rats which had consumed saccharin at a 5 percent dietary level. In another study, Purdom, Hyder and Pybas at the North Texas State University reported in December 1973 that some rats, fed saccharin making up 5 percent of their daily intake, had also developed bladder tumors. In the same study, no extreme alterations in growth, protein synthesis, blood glucose or cholesterol levels attributable to the saccharin were found. Of course, further studies are needed to clarify saccharin's effect on these processes and especially in lipid metabolism and lipid-protein complexing. But based on the present carcinogenic evidence, the FDA has recently removed saccharin from the GRAS list of food additives.

Saccharin's continued presence in widely used dietetic products has stirred up some concern about the body's storage of this sweetener. Studies, such as the one performed by Byard et al. at Albany, New York, indicate that 95 to 98 percent of ingested saccharin is excreted unchanged in the urine and feces within seventy-two hours and that about half of the saccharin is excreted in just six hours. The remaining 2 to 5 percent is stored (or destroyed) within the body. The implications of this storage must be determined, but some evidence already suggests that one week's abstinence from saccharin intake can eliminate the stored sweetener from the body.

Cyclamates: Sodium and Calcium Salts of $C_6H_5NHSO_3$

The cyclamates (sodium and calcium cyclamate) are about thirty to forty times as sweet as sugar and one-tenth as sweet as saccharin, but they do not have saccharin's bitter aftertaste. The cyclamates were discovered in 1944 and took hold of a large portion of the artificial sweetener market. Some manufacturers made exaggerated claims of weight loss resulting from cyclamate use.

By 1968 the FDA accumulated evidence that cyclamates caused bladder cancer, birth defects and mutations in animals. The debate was a long one. In April 1969, the FDA recommended that people voluntarily restrict their intake of cyclamates. As a result of mounting evidence of possible carcinogenicity, cyclamates were banned in October 1969, but the FDA reversed its decision in February 1970, ruling that cyclamate-containing foods were to be labelled "drugs." However, it reversed itself again after much scientific, congressional and public pressure and banned cyclamates totally from foods on 14 August 1970.

After an exile of nearly five years, cyclamates are again being reconsidered. They may possibly reappear on the market. It is therefore worthwhile to review the experimental literature pertaining to the ban on this sweetener.

Abbott Laboratories, the world's largest cyclamate manufacturer, sponsored research in 1969 which revealed bladder tumors in a few of the cyclamate-fed animals. A few other studies were conducted, some supported by the competitive sugar industry, but the Abbott study was the main one responsible for the ban on cyclamates. This major producer now contends, after much lengthy research, that use of cyclamates at a rate or amount producing no pharmacological effect represents reasonable safety levels for human consumption.

One aspect of the cyclamates which needs further research is their potential for degrading into the compound cyclohexylamine (CHA) which is toxic in experimental animals. About 10 percent of humans are estimated to produce CHA from cyclamates, but some evidence suggests that intestinal flora can begin to metabolize a cyclamate after its continued intake. Furthermore, research has indicated that in human subjects both cyclamates and CHA are almost completely eliminated in urine and feces with no observable retention, even with 5-gm doses.

Some scientists, including England's illustrious Dr. John Yudkin, have criticized the design of the experiments used to condemn the cyclamates, wherein a few of the animals showed evidence of the beginning of bladder cancer. Because the cyclamates are about thirty times sweeter than sugar and the rat's lifespan is very short, the amount of cyclamate fed to the rats for two years would be the equivalent, in an adult human, of consuming 10 to 12 pounds of sugar every day for forty or fifty years.

In reality, much smaller quantities are used—something like one-fiftieth of the equivalent dose in the human. The dietary levels used in the saccharin experiments in which the detrimental evidence was obtained were similar to those used for cyclamates; but saccharin is ten times stronger than the cyclamates, and thus the equivalent level for saccharin should have been one-tenth that used in the cyclamate experiments. The level of a substance needed to obtain a deleterious effect should be determined realistically and, taking a wide margin of safety into consideration, this level should be evaluated in relation to the possible human consumption level.

Dr. Yudkin has reported experiments indicating dangers from sugar in the body, using 15 ounces of sugar a day or less. These amounts have been criticized as being abnormally high and his results thus as invalid. However, these quantities are, in fact, not ridiculously high and have been consumed. They are, furthermore, much less than the equivalent amount of cyclamates needed to demonstrate their danger. Some of the experiments sponsored by the sugar industry used cyclamates as 5 percent of the diet, which is equivalent in sweetening power to 150 percent of dietary sugar. Yudkin contends that no one should be surprised that rats on this diet did not thrive, and in fact did not grow as well as those rats without cyclamates. He states that even if cyclamates made up only 2 percent of the diet, it would be the equivalent of a person consuming 13 ounces of sugar a day, which is close to the amount (15 ounces) that Yudkin has shown to produce harmful effects on people and animals.

The Delaney Clause in the American Food and Drug laws, which determines the GRAS list of additives, states that any substance that causes cancer in any dose in any animal must not be used in human food. Perhaps this clause should be revised, since many substances are relatively safe in small doses but harmful at higher levels. Iron and copper, two of the metals needed by the body, can cause problems (schizophrenia, for one) when present at too high a level. The same is true of the requirement for and toxicity of vitamins A and D. Other substances, such as sugar, have been cited. The toxicity of each substance must be evaluated relative to its consumption level.

Sorbitol

Sorbitol is a chemical relative of the sugars which is about 60 percent as sweet as sugar. The body converts sorbitol slowly to sugar, and thus sorbitol was used by diabetics before the introduction of insulin. However, "dietetic" products using sorbitol contain as many calories and as much carbohydrate as those using sugar. Therefore, they are worthless for restricted-carbohydrate diets and for weight-reduction diets.

This sweetener has a pleasant taste with no bitter aftertaste. Sorbitol is used widely in chewing gums and candies, and in low-calorie foods and drinks to cover up the aftertaste of saccharin and to add the "body" usually provided by sugar. It is relatively noncariogenic—that is, it does not provide a good medium for tooth decay—and many studies on animals and humans have indicated that it is probably entirely safe.

Aspartame

With cyclamates still banned and saccharin off the GRAS list, many who cannot, or do not want to, use sugar are wondering what they can use as an alternative.

A new sweetener has been discovered and will soon be on the market shelves. Aspartame, the generic name of the new compound, was discovered by accident in 1965 by James Schlatter, a chemist at G. D. Searle and Company. Aspartame is made up of the two amino acids, phenylalanine and aspartic acid, and it is metabolized by the body in the same way as the amino acids found naturally in protein foods.

On 28 July 1974, the FDA approved aspartame for sale by Searle. The new sweetener is 180 times as sweet as sugar. It gives the same number of calories as sugar or protein (four calories per gm) but because of its intense sweetness, it will provide sweetening equivalent to that of sugar at 1/180th of the calories. If used like sugar, the estimated maximum daily intake will be one gram per person (about four calories a day), constituting an insignificant contribution to caloric intake.

At first, aspartame's approved use will be in dry packaged goods and as a table sweetener for coffee and tea. It cannot now be used in soft drinks and canned goods because it tends to lose its sweetness gradually after prolonged shelving in liquids. In addition, aspartame is not as yet usable in baked goods because, like saccharin, it loses its sweetness when exposed to high temperatures. When heated, it breaks down into a diketopiperazine (a condensation derivative of amino acids), but tests of this compound have not yet indicated any safety problems. One of aspartame's great virtues is the lack of the bitter aftertaste experienced with the use of large doses of saccharin.

Since 1965, when aspartame was discovered, the G. D. Searle Company has conducted extensive safety studies, including feeding studies on rats and dogs for two-year periods and one in which rats were exposed to the compound in the uterus and subsequently fed aspartame throughout their lifetimes. Even with daily doses as high as 1/500th of total body weight, no effects on the animals were found. Allowing for an extra safety margin, the acceptance level of use by humans as set at 1/600th of body weight, which would be less than 1/15th of an ounce (2 gm) per day. Lifetime studies in rats and mice, a multigenerational study in rats, studies of deformation and mutation effects in three species, and bladder implant studies of the same type used for cyclamates and saccharin have all produced no adverse effects.

In spite of all the promising evidence for aspartame's safety, Dr. John Olney, a neurophysiologist at Washington University Medical School, has drawn attention to potential dangers. He has noted that aspartic acid and glutamate are both di-acidic amino acids, bearing a chemical resemblance to one another and that aspartame may produce the same kind of brain damage that glutamate (as in monosodium glutamate, MSG) has been found to cause in very young animals. Olney has stated that consuming aspartame in addition to glutamate (which is already present in so many foods) is like doubling the amount of glutamate on the market; if both were being regularly consumed, they might have a combined effect. Further research into this theoretical danger is needed.

Another danger, according to Dr. Olney, lies in aspartame's second component, phenylalanine. For the one in ten thousand humans born with the error in metabolism known as phenylketonuria (PKU), ingesting phenylalanine leads to irreversible mental retardation. However, these persons can be warned against phenylalanine content in nonprotein foods sweetened with aspartame by the presence of a label on the product.

Isomerose 100 and Isosweet 100

The use of artificial sweeteners in place of sugar falls short in one major respect. Artificial sweeteners (except for sorbitol) cannot mimic sugar's other qualities, such as its bulkiness or "body." Thus, they have not been effective sugar substitutes in "foods" such as candy, chocolate, and ice cream. As a result, some food producers have taken a different course in their search for new sweeteners.

Soft-drink producers, worried that the need for 300,000 tons of sugar per month will price their products off the market, have adopted a corn-syrup sweetener, described as a "high-fructose product." The corn syrup is treated with a special enzyme, glucose isomerase, which converts the glucose into fructose, a sugar which is 50 percent sweeter than sucrose. The new corn-syrup sweeteners are being produced under the trade names Isomerose 100 and Isosweet 100 and are used in the proportion of one part to about three parts of sugar.

The use of fructose to replace sucrose may be a good idea because fructose is absorbed slowly, it does not stimulate insulin release, and it is less cariogenic. Also, the potential dangers of sucrose excess are numerous. Since 35 percent less fructose would be required due to its greater sweetness, one can only wonder why the food manufacturers could not replace all of the sucrose in their products with fructose. However, the best approach of all would be to reduce the amount of any sweetener used, since most products are already too sweet. As soft drinks are now marketed, the consumer often loses out. He may get too much sucrose or he may get too much of an artificial sweetener of doubtful safety.

Thaumatin and Monellin

With the safety of cyclamates and saccharin in doubt, the price of sugar having skyrocketed, and the demand for low-calorie sweetening agents increasing, new sucrose substitutes are actively being sought, especially from natural sources.

Thaumatin and Monellin are two sweet-tasting proteins derived from the miracle fruit and the serendipity berry of Africa. The miracle fruit has the ability to affect taste receptors so as to cause acidic foods to taste sweet after the fruit has been in the mouth. By weight, Thaumatin is 1,600 times as sweet as sucrose, and Monellin, 2,000 times as sweet; their intense sweetness makes their caloric contribution low. However, the sensitivity of the proteins to high temperature, low pH, and the splitting of disulfide bonds limit the potential use of these substances as sucrose substitutes in foods.

Miraculin, a related glycoprotein obtained from a tropical fruit, is available from the Miralin Company as a chewable tablet which will change the taste of sour substances for one to two hours after the tablet is taken. The discovery of sweet-tasting proteins and a taste-modifying glycoprotein provides a precedent for new sweet-tasting substances of natural origin, and opens new possibilities for studying the molecular mechanisms regulating the behavior of taste receptors.

The artificial sweeteners have aided many Americans who must avoid sugar or reduce weight. These sweeteners are relatively safe if their use does not exceed the low recommended levels. A substance's toxicity must be evaluated relative to its human consumption level. (This kind of evaluation should also be applied to other chemical food additives.)

Compared to other chemical additives, the artificial sweeteners are safer because of the greater control one has over the amounts ingested, especially if they are only used as table sweeteners. Clinical studies are continuing to examine the long-range effects of the artificial sweeteners in man.

Saccharin Warning Makes Sweet Sense

The warning printed on saccharin-sweetened products tells one that saccharin is a "nonnutritive sweetener for use by persons who must restrict their intake of ordinary sweets." Ironically, however, this refers to everyone! With the knowledge we now have concerning the dangers of the unlimited sugar intake which is rampant in the United States, neither you nor I should partake of refined white crystals of any kind.

Sugar and artificial sweeteners dull one's sense of taste; even after discontinuing their use, it takes a few weeks to be able again to enjoy Nature's natural sweet flavor, as found in her fruits. We would all be better off if we curtailed our dependence on sweetened foods in any form, "natural" or "artificial."

References

Blank, M. A sweet tasting protein. *Europ. Scient. Notes.* Offices of Naval Research 28, 10:356, 1974.

Byard, J.; McChesney, E.; Goldberg, L. and Coulston, F. Excretion and metabolism of saccharin in man. *Fd. Cosmet. Toxicol.* 12:175, 1974.

Coming up: new artificial sweetener. *Med. World News:* 52G, 13 August 1974.

Hackler, D. Artificial sweeteners, old and new, and new exotic natural sweeteners being studied as sugar prices climb. *Worthington's World* 3,1:3, 1974.

Holsendolph, E. Big sugar users study substitutes. *New York Times*, 13 August 1974.

Jacobson, M. *Eater's digest*. Garden City, New York: Anchor Books, 1972.

Purdom, M. E., Hyder, K. and Pybas, M. D. Effects of saccharin on rats fed chemically defined diets.. *J. Amer. Diet. Assoc.* 63,6:635, 1973.

Schneck, H. M., Jr. F. D. A. to approve a new sweetener. *New York Times*, 26 July 1974.

Was the cyclamate ban ill-considered? *Med. World News*, 74T.

Yudkin, J. *Sweet and dangerous*. New York: Bantam Books, 1973.

CHAPTER 8

Vegetarianism: Its Advantages and Shortcomings

Current medical and scientific evidence indicates that, statistically, vegetarians in the United States are thinner and healthier, and that they may live longer than meat eaters. When Danes virtually gave up meat during World War I, nutritionists found that their general health had significantly improved. During World War II, Norwegians had a significant drop in heart disease when they had to adopt a vegetarian diet. Both countries returned to meat diets after the crises, with a subsequent decline in their temporary health gains.

At this point, you may be confused: Isn't a vegetarian diet supposed to be nutritionally unsound?

It can be, but it doesn't have to be. Man can subsist very well on a properly managed nonflesh diet. It's simply that we Americans have been conditioned to believe that only a meat-based diet can meet our nutritional needs and maintain our health. This chapter will examine the advantages and problems of vegetarianism, explain how a proper vegetarian diet can meet one's needs and uncover possible reasons for the good results that have been obtained on some vegetarian diets.

A Bit of History

Vegetarianism, or abstinence from meat, first became popular in Europe in the eighteenth century. Its advocates believed that eating meat excited animal passion, whereas a vegetable diet resulted in peaceful health, tranquility and virtue. There were claims that a vegetarian diet could produce clarification of intellect and even flashes of genius.

Are vegetarians calmer and more tranquil than other people?

Meat-eating animals (carnivores) such as wolves, lions, and tigers are aggressive, while vegetable-eating animals (herbivores) such as rabbits, cows and horses can be more easily domesticated. In between are the omnivores such as man, dog and pig, which will eat both vegetables and meat. The young baby might not be safe if left with a large, aggressive watchdog; but if the baby were made of lettuce, would you leave him with a rabbit? Among human tribes, vegetarians such as the Hindus are not necessarily more peaceful than the Eskimos who subsist primarily on meat products. Wars among the Eskimos have been rare and, if anything, the Eskimo typically is too friendly for his own good.

Vegetarianism was introduced to England by Dr. William Lambe, a Cambridge graduate, who gave up meat in 1806. He was convinced that his action had restored his health and that a vegetarian diet could cure almost all disease. On his death in 1847 at age 82, the London Vegetarian Society was founded.

American vegetarianism has produced such patrons as the Reverend Sylvester Graham and William Fletcher. In the early nineteenth century, Graham, the self-styled doctor of medicine after whom graham crackers and graham flour were named, extolled the virtues of his special dietary regime (abstinence from meat and alcohol and consumption of dry, stale, whole-meal, wheaten bread) and other hints for health such as open bedroom windows, hard mattresses and cold showers. At the beginning of this century, William Fletcher (the founder of Fletcherism) reiterated the need, first proclaimed by Graham, for prolonged chewing of every mouthful of food.

In the 1890s, Charles William Post, while regaining his

health at the Battle Creek sanatorium directed by Dr. John Henry Kellogg, created a cereal coffee substitute called Instant Postum. Then, in collaboration with Dr. Kellogg, he developed several breakfast cereals which were the foundation of the giant General Foods Corporation.

Reasons for Becoming a Vegetarian

The United States Department of Agriculture (USDA) estimates that less than 5 percent of the United States population is predominantly vegetarian, but even that small percentage figure represents more than ten million people. Most Americans, however, cannot understand why anyone would *want* to give up that great steak, or the all-American hamburger or the Thanksgiving turkey.

People turn away from meat for a variety of reasons. The majority of the world population seldom eats meat, more out of necessity than choice, since meat is the most expensive of foods. In the Far East, religious teachings have led to vegetarian macrobiotic diets. A minority of vegetarians are against killing animals for clothing as well as for food.

A large proportion of the vegetarians in this country have had a meatless diet creep up on them, not so much by choice as because of the rising cost of meat. As meat prices have gone up, meat consumption has declined.

Many present-day vegetarians have chosen a no-meat or a low-meat diet because of environmental and/or health concerns. In *Diet for a Small Planet*, for example, Frances Moore Lappé presents guidelines for eating from the earth that maximize the earth's potential and, simultaneously, minimize interference with the earth's resources.

Cautions Concerning Meatless Diets

Vegetarians are classified into three major categories. Complete vegetarians, or vegans, eat no meat or other animal-related foods. Lacto-vegetarians will drink milk and eat cheese and butter (dairy products). The lacto-ovo-vegetarian also eats eggs in addition to dairy products.

Today we possess an understanding of biochemistry which can enable us to follow a vegetarian regime knowledgeably. Some vegetarians are careful about balancing their diets and often use food supplements. However, many make the switch to a meatless diet without adequate nutritional knowledge. This can result in nutrient and protein deficiencies. A seventh-stage macrobiotic diet, for example, can cause hypoproteinemia, anemia, scurvy, hypocalcemia, emaciation and loss of kidney function. Other ill-advised vegetarian diets have produced kwashiorkor (a protein-deficiency disease commonly seen in other parts of the world), marasmus (a protein- and calorie-deficiency disease also rare in the United States), beriberi, rickets, pellagra and other severe vitamin deficiencies.

The major concern in connection with vegetarian diets has been with respect to adequate protein. Protein is needed by the body for growth, for maintenance of tissues and bones and for certain metabolic reactions. The RDA is 55 to 65 gm of protein a day for an adult, 65 during pregnancy, 75 during lactation, and 25 to 40 for children. (Protein is probably one of the few nutritional factors for which the RDA does not underestimate our need.) Signs of severe protein deficiency include falling hair, lassitude, depletion of plasma proteins, edema (abdominal enlargement due to fluid accumulation) and negative nitrogen balance. A well-planned vegetarian diet easily meets the protein requirement, and of the three types of vegetarians, the vegan is usually the only one who need be concerned about this.

The next common warning against vegetarianism is with respect to vitamin B-12, which is found only in animal products; thus B-12 deficiency is inevitable for the vegan unless he takes a B-12 supplement. The consequences of this deficiency are megaloblastic anemia and perhaps degeneration of the spinal cord. Green vegetable diets contain adequate folic acid, which masks the symptoms of B-12 deficiency, and thus the deficiency may go unnoticed by the individual until irreparable nerve damage has occurred. Most vegetarian diets also contain little vitamin D, so the vegetarian again may have problems especially if he lives in a city where sunlight doesn't penetrate the smog.

Another important nutrient that may be lacking in a vegetarian diet is zinc. Most vegetarians not only swear off meat, a good source of zinc, but usually accompany this with increased consumption of foods rich in phytates (beans, legumes and grains) which bind zinc, calcium and other minerals in the digestive system. This can become a major problem if large quantities of phytate-rich foods are consumed. However, the addition of leaven or yeast to grains in bread destroys the phytates by fermentation. Also, sprouting neutralizes the phytates, even in soybeans. Sprouted grains, beans and seeds are most nutritious and should be a part of everyone's diet.

Adding to the danger of low zinc status is the declining trace mineral content of edible plants, especially grains, as a result of soil exhaustion (without replacement) and overuse of nitrogen and phosphorus fertilizers.

Zinc insufficiency is one of the greatest and least-known dangers of vegetarianism. The individual who does not eat meat must be careful to fulfill the need for zinc adequately, probably through a tablet supplement. The light-headed feeling of detachment that enshrouds some vegetarians can be caused by hidden zinc hunger, rather than by some mystical quality of the brown rice or other food consumed.

Some vegetarians may ingest an excess of vitamins and iron. Over several years, excess iron can result in a systemic iron overload that may damage the muscular tissue of the heart and liver, especially when eaten in conjunction with a protein-deficient diet.

The individual who pursues a meatless diet for economic reasons is the least likely vegetarian to be positively health-minded or knowledgeable about proper nutrient intake. The poor are probably the least likely to eat more fresh fruits, vegetables and seed sprouts, all of which are low in phytates. They will be the most likely to continue to consume refined foods, processed snacks, white bread, sugar, additives and alcohol (very efficient in flushing zinc from the human system), instead of more nutritious foods.

A vegetarian diet, or at least a diet in which meat consumption has been reduced, can, however, be planned with these cautions in mind. Emphasis should be placed on natural and unprocessed foods and the vegan, and probably the lacto- and lacto-ovo-vegetarians (to be safe), should take, at the very least, B-12 and zinc supplements.

Balanced Protein Intake

When laymen and even some nutritionists speak of protein, they divide protein sources into two distinct classes, animal and plant, and consider the former far superior to the latter in quality. Actually, this is not always true. Proteins should be viewed more as a continuum with consideration given to both quantity and quality. A few plant foods have a higher *quantity* of protein than meat. The proteins in eggs, milk, fish, cheese and whole rice are of better *quality* than those in meat. Why, then, is such great importance placed on meat in the American diet?

Meat is erroneously believed to be the best food for health, and is indeed tasty. Meat consumption is associated with status in this country, and we consume an average of one-half pound of meat per person every day. Americans eat about twice as much beef and veal and about 2½ times as much poultry as they did forty years ago.

Despite the fact that North Americans make up only 7 percent of the world's population, they consume 30 percent of the world supplies of animal protein and devour thirty times as much meat as the Japanese and sixty-six times as much meat as the average Asian. Since some Americans do not receive enough protein, many of the others must be very much overloaded. The average American has been estimated to consume from 10 to 12 percent more protein than his body can use for growth, maintenance of tissues and metabolic reactions. The leftover protein gets stored as fat or burned as fuel for energy, which requires additional pyridoxine (B-6) and calcium. This overconsumption of protein, especially from animal sources, might not matter if it were not for the misuse of and imbalance in the environment which is required to provide the unneeded protein.

The myth of red meat as the key to health and as vastly superior to plant protein can be dispelled if protein balance is understood. Proteins are composed of amino acids in different combinations. There are twenty-two amino acids that can go into proteins, eight of which (nine in the case of children) are considered essential because they cannot be synthesized by our bodies and must be obtained from foods.

The body can only use the essential amino acids in specific patterns; certain ones must be present simultaneously (at the same meal) if protein synthesis is to take place in the body.

The extent to which the amino acid pattern matches that which the body can use is reflected in the "biological value" of food. The net protein utilization (NPU) reflects the biological value and the digestibility of a protein—in other words, how much of the protein we eat is finally available to our bodies. No food corresponds exactly 100 percent with the body's required pattern, but the protein in eggs comes closest and therefore other proteins' NPUs are rated in relation to that of the egg.

All proteins, in varying degrees, are of lower quality than that of the egg, and this constitutes the protein continuum. In each food, only one or two essential amino acids are deficient or totally lacking, and these are called the "limiting amino acids" for that food. The protein will be utilized by the body as protein only to the extent that the limiting amino acid is present. The excess of the other amino acids will be wasted, or rather, burned for energy.

The amino acid patterns closest to that of the egg are found in milk, fish, cheese, whole rice, red meat and poultry, in that order. But there is a greater disparity in quality between meat and eggs than between meat and most plants (grains, legumes, nuts and seeds). Green vegetables and fruits are not considered because of their negligible protein content. The most commonly lacking essential amino acids in plants are lysine, tryptophan and methionine. All cereals are deficient in lysine; corn and rice are also low in tryptophan and threonine. Soybeans and seed oils are low in methionine. Legumes are short on methionine and tryptophan; peanuts are deficient in methionine and lysine.

The other criterion used in evaluating protein sources

is quantity, or the proportion of useable protein to total weight. Meats are 20 to 30 percent useable protein, ranging from lamb at the bottom to turkey at the top. Soybean flour is 40 percent protein, most cheeses 30 to 35 percent protein, many nuts and seeds between 20 and 30 percent, and peas, lentils and dried beans between 20 and 25 percent. Whole grains contain a fairly small quantity of protein (12 percent), but so do milk (4 percent) and eggs (13 percent). Thus, in evaluating the value of a protein source, both quality and quantity must be considered.

In general, animal proteins are more complete than plant proteins, so one usually needs to eat proportionately less meat than grains to obtain the same amount of useable protein. But, proteins from nonflesh foods are perfectly adequate nutritionally; people do not have to rely on meat for the correct supply of amino acids. Plant and animal protein sources (such as cereals and dairy products) can be combined in the same meal. And different plant foods which have mutually complementing amino acid patterns (where the amino acid deficiency of one food is supplemented by the amino acid contained in others) can be eaten together. Such a pair is rice with beans, or wheat and beans.

Complementing two or more plant proteins will result in an increase of the protein value of the meal. The whole (complemented protein value) is greater than the sum of its parts (the individual protein value of each plant food). Thus plant foods, when eaten in combination, can be planned to far exceed meat in protein value. For details about complementing proteins, you might refer to *Diet for a Small Planet* which contains excellent suggestions. Once the major limiting amino acids for various families of plants are learned, complementing them will become routine.

Maximizing Nature's Potential

Livestock such as cows are able to produce high-quality protein for human consumption from otherwise inedible sources such as cellulose and low-quality protein in plants. At present, however, full advantage is not taken of this ability to convert grass to human food in highly industrialized countries.

Large quantities of high-quality, human-edible foods are

fed to animals. One-half of the harvested agricultural land in the United States is planted with feed crops. Three-quarters of the grain is fed to animals (the largest proportion in any country in the world). In 1968, U.S. livestock, excepting dairy cows, consumed twenty million tons of protein, primarily from sources edible directly by man—that is, grains such as corn, sorghum, oats, barley, soybeans, wheat and rye, and fish products.

Furthermore, livestock are very inefficient in their conversion of plant protein to meat protein. The average protein-conversion ratio of all livestock is eight to one. Cows are least efficient, requiring 21 pounds of plant protein to produce 1 pound of animal protein. Plants produce much more protein per acre than livestock: an acre used for cereals can provide five times as much protein as an acre used for meat production, an acre used for legumes ten times as much protein, and an acre used for leafy vegetables fifteen times as much.

These impressive statistics make clear the inefficient use of agricultural land and of food resources in this country. This is especially important in light of existent malnutrition in this country and of the food shortages which affect millions of people in other parts of the world. F.M. Lappé estimates that every year eighteen million tons of plant protein become unavailable to man, an amount equivalent to 90 percent of the yearly world protein deficit, and also enough protein for 12 gm a day per person in the world! The Dean of Agriculture at Ohio State University has estimated that 40 percent of world livestock production is obtained from vegetable sources suitable for human consumption.

If this protein were made available to man directly, the world food supply could be increased by 30 percent. Lyle P. Schertz, an administrator in the USDA, has stated that "the billion people in the developed countries use practically as much cereals as *feed* to produce animal protein as the *two* billion people of the developing countries use directly as *food*."

Concerned people such as Lappé advocate eating lower on the food chain, or at least lowering one's consumption of meat and returning the grains used for feed to humans. Animals like cattle, sheep and goats do not need to eat protein to produce protein. They are able to live well on marginal arable land. Furthermore, America is importing meat from protein-deficient countries to further feed her protein-sufficient citizens. Animal waste, unfortunately, is not adequately used as fertilizer and ends up contaminating our sewage systems. Much land is wasted on producing nonnutritional money-making crops such as coffee, tea, rubber, cocoa and fibers. The concentrated use of agricultural land depletes our soil and results in agricultural products of lower quality, notably lower protein levels in grains.

With respect to environmental concerns and protein needs of the world population, research is already under way and innovations are being practiced. The Ceres Land Company in Colorado can now process manure by sterilization and treatment with chemicals to produce a powder containing 25 to 35 percent protein and roughage. This recycled manure is being used in animal feed. The limiting factor is the high level of the heavy metals—lead, mercury, cadmium and copper.

Scientists of the "Green Revolution" of the 1960s obtained high-yielding wheat and other grains. However, these crops require greater amounts of fertilizer, which can cause accumulation of algae and other clogging vegetations in waterways. High-yield crops may be more profitable than lower-yield, protein-rich crops, but efforts to improve yields have tended to reduce the protein content of the crop, and efforts to improve the protein quality (by better amino acid balance) have usually lowered productivity.

Researchers have not yet been able to improve the protein content or quality of cereals and legumes without losing productivity. However, strains of corn, barley and sorghum have been selected for higher lysine content. Opaque-2 corn is a step in the right direction. This corn kernel has adequate lysine and tryptophan, but the yield per acre is 10 percent less than for other corns, and the soft white kernel is more easily penetrated by boring insects. By crossing this corn with others, an ideal hybrid may be obtained.

In the effort to find alternate suitable protein sources with which to feed the world, researchers have come up with textured vegetable protein (TVP), chunks of spun soybean fiber flavored to imitate chicken, ham, bacon and hamburger. The protein quality is enhanced by fortification with methionine, the limiting amino acid, or by addition of egg protein. Studies have found TVP to be high-quality protein and efficient for maintaining nitrogen balance. TVP has little or no fat and no cholesterol and, unlike meat, it does not shrink in cooking. Soybeans are 40 percent protein, and these new meatless meats are cheaper than actual meat. An acre of land planted in soybeans can produce ten times as much protein as animals grazing on an acre of land. TVP is starting to make inroads in the sale of meat, and consumption is expected to rise to 15 or 20 percent by 1980.

At first glance, TVP sounds like a great discovery. However, soybeans have two faults. They do not contain the good combination of trace minerals that meats have. The zinc content of soy protein is much lower than that of meat, and copper is much higher. To complicate matters, soybeans, as well as other types of beans and whole grains, are rich in phytates which tie up zinc and other minerals; thus, not only is the small amount of zinc in the soybeans made unavailable, but some of the zinc from other foods consumed gets tied up with the phytates.

Recently, another potentially valuable protein source has been extracted from cottonseed. This high-protein cottonseed concentrate, manufactured in the form of a flour, may assist in filling the world protein gap.

Cautions Concerning Use of Some Plants

The benefits and delights of plant food sources are many, and the varieties of preparation are infinite. Many fruits and vegetables need no cooking and are, in fact, more nutritious when eaten raw. However, care must be taken with some vegetables because of plant toxins.

The legume family (lima beans, lentils, soybeans and other beans) contains a variety of dangerous toxins which become harmless when cooked or sprouted: (1) trypsin inhibitors, which inhibit the action of the enzyme trypsin in the digestive tract, thereby inhibiting growth; (2) hemagglutinins, which inhibit growth by combining with the cells lining the intestinal wall, thus blocking intestinal nutrient absorption; (3) goiterogenic factor, which is believed to block the uptake of iodine by the thyroid, thus resulting in goiter; (4) a complex glycoside factor in lima beans and some forage plants that yields hydrocyanic acid, a deadly poison. Green peas and chick peas contain a trypsin inhibitor not neutralized by heat, and green peas also contain a hemagglutinin resistant to heat. These toxins are present in very small amounts in these peas, and many people eat both types without bad effects. Raw lima beans and other legumes, however, have been reported to cause death.

Uncooked fava beans can cause hemolytic anemia, a characteristic of favism. Other symptoms include fever, abdominal pain, headache and coma. This disease is common in some Mediterranean countries, and susceptibility to it seems to be hereditary. Seeds or seed meal from several species of pealike legumes known as vetches can produce lathyrism, a neurologic disease at one time responsible for many deaths and disabilities throughout Europe, Africa and India; it characteristically paralyzes the lower limbs.

Some of the brassica family of vegetables, if eaten raw, have the property of contributing to goiter. This family includes cabbage, Chinese cabbage, watercress, kale, rutabaga, turnip, rape and mustard. Drinking milk from cows which have eaten brassica plants can interfere with thyroid function.

There are still other plant toxins. Rhubarb leaves have a high oxalic acid content. Excessive oxalic acid blocks the absorption of calcium and can cause severe kidney damage and also death. Rhubarb leaves should not be eaten. Raw nutmeg (15 to 25 gm) is a psychedelic drug which can cause hallucinations and other psychiatric symptoms. The intoxication usually lasts only a few days but death has been known to occur with overdosage.

Beet- and carrot-juice cocktails are to be eaten sparingly because the carotene can be deposited in the human skin and turn the skin yellow. The yellow color is most evident in the palm of the hand. Fortunately, no harm is done, and when celery cocktails are substituted, the yellow pigment slowly disappears.

Advantages of Consuming Less Meat

There are several advantages to relying on protein sources

other than meat. In addition to factors of environmental efficiency, there is evidence that eating low on the food chain is healthier. Pesticides, especially of the chlorinated phenyl and organic mercury types, are a major concern of many today. Carnivores are more likely to accumulate these potentially harmful contaminants than are herbivores because animal meat is higher on the food chain than plant life, and thus contains more pesticide residues. For example, people have been poisoned by eating large-sized fish high in methyl mercury. Many meats also contain sodium nitrate and hormone residues, the effects of which are potentially dangerous. And there are indications that meat is highly susceptible to bacteria growth and food spoilage.

Some studies indicate a strong correlation between a meat diet and cancer of the colon. Equally important is the finding that vegetarians have lower serum cholesterol levels than meat eaters. Forty percent of the fats in our diets comes from meat, which is about 4 percent saturated fat or cholesterol. Except for eggs, nonflesh foods have no cholesterol. Heart diseases and many forms of cancer appear to be Western diseases; they are practically unknown in some underdeveloped countries where meat is seldom eaten. (That lower incidence, however, may be due to other factors such as consumption of less sugar and processed foods, and a very different lifestyle.)

You will remember from the previous chapter that consumption of plant foods or whole natural carbohydrates maintains lowered blood cholesterol levels. This is due to the roughage or fiber in the form of bran and cellulose in plants. Furthermore, this roughage is indigestible by the human body, passes on through, and in this way is also essential to proper digestive and eliminative functions. People who are predominantly meat eaters are not uncommonly bothered by poor absorption and elimination. Food with a low fiber content, such as meat, is sluggish in its movement through the digestive tract, resulting in dry and hard-to-pass stools. Vegetables and other natural plant foods retain moisture and bind waste bulk for easy passage.

At the beginning of the chapter, we noted that vegetarians tend to be thinner than meat eaters. Most vegetarians who eat a proper diet meet, but do not significantly exceed, their protein and caloric needs. (Fiber does not provide calories.) Most meat eaters, on the other hand, consistently exceed their needs, and therefore tend to weigh more.

Anthropological field investigations have documented the excellent health and longevity characteristic of certain nonmeat cultures. And it should not be forgotten that plants provide, on the average, in Britain and America, more than twice the amount of vitamins and minerals provided by meat and fish. The only required nutrient restricted totally to animal sources is vitamin B-12. Riboflavin (B-2) and calcium are provided mostly by dairy products and eggs, but not by meat. Another advantage to eating less meat and more plant foods is that the latter are cheaper.

At first, planning a diet in which nonflesh foods play a larger role may be difficult and require some imagination. Balanced against this, however, are the benefits to be gained from plant food sources and the disadvantages of a heavily meat-laced diet. For ecological, health and economic reasons, investigating plant sources of protein as alternatives to meat is advised. Doctors seldom recommend complete abstinence from meat, since meat is a good food; but meat certainly is not needed more than once a day at the most. Neither is a complete vegetarian diet (no eggs or dairy products) advisable, especially for children with their higher protein requirement. However, ample vegetables and fruits are needed by the body. Vegetarians must expertly manage their diets as outlined and take care to get adequate B-12 and zinc and proper amino acid combinations in the same meal.

Hypoglycemics should be advised not to become *complete* vegetarians (vegans); they would be able to obtain adequate protein for body maintenance and even some for energy, but their carbohydrate intake might be too high because the starchy vegetables (especially some grains and legumes) are high in carbohydrates.

Certainly, a varied diet in which meat does not play an overemphasized protein role is healthful and adequate for everyone.

References

Arehart-Treichel, J. Green revolution: phase 2. *Sci. News* 103:42, 1973.

Grott-Kurska, D. Before you say "baloney" . . . here's what you should know about vegetarianism. *Today's Health* 18 October 1974.

Lappé, F. M. *Diet for a small planet.* New York: Ballantine Books, 1971.

Maxton, C. Some foods must be cooked. *Prevention* 161 July 1974.

Robb-Smith, A. Doctors at table. *JAMA* 224:28, 1973.

Rodale, R. Creeping vegetarianism creates zinc hunger. *Prevention* 21 July 1974.

Turk, R. E.; Cornwell, P. E.; Brooks, M. D. and Butterworth, C. E. Adequacy of spun-soy protein containing egg albumin for human nutrition. *J. Amer. Diet. Assoc.* 63:5, 1973.

Vegetarian diets. *The Medical Letter* 15:30, 1973.

PART TWO

The Vitamins

INTRODUCTION

So far, we have dealt with nutritional problems. We shall now focus on the biochemicals themselves.

Everything in the universe is technically a "chemical," and many of these are good biochemicals, like human beings. We are biochemicals, if you'll pardon such a pragmatic definition. Some of the most beneficial biochemicals, by our standards, are contained in our food, air and water. These are the nutrients that evolved with life, the vitamins and minerals natural to our food and bodies.

Parts Two and Three deal with those vitamins and trace elements which are most needed by or have measurable effects on the human brain.

A great gap in knowledge exists between the initial rat-guinea-pig studies and the ultimate human studies. Even the available human studies are usually conducted on young men living in a dormitory in a cozy nonstressful situation. These human data are not transferable to everyday life with its stresses. The pregnant woman, the growing adolescent, the aging individual, the vegetarian, the fasting individual, the "dietary dub" and the child allowed to eat inadequately fortified sweet junk food for breakfast are among those who are subject to stressful situations and who may therefore derive special benefit from the vitamins and trace elements discussed in these sections.

The aspects to be discussed include history of usage, metabolism, and occurrence in foods and natural systems. Finally, food sources for the vitamins and essential trace elements are listed.

CHAPTER 9

Niacin and Megavitamin Therapy

In the early 1900s, Goldberger, noting the many people with pellagra and mental illness in the southern part of the United States, remarked that "if poor people subsist on a diet of cornbread, cane syrup and pork fat they will inevitably get sick." He later noted a similarity between black tongue in dogs and pellagra in man. Goldberger published nutritional studies on pellagra in 1928 but unfortunately died in 1929. Pellagra is characterized by diarrhea, dementia and a dermatitis marked by a pigmentation of the skin exposed to the sun. Death can result.

Following Goldberger's work, Elvehjem at the University of Wisconsin became intrigued with Goldberger's attempts to find a cure for pellagra. Knowing that liver extract would protect dogs against black tongue, Elvehjem tried various chemicals that occur in liver and finally in 1937 found the protective substance—nicotinic acid. Vitamin B-3, nicotinic acid (niacin) was the vitamin missing from the diets of poor southerners.

In 1938, Tom Spies et al. reported that seventeen patients were cured of their physical symptoms (pellagra) after the administration of nicotinic acid or nicotinamide. This study was followed by a more thorough investigation of seventy-three patients in which it was noted that with reduction of physical symptoms there also occurred complete relief of accompanying mental problems. Pellagra is probably a combined deficiency of the vitamins B-3 and B-6 and the amino acid tryptophan which the body can convert to B-3.

In 1939, H. M. Cleckley and colleagues reported excellent results in the treatment of pellagra psychoses with niacin. Out of eighteen cases, vitamin therapy contributed greatly to the improvement of four, while the other fourteen were dramatically cured.

Then, in 1951, Drs. H. Osmond and A. Hoffer of the University of Saskatchewan studied mescaline psychosis. Their studies triggered an entirely new biochemical hypothesis concerning schizophrenia which is based on a similarity of the delirium in pellagra to that seen in psychotics and schizophrenics. (They were familiar with the fact that since niacin had been added to the processed flour in the United States, pellagra and its psychosis had almost disappeared.) With the idea that schizophrenics might need more than normal amounts of niacin, they treated their first schizophrenic in February 1952 and obtained dramatic results. Since then, they have done double-blind studies with niacin which have confirmed the outcome of their original study. Others, in smaller blind studies, have confirmed the findings of Hoffer and Osmond. Results of a recent study in Ireland on megadoses of niacinamide were negative, however, as were those of a double-blind study at Marlboro Hospital in New Jersey.

The now famous "megavitamin therapy" evolved from these early studies. At its core are niacin and vitamin C in doses of 3 gm each per day. Megavitamin therapy has had an interesting history: despite the publication of two double-blind studies, thirty papers and several pamphlets and books prior to 1966, the medical profession in general regarded this therapy with indifference and sometimes hostility. In the middle 1960s, its use began the first marked upward swing on what appears to be a soaring curve of rehabilitation in the schizophrenias. But even today most medical associations, naturally conservative and wary of novel ideas, do not acknowledge the value of megavitamin therapy. One doctor asked, "If it's so damned good, why isn't everyone using it?" Dr. Abram Hoffer believes the answer is, "It's so damned good, no one believes it!"

Niacin, part of the B complex (B-3), is synonymous with nicotinic acid. As a coenzyme, it assists in the breakdown and utilization of fats, proteins and carbohydrates. The niacin-deficiency disease, pellagra, produces such symptoms as weakness, diarrhea, dermatitis and nervous-mental disorders. Niacin is most effective when used in conjunction with other vitamins of the B complex. Niacin, or its amide, niacinamide, is widely distributed in foods. Lean meat, eggs, liver, fish, wheat germ and even beer have appreciable amounts. Corn, however, is low both in niacin and tryptophan. Average "normal adults" excrete 2 to 8 mg of B-3 daily, mainly as the niacinamide methochloride. This excretion product uses carbon atoms or methyl groups, and this may be in part the mode of action of large doses of niacin since excess methylation may produce hallucinogenic substances.

Niacinamide (or nicotinamide), another form of vitamin B-3, differs from niacin in that it has a substituted amide group whereas niacin has an hydroxyl group. Niacin may cause redness and itching in the blush area when taken in large doses, and niacinamide is often used as an alternative in equal doses to the niacin in patients who cannot tolerate this red flush. The niacinamide, however, may cause psychiatric depression in some adults.

In its role of coenzyme, niacin helps in the oxidation of sugars and is essential to proper brain metabolism. In this way, it also helps regulate the blood sugar level in the hypoglycemic patient. In 1966, Pfeiffer and Iliev discovered the possible role of histamine in the schizophrenias and noted that niacin, in conjunction with other vitamins, raised blood histamine and thus helped to relieve such symptoms as paranoia, hallucinations and other disperceptions. Schizophrenic patients who are high in histamine or have pyroluria (mauve factor) are not benefited by niacin therapy.

Niacin is also effective in treating some alcoholics, many of whom are basically schizophrenic. One study, which ran for

1½ years, by Dr. Russel F. Smith of Guest House, Lake Orion, Michigan, and Brighton Hospital, Detroit involved 507 alcoholics treated with niacin. Niacinamide was used in the few cases where niacin could not be tolerated. Of these patients, 103 were classified as excellent results, 240 good, 98 fair, and 66 poor. Among the hard-core alcoholics placed on an average of 6 gm of niacin per day, 87 derived benefit. Twenty percent of this group maintained complete abstinence which, despite other rigorous therapies, had been impossible before beginning the treatment with niacin.

The study showed that niacin far surpassed all other therapeutic agents commonly used in the treatment of alcoholism. Some of these, unlike niacin, have a high potential for abuse and also represent a suicide risk. (Dr. Hoffer once had a patient who tried to commit suicide by taking about 90 gm of niacin. The only result was nausea, vomiting and diarrhea. Aspirin at this megadose would have been much more toxic.)

Niacin also helps to alleviate the pain and other problems of arthritis and other joint dysfunctions. In 1941, Dr. William Kaufman began using niacinamide in large doses for his arthritis patients. He found that their joint mobility increased, that their stiffness decreased and that joint deformity and pain was alleviated. In 1955, Kaufman reported extensively on his use of nicotinamide on 663 patients. Those who took adequate doses of the vitamin continuously, he reported, experienced additional benefits such as gains in muscle strength, decreased fatigue and relief of chronic emotional disorders.

Dr. Abram Hoffer has also observed the effects of B-3 (niacin and niacinamide) on his arthritic patients and has summarized his observations in a paper published in the *Canadian Medical Association Journal* of August 15, 1959. While the effect of B-3 on arthritis can be immediate, even seemingly miraculous, most cases require long-term treatment to achieve maximal results. In any event, niacin does not produce the variety of undesirable physiological side-effects that can occur with cortisone, the commonly prescribed therapy for arthritis.

Niacin, as an acid, competes with release of free fatty acids and thus helps keep blood cholesterol down. It has been used in large doses (i.e., 3 or 4 gm daily) to treat fat-induced hyperlipemia, hypercholesterolemia and occlusive vascular disease. Dr. Edwin Boyle, Research Director of the Miami Heart Institute, has used niacin in more than a thousand cases. In one group of 600 patients, insurance company actuarial mortality tables predicted 62 deaths over a ten-year period. Among these patients, all of whom took large doses of niacin during the period, only 6 deaths occurred.

Niacin is also known to decrease the effects of the hallucinogens such as LSD and mescaline, to help smokers reduce their use of nicotine, and to increase the effects of tranquilizers so that, thereafter, the dosage can be reduced.

The initial flushing which occurs in some patients using niacin can be frightening, particularly if the physician has not instructed his patient concerning this beforehand. If severe skin redness in the blush area is continuous, cold milk should be taken with the niacin after meals. Periactin (4 mg) may also help.

Precautions

Massive doses of niacin have been given during the last twenty-five years without evidence of any serious or sustained damage to the body organs. This is not true for niacinamide, which may produce liver damage in doses as low as 3 gm. daily.

Several precautions should be observed in administering niacin.

1) The severe redness and itching in the blush area usually passes in an hour's time. Where this is a problem, we recommend using smaller doses after meals and building up slowly.

2) Niacin may precipitate an attack of gout because nicotinic acid competes with the excretion of uric acid. Acute nausea and vomiting may occur with the rapid rise in uric acid.

3) Hyperkeratosis (dark thickening of the keratin or horny layer of the skin) may occur with prolonged large doses of niacin. The front of the arm near the elbow, the armpits and the abdomen are usually the first places for hyperkeratosis to ap-

pear. We have not seen this for the past three years and have theorized that this skin thickening may occur only in pyroluric (mauve-factor) patients, who should be getting large doses of B-6 rather than niacin.

Niacinamide (which is recommended by some because it does not cause redness) may cause depression in some adults. Although niacinamide may be used in children without producing psychiatric depression, children usually need zinc and vitamin B-6, rather than niacin or niacinamide.

Administration

Niacin is usually given with equal doses of vitamin C. It should be administered after meals to minimize flushing and nausea. Dosage can vary from 50 mg to a maximum of 3 gm daily. In our present state of knowledge, it appears that the patient should be placed on adjuvant therapy such as folic acid and B-12 injections to reduce high doses of niacin to lower levels that we know are safe, namely 3 gm or less per day. The schizophrenic patients who will respond are those who are low in histamine (histapenic). These constitute half the patients now called schizophrenic. The response of those who are improved is frequently much better than that obtained by conventional tranquilizer therapy.

An amino acid, tryptophan, can be converted into niacin by body chemistry. Thus niacin may be obtained from tryptophan-containing foods like eggs, meats, poultry and dairy products. Sixty milligrams of tryptophan yields 1 mg of niacin, and tryptophan may provide all of the daily niacin requirements if only small amounts are required. However, the need for niacin, as for all vitamins, can vary greatly from individual to individual. The RDA or minimum daily requirement (MDR) can be misleading in this sense. For someone on a 2,000-calorie diet, the National Research Council recommends 13.2 mg of niacin or niacin equivalent; yet the histapenic schizophrenic may require two hundred times this amount as a bare minimum. This niacin-dependent patient cannot rely simply on the niacin or tryptophan content of his food. He must supplement his intake with niacin tablets.

We might conclude, then, that "megavitamin" is a poor name for the type of vitamin treatment involving niacin. A person taking niacin treatment is not necessarily taking a "mega" dose at all, but merely the minimum daily requirement of his or her particular body chemistry. "Mega" also has some undesirable connotations as a prefix, implying something explosive (i.e., megaton hydrogen bomb) or of great debilitating potential. Granted, there are some vitamins (A and D) which in "mega" doses may have some "mega" effects of a debilitating kind, but niacin, and the vitamin C which is used in conjunction with it, are not mega poisons. The only things which niacin may "blast" away" are the symptoms of schizophrenia or arthritis or alcoholism.

The development of niacin therapy (niacin used in conjunction with vitamin C) is one of the great advances in medicine, heralding a new age in biochemical treatment of the schizophrenias. It is far more effective when used with tranquilizers than tranquilizers used alone, and thus permits use of lower doses of these powerful drugs with a consequent reduction in the incidence of side-effects. However, now we can go even further in including niacin therapy within the broad spectrum of nutrient therapy, which involves the deployment of trace metals, vitamins and other nutrients in addition to niacin, and is more far-reaching in the number of mental disorders that can be alleviated.

References

W., Bill. The vitamin B-3 therapy. (A second communication to A.A.'s physicians.) Privately printed. Box 451, Bedford Hills, New York 10507. February 1968.

Denson, R. Nicotinamide in the treatment of schizophrenia. *Dis. Nerv. System* 23. March 1962.

Hawkins, D. and Pauling, L., eds. *Orthomolecular psychiatry: Treatment of schizophrenia.* San Francisco: W. H. Freeman, 1973.

Hoffer, A. and Osmond, H. *How to live with schizophrenia.* New Hyde Park, New York: University Books, 1966.

———Treatment of schizophrenia with nicotinic acid. *ACTA Psych. Scand.* 40:171, 1964.

Spies, Tom et al. The treatment of subclinical and classical pellagra. *JAMA* 111:584, 13 August 1938.

CHAPTER 10

The Sleep Vitamins: Vitamin C, Inositol and Vitamin B-6

Vitamin C

Vitamin C (1-ascorbic acid) has been the subject of much medical controversy in the past few years, specifically as a postulated cure for the common cold. Linus Pauling, who first publicized the "miraculous effects" of large doses of this vitamin, has been under constant attack from some members of the medical establishment for his so-called unsubstantiated claims that 2 to 4 gm a day of vitamin C will reduce the incidence of cold-related symptoms.

Aside from its possible beneficial effects on head colds, vitamin C is known to be essential for many biochemical functions and, more recently, has been found to have an antianxiety effect (as shown by the quantitative EEG) which has proven advantageous in the biochemical treatment of the schizophrenias. Vitamin C also mobilizes heavy metals such as copper, lead and mercury and allows their excretion by the kidneys.

If asked what vitamin C does, most people will answer, "It prevents or cures scurvy." This is an accurate but inadequate reply. Perhaps a better understanding of the functions of vitamin C will alert individuals to the necessity of having optimal amounts at all times within the body.

Many animals synthesize vitamin C in their livers but some cannot do this. Among the species that have lost the ability to make ascorbic acid are man, other primates and the guinea pig. The evolutionary process has rendered them incapable of manufacturing this vitamin due to the lack of liver enzyme (1-gluconolactone oxidase) necessary for its formation. Without this enzyme, the biochemicals cannot combine to produce the 1-ascorbic acid. As a result of this inability, failure to ingest at least a small amount—as little as 10 mg a day (¼ glass of orange juice)—will cause biochemical complications that may eventually cause scurvy, a deficiency disease that has many serious side-effects.

Historical Background

> A large number of men in our army were attacked also by a certain pestilence, against which the doctors could not find any remedy in their art. A sudden pain seized the feet and legs; immediately afterwards the gums and teeth were attacked by a sort of gangrene, and the patients could not eat any more. Then the bones of the legs became horribly black, and so, after the greatest patience, a large number of Christians went to rest on the bosom of the Lord.

Thus wrote Jacques de Vity in the thirteenth century. He gave us the first concise account of scurvy in his history of the Crusades. The Crusades frequently took the Europeans to the dry countries of Eastern Europe and Southern Asia. These arid countries have fewer green vegetables available for forage. Also, the strange plants of an arid land may be edible or poisonous, and only by dangerous experimentation can the explorer determine the useful plants. This sampling takes time, and, during the period without vegetables or plants, the Crusaders fell ill with scurvy and their legs turned black and blue from subcutaneous bleeding.

The credit for the discovery of a treatment for scurvy is usually given to Dr. James Lind (1716-94), but history shows that Jacques Cartier, the French explorer and first European to explore the St. Lawrence River, had earlier found a specific remedy in the form of *Annedda* which was promptly called *arbor vitae* because of its life-saving properties. Modern classification lists *Annedda* as white cedar *(Thuja occidentalis)*, and modern chemical analysis shows that the needles of most evergreens are high in ascorbic acid (vitamin C) content. The actual content of C is from 27 to 31 mg percent. In comparison, lemon juice has 27 mg percent, lime juice 27 mg percent, orange juice 42 mg percent, fresh green peppers 120 mg percent and fresh rose hips about 500 mg percent.

In 1747, Lind conducted a test aboard a British naval vessel, using twelve sailors afflicted with scurvy as his subjects. He divided them into two-man teams, with each of them receiving a different antidote—cider, diluted sulfuric acid, vinegar, sea water, various drugs, or two oranges and a lemon a day. The citrus subjects recovered in six days, while none of the others improved. After further experimentation Lind published *A Treatise on Scurvy* (1753). He also reported on the use of lime and lemon juice in his *Essay of the Health of Seamen* (1757), but many years passed before the treatment was officially adopted by the Royal Navy. The required use of limes while at sea gave the nickname "limey" to the British sailors. The citrus juice was prepared for use on long voyages by evaporation of the juice to a thick syrup in an open earthen vessel; alternately, the citrus juice was mixed with enough rum so that the alcohol would act as a preservative of the juice and vitamin.

An insufficient supply of ascorbic acid will result in scurvy with accompanying symptoms of subcutaneous bleeding, tenderness of the joints, loss of appetite, anemia and slow wound healing. The odontoblasts (bony cells between the root canals) of the teeth will shorten and separate from the dentine; the tooth then becomes porous and decays. The gums become spongy, but with 50 mg vitamin C per day healing occurs in two weeks. Psychological symptoms manifest themselves as fatigue, lassitude, depression and an increased incidence of Minnesota Multiphasic Personality Inventory (MMPI) ratings of hypochondriasis, depression and hysteria. If left untreated, scurvy can cause rapid death. On a C-free diet, the guinea pig, which (like man) makes no C, will show severe symptoms of scurvy in two weeks and die at the end of four weeks.

At present, scurvy predominates in populations ravaged by starvation and severe malnutrition. In the United States, scurvy is found among infants six to twelve months old who are fed a formula without vitamin supplements and also among middle-aged single people who, for convenience, subsist on junk foods.

Specific Sources, Functions and Uses

Although a cure for scurvy was discovered and used in the sixteenth century, the active substance, ascorbic acid, was not chemically identified and synthesized until the work of Szent-Györgyi et al. in 1933. Since then, synthetic vitamin C has been found to be equal to natural vitamin C for human body functioning. Ascorbic acid is normally present in both the blood plasma and cells, and any excess is excreted via the urine. Vitamin C occurs in large concentrations in both parts of the adrenal gland and is essential in the formation of noradrenalin and adrenalin, which are used to mobilize quick energy in emergencies. With stress of any kind, an increased secretion of adrenocorticosteroids occurs, and a rapid decrease also occurs in the level of adrenal ascorbic acid and cholesterol. This indicates synthesis of adrenal steroids.

The main food sources of vitamin C are fruits and green vegetables, with the richest sources being citrus fruits, peppers, tomatoes, turnip and broccoli greens and brussels sprouts. Vitamin C produces and maintains intercellular material, such as collagen, which cements individual cells into a tissue or organ functioning as a whole. Without enough vitamin C the tissues of the entire body are affected, the blood vessels become porous and let the blood through, muscles weaken and may even grow paralyzed, mineral salts drain away from bones and teeth, ligaments grow so weak that they will not hold the joints together, anemia develops and wounds refuse to heal. In addition, C has other specific actions. Some of the lesser-known effects are:

1. Vitamin C is one of the body's strongest reducing agents in a chemical sense. It may therefore be safely used to keep

drugs that are easily oxidized in a reduced or stable state. Conversely, vitamin C can itself be easily oxidized by metal contamination during the processing of foods. A steel knife quickly becomes dull if used for slicing lemons. (The iron ends up in the lemon juice!) Stainless steel is better, and a plastic knife is best. Citrus juice free of copper or iron contamination provides the highest level of vitamin C activity. Patients who have high levels of copper or iron in their blood have the lowest levels of vitamin C and need a larger intake.

2. In general, the metabolism of amino acids (which are the building blocks of proteins) is affected by several vitamins. In a way that is not yet clear, vitamin C is an essential constituent in the specific metabolism of the amino acids phenylalanine and tyrosine. An imbalance of these amino acids may result in stress which increases the need for ascorbic acid. The protein collagen as well as some mucoproteins are not properly formed and maintained in C deficiency.

3. Conversion of the vitamin folactin to folinic acid as related to the manufacture of blood. The folic acid coenzymes require both C and vitamin B-12 for continued activity in maintaining the folic acid coenzymes in the reduced or active state. These compounds mediate the transfer of certain carbon groups to organic compounds which are undergoing synthesis in the cells. Patients with megaloblastic anemia—who have some large nucleated red corpuscles—have been observed to have mixed deficiencies of folic acid, vitamin C and B-12.

4. Vitamin C regulates the respiratory cycle in the cell parts called mitochondria and corpuscles.

5. In human studies, the intestinal absorption of iron has been shown to be greatly increased by the addition of vitamin C or foods rich in vitamin C. Increased iron absorption has also been noted in the treatment of anemia in infants and children. Further, in experiments with rats it was found that iron with vitamin C caused the most rapid red blood cell formation with the highest hemoglobin concentration. McCurdy and Dern found that this enhancement of iron absorption persists with amounts of iron up to 120 mg. Vitamin C aids in the movement of plasma iron to storage depots in the tissues; its function is to reduce and release the ferric ions, enabling them to form tight linkages with the plasma proteins. However, vitamin cap-

sules *plus iron* can result in the absorption of too much iron, and hemosiderosis or siderosis can result. This excess accumulation of iron in the tissues occurs among the Bantu in Africa. They prepare, in iron vessels, a drink strong in C. Their drink ends up heavy in iron, and they fall ill with siderosis, which is characterized by iron deposits in all the tissues of the body. The organs are impaired by the iron deposits.

6. During stress, C is depleted from the tissues, particularly the adrenal cortex. Dietary supplementation with vitamin C will prevent stress reactions such as those which may occur if an animal is exposed to cold for a prolonged period. In general, vitamin C seems to operate as an antistress factor, enabling the organism to adapt to rapid environmental changes. (Dr. John H. Crandon has found in 150 patients that ascorbic acid levels dropped 18.5 percent immediately after surgery.)

7. Wound healing is promoted by adequate vitamin C. Deficiency reduces the rate of collagen synthesis, which is important in normal healing. Animal studies show that vitamin C concentration in the center of a wound is greater than at areas distant from the wound, indicating that vitamin C is mobilized in the wound to meet specific needs. Animal studies have also demonstrated that calcium and ascorbic acid, when administered together, produce earlier and quicker healing of fractures. The strength of the bone is significantly increased, and healing time is reduced by about 30 percent. (However, *calcium salts and C in combination may cause calcium oxalate kidney stones.*)

In clinical studies James Greenwood, Jr. of Baylor Medical College has reported that vitamin C is of substantial value in low back pain, and its use can often avert spinal disc operation. This points to the significance of C in maintaining the health of bones, cartilage and connective tissues. The arthritic requires more than the normal amount of vitamin C to remove the heavy burden of iron and copper in the joints.

8. Antibiotic therapy with tetracycline can be more effective (with lessened dosage) if there is adjunctive use of vitamin C. A great amount of research on this has been done by the Russians, who have also reported on the extended use of vitamin C in retarding the aging process. They also use it as a muscle builder for their athletes in training.

Recent studies have shown vitamin C to be necessary for cholesterol regulation. Dr. Constance Spittle has reported that she noticed that her own serum cholesterol was lowered from 230 to 140 mg percent when she took vitamin C. She then did a clinical study on various groups of individuals. In normal, healthy patients, aged twenty-five, cholesterol levels tended to fall when 1 gm of C per day was added to an otherwise normal diet. In atherosclerosis patients, however, serum cholesterol increased in the weeks with vitamin C supplements, possibly due to the mobilization of the arterial cholesterol. She suggests that atherosclerosis may be a long-term deficiency (or negative balance) of vitamin C which permits cholesterol levels to build up in the arterial system.

In confirmation of Dr. Spittle's work, Dr. Ginter found that daily doses of less than 1 gm of ascorbic acid over a period of forty-seven days lowered the blood cholesterol level by approximately 10 percent in men over forty. Dr. Sherry Lewin feels that depression of blood cholesterol, as well as the more rapid conversion into bile acids, may be a direct effect of ascorbic acid. Results have indicated that as adrenocortical activity increases, the concentration of ascorbic acid and cholesterol in the adrenal gland decreases. Thus, it appears that ascorbic acid may be involved in the synthesis of steroid hormones from cholesterol. Guinea pigs with chronic latent hypovitaminosis C showed an increase in the amount of tissue cholesterol. Latent hypovitaminosis C may cause hypercholesterolemia in humans and may also play a role in the pathogenosis of atherosclerosis, a major factor in the aging process.

9. Recent work of Indian scientists suggests that vitamin C metabolism is slowed when excessive amounts of protein or trace metals are taken into the body. This indicates that patients who are hypoglycemic and on high-protein diets should take extra amounts of vitamin C. When, for example, 150 parts per million of zinc are added to the diet, vitamin C metabolism is improved. The same is true of copper at 25 ppm and chromium and tungsten at 5 ppm. However, high dietary levels of zinc and copper decrease vitamin C content and lower enzyme activity.

10. If toxic substances enter the body, adequate vitamin C often detoxifies them, rendering them harmless. Its effective-

ness has been shown in correcting the toxic effects of lead, iron, copper, bromide, arsenic, benzene and the pesticides DDT, dieldrin and lindane. Vitamin C also reduces the action of cancer-producing compounds.

11. The common practice has been to cure meats with nitrites and nitrates, but nitrites can combine with other substances to form nitrosamines, a group of chemicals which are potent carcinogens. Many of our smoked meats and bacons may possibly have carcinogenic effects. Thus nitrites should not be used. Unfortunately, until recently, no other meat additives have been able to prevent botulism.

Preliminary studies have shown that vitamin C will prevent the formation of nitrosamines in cured meats if used at levels of 1,000 ppm or greater, but government regulations have not yet allowed these levels. If vitamin C does become a food additive for meats, the American bacon-and-egg breakfast will gain a few more points in its favor.

Other industrial uses of vitamin C, as reported by a spokesman for the Hoffman-LaRoche Company, are as follows: (1) as an aid to the manufacture of polyvinyl, acrylic and polystyrene plastics; (2) as a retardant of yellowing in the storage of plastics; (3) as a good dough conditioner; (4) as a method of increasing shell strength in hen's eggs, thus reducing egg breakage in handling and lowering egg costs.

How Much Vitamin C is Needed by Man?

Vitamin C may prevent or cure scurvy, but, as previously shown, its effects are ubiquitous and this must be taken into consideration when deciding an individual's optimal dosage. The problem of the optimal dosage in man has not been solved, as is evident from the fact that different recommendations have been made in various countries. For example, the British Medical Association recommends 30 mg daily for adults; the Food and Nutrition Board of the United States 60 mg and the German Society of Nutrition 75 mg. Linus Pauling considers that 2,300 mg are needed. The reason for these differences lies in the fact that we still do not know all of vitamin C's essential functions and therefore we cannot assess directly the optimal daily intake. However, because vitamin C is needed only by man and a few other animal species, one can obtain from biochemical studies in animals which synthesize C some knowledge of the actual need in man. The rat makes 42 mg per body weight per day, which is equivalent to Pauling's 2.4 gm per day. The gorilla obtains about 4.5 gm per day on its diet of succulent greens.

In the 1930s it was believed that in those animals that manufacture vitamin C the tissues are saturated with the vitamin. At that time this provided the rationale for selecting the 60 mg daily dose, on the assumption that with this dose saturation of the human organs would be achieved. However, this has not been proven. Also, the finding that with increased consumption of vitamin C urinary output is increased does not mean that the body tissues are saturated. This is especially important because in some schizophrenics increase in urinary excretion does not occur even after administration of enormous doses of vitamin C, a fact which would indicate that the vitamin has been retained by the tissues and utilized for specific needs.

Blood studies in man have shown that after a single-dose administration the biological half-life of ascorbic acid is only a few hours and that the plasma level will return to its normal value in about twelve to thirteen hours, no matter how much is taken. This would indicate that in order to maintain equilibrium of the serum C level, the vitamin should be taken several times daily. The liver is the organ which releases C into the blood. In guinea pigs, after *only* twelve hours of starvation, almost 50 percent of the liver C is utilized. Subclinical deficiency of C, as defined by low dietary uptake and low blood levels, is quite common. Under normal conditions a low intake is harmless, but in time of stress with increased utilization of C by the tissues, supplementation is needed.

The Schizophrenias

Several clinicians have observed that ascorbic acid in large doses has a therapeutic effect in some schizophrenics. This suggests a biochemical abnormality in the utilization of C in some patients. Studies with animals have demonstrated that the ascorbic acid content of the adrenal glands decreases when animals are stressed. Iliev and Pfeiffer have postulated that both the increased demand for and utilization of ascorbic acid are related to an increased consumption by the adrenal glands during stressful situations. Milne found that psychiatric patients have an unusually high demand for ascorbic acid. While on a placebo, the mean twenty-four hour urinary excretion of ascorbic acid was 15.2 mg—the lower limit for normals. When given one gram of C daily, it took the psychiatric patients six days to reach their saturation point. (It only took normals twenty-four to forty-eight hours.) Following achievement of saturation, there was a statistically significant improvement in patients suffering from depressive, manic and paranoid symptom complexes.

In 1966, Harry Vanderkamp reported studies on the urinary spillage of C in schizophrenics after administration of large doses. He proposed that because of constant brain stimulation, the schizophrenic has more internal stress than normals do and thus needs more ascorbic acid. In studying the urine of a group of schizophrenics, he found abnormal metabolites indicative of vitamin C deficiency.

Commenting on the beneficial effect of ascorbic acid in patients, Vanderkamp states: "All patients who received the vitamin in large doses made definite clinical improvement, predominately in the area of socialization. The patients expressed a feeling of well-being. The anxious, tense facial expressions were replaced with a smile and friendliness. The patients stated that they did not feel so spacially constrained. Those who were shy, reclusive, and withdrawn began to participate in ward activities, in conversations with other patients, and ward personnel." The pioneer work of Hoffer and Osmond has demonstrated the same results and, more recently, vitamin C has been made a vital component of all nutrient therapy. In the schizophrenic this extra vitamin C is needed to get rid of the accumulated copper.

Estrogen and Vitamin C

Any biological state which elevates the serum copper is likely to increase the need for C. The schizophrenic state, late pregnancy, excessive smoking of tobacco and, particularly, the use of the contraceptive pill produce states of elevated copper.

Natarayan Saroja administered mestranol (an estrogen) to guinea pigs with a resulting marked reduction (23 percent) in the ascorbic acid concentration in their blood plasma and an even greater reduction (38 percent) in their visible blood capillaries. Rivers and Devine found that in controls the total ascorbic acid concentrations were highest at ovulation and lowest during the menstrual period. All subjects had higher copper concentrations at the menstrual period, even when they were not on the drug. The results of the study indicate that oral contraceptives effectively alter the cyclic changes in plasma and total ascorbic acid levels and prevent the normal sharp increase in plasma ascorbic acid at the time of ovulation. With normal pregnancy, Mason and Rivers have found that the mean level of total serum ascorbic acid falls steadily. Thus, as all research to date has shown, drugs or situations which cause a rise in serum copper demand extra ascorbic acid. Research is now needed on other trace metals such as iron, which is known to oxidize vitamin C. Such studies on iron should be designed to correlate changes in blood serum levels with iron levels and iron balance.

Controversy over the Common Cold

Since the publication of Linus Pauling's *Vitamin C and the Common Cold* in 1970, vitamin C manufacturers have been busy indeed! Careful studies on human volunteers in a dormitory who were given massive inoculations of virulent cold or flu virus, however, have shown an equal incidence of colds when 3 gm per day of C or a placebo was used.

It is important to recognize that this does not test the vitamin's preventive effect. Pauling, who advocated 2 to 4 gm of C a day, argues that these studies have failed to take into account the stresses of everyday life and the minimal amount of virus which might be handled by the tissues if adequate vitamin C were present.

A survey of the literature has led Pauling and others to

believe that taking the vitamin in large quantities is "virtually nontoxic" and can, indeed, lower the incidence and symptomatology of the common cold. His hypothesis, as yet untested, is that ascorbic acid provides protection against viral disease by allowing the synthesis and increasing the activity of interferon in preventing the entry of virus into the cell.

Pauling cites in favor of his theory a study done by Baker et al. which indicated a statistically significant difference in the average incidence of colds between students taking 250 mg of C—a dose Pauling believes is too low to be very effective—and students not taking it. Other studies have reported the same results with 250 mg or more. In one double-blind study which involved 818 subjects, a significant difference was found in the two groups as to "days confined to the house." The group taking the vitamin averaged 1.3 days while the non-C group averaged 1.87 days. In another study, Joseph Barboriak found that 26 percent of the subjects taking supplementary ascorbic acid remained free of cold symptoms while only 19 percent not taking it remained symptom-free. Barboriak suggested that the mechanisms by which large doses of vitamin C might modify cold symptoms are either reduction of the disulfide bridges in the bronchial mucus with subsequent thinning of the material and easier expectoration, inhibition of histamine-inducing bronchoconstriction, or, with large doses, a vitamin-sparing effect, particularly on the B complex, which would delay or prevent metabolic impairments associated with other vitamin deficiencies. These are speculations, but as Thurber once said, "Speculations, if confined to certainties, are robbed of their wonder and warmth."

What is now needed is a study on a large, diverse group of individuals to provide conclusive evidence that vitamin C does indeed reduce the body's susceptibility to cold-inducing viruses. As T. W. Anderson recently indicated, the incongruous results obtained by various researchers may be due to different tissue saturations at the onset of the studies. The average level of vitamin C in the blood of the general population may be about 40 to 50 mg, but any subpopulation, due to high interest in nutrition, may have a greater level of vitamin C in the blood prior to the study. Supplementary C would then increase the already high level and tend to show more positive results. Thus, it is advocated that a massive study should control for this factor and thereby present a more valid picture of vitamin C's therapeutic properties.

Factories which provide their employees with free C tablets during the winter have less sick leave for any reason. This may, however, be an index of better employee relations in the plants of some progressive employers.

Certainly no harm is done with oral doses of 3 to 4 gm per day of C, although some risk of calcium oxalate kidney stones is present when the female patient takes high doses of both vitamin C and calcium. If magnesium is used with the calcium, however, this hazard is negligible.

Whatever validity Pauling's hypothesis may have, we do know that vitamin C is needed by the body for normal functioning and that any extra vitamin C will be harmlessly discharged. The patient will have a lower blood cholesterol and absorb more iron. In addition, heavy metals such as lead, mercury, cadmium and copper will be mobilized and slowly eliminated. These pluses for vitamin C are not to be sneezed at!

Natural and Synthetic Vitamin C

The food purist may extoll the virtues of rose-hip vitamin C over synthetic, and it is true that natural C in natural packages has a distinct advantage. Oranges provide calcium, trace elements, bioflavonoids and pectin while synthetic vitamin C tablets are only pure vitamin C. Rose hips eaten from the rosebush undoubtedly provide similar advantages. However, pure rose-hip vitamin C, when available, is five to ten times as expensive as synthetic vitamin C. When large daily doses are needed, as in modern family medicine, then rose-hip vitamin C is too expensive for the family with an average income.

On careful reading of the labels of some rose-hip-containing products, we find that rose hips are used *only* to flavor a synthetic product. The hidden fact is that the vitamin C is synthetic ascorbic acid and that most of the additional C advertised as present in rose-hip products originates as ascorbic acid, not from rose-hip powder or any other similar form of rose-hips. The deceptive labeling of this product as natural rose hips is legal because the Food and Drug Administration requires only that the proper amount of ascorbic acid be listed, not its sources. Rose-hip powder contains 500 mg percent vitamin C. You can save money by buying the manufactured ascorbic acid, which is pure vitamin C. (Synthetic vitamin C is manufactured from corn sugar, however, so that patients who are allergic to corn may show an allergic reaction to synthetic vitamin C.)

Vitamin C—the Sleep Vitamin

A last and most interesting effect which vitamin C has in man is that of an antianxiety agent useful in neuroses. Dr. Pfeiffer and his colleagues conducted a study of possible biochemical stimulants and sedatives, among them ascorbic acid (Table 10.1). The method used was the quantitative EEG (electroencephalogram) which allows the assay of stimulants, sedatives, hypnotics and antipsychotic drugs in man and has provided a dose-response curve for many drugs which act on the central nervous system (CNS) (Table 10.2). The action of large doses of vitamins on the CNS is most interesting (Table 10.3): thiamine and ascorbic acid have an antianxiety or sedative effect, characterized by a significant decrease in the mean energy content (MEC) of the EEG and an increase in the coefficient of variation (CV) which is the standard deviation when all means are mathematically transformed to 100 percent. By use of this method they found that the effect of vitamin C lasts for a full six-hour test period and that it was the most effective substance at the dosage used. Vitamin C is now used in the general nutrient therapy program to treat patients who show excess copper or nervousness.

Inositol

To compensate for the fact that few, if any, books on biochemistry and nutrition provide much information on this topic, our treatment of inositol will be more detailed than some of the other discussions in this book.

Chemistry

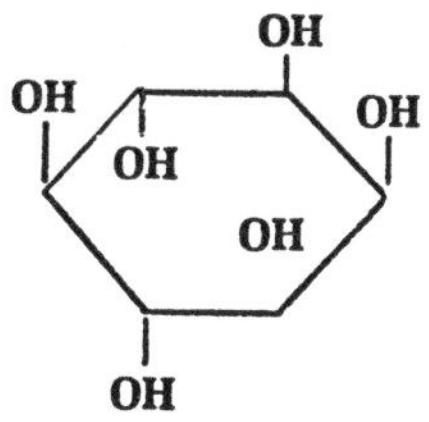

Free inositol.

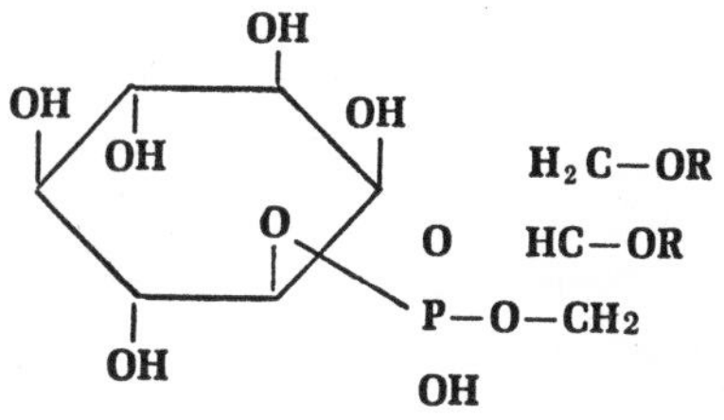

Inositol phosphatides.

Phytic acid is inositol hexaphosphate when every OH group is attached to a phosphate group. Phytic acid occurs in cereals and prevents the absorption of zinc and other trace metals from the gastrointestinal tract.

In plants, phytic acid may account for 86 percent of the phosphorus present in seeds. This is slowly liberated by the germination process. Thus seed *sprouts* may be a better source than seeds of both phosphorus and inositol.

Approximately 80 percent of the phosphorus in corn exists as phytate, corn having been reported to have a content of phytic acid phosphorus which varies from 0.199 to 0.270 percent, compared with a variation in total phosphorus of 0.248 to 0.330 percent. Among the other foods in which phytic acid has been found are wheat, rye, oats, peas, beans, barley, rice, cottonseed, flaxseed, soybeans and peanuts.

In extracting the phytate from the plant materials, investigators have used dilute hydrochloric or sulfuric acids to treat the whole seed or individual fractions of the seed. From these extracts, various phytate salts have been precipitated and free inositol obtained by hydrolysis of the phytate salt. This is the main commercial source of inositol. Corn is steeped in water to burst the kernel and release the starch and oils.

By virtue of its ability to form insoluble salts, phytic acid reduces the absorption of zinc and calcium from the intestines of animals and human beings. Farina is low in phytate, but oat-

TABLE 10.1

Outline of possible biochemical stimulants

Potentially stimulant precursors of neurohumors	**Deanol, acetylcholine, tyrosine, norepinephrine, tryptamine, 5 HT, histidine, histamine**
Inhibitors of amine oxidation or conjugation	**MAO inhibitors**
Potentially stimulant amino acids	**Glutamic acid, Na glutamate, glutamine, asparagine, methionine, tryptophan, 5 OH tryptophan**
Potentially stimulant or sedative vitamins	**Thiamin, riboflavin, pyridoxine, ascorbic acid, cyanocobalamine, pantothenate**
Combinations of vitamins with similar actions	**Niacin, folate, vitamin B-12 (raise histamine level)**
RNA and purines	**Adenosine, inosine, hypoxanthine, guanosine, etc.**
Metabolic hormones	**Thyroid, insulin, corticoids**
Increasing lipid solubility of amine stimulants	**Alpha methylation, amine methylation, primary amine alkylation with acetaldehyde or pyridoxal**

Source: C. Pfeiffer, L. Goldstein, H. Murphree and R. Nichols. A critical survey of possible biochemical stimulants. *Psychopharmacology*, 1968.

meal may be high. For instance, Bronner demonstrated that the uptake of radioactive calcium by boys fed an oatmeal breakfast was 74 percent of that of boys fed a farina breakfast, while the uptake of calcium by those boys fed farina containing added sodium phytate was only 45 percent. A similar result was obtained by Sharpe, who compared the uptake of radioiron by children who had received farina, oatmeal or farina plus sodium phytate. Various disorders due to magnesium deficiency were shown to occur when young rats were fed sodium phytate. The phytic acid in soybean protein has been shown to render zinc unavailable for chicks. This is even more important when the copper-high soy protein is substituted for beef, which is a good source of zinc. Excess copper means less zinc effect in the body.

TABLE 10.2

Drug actions measurable in man by means of the quantitative electroencephalogram

Type of drug effect	*Mean energy content*	*Coefficient of variation*	*Wave form change*
Stimulant	**Decrease**	**Decrease**	**Decreased amplitude of alpha**
Antianxiety (sedative)	**Great decrease**	**Increase**	**Flatness with periods of normal alpha**
Sleep producing (stage IV)	**Great increase**	**Increase**	**Slow waves of high amplitude**
Antipsychotic (initial effect)	**Great increase**	**Normal range**	**Increased amplitude of all wave forms**

Source: C. Pfeiffer, L. Goldstein, H. Murphree and R. Nichols. A critical survey of possible biochemical stimulants. *Psychopharmacology*, 1968.

Lipotropic Effect of Inositol A number of dietary variables can lead to deposition of unusual amounts of fat-like lipid in the liver. Certain nutrients favor this deposition, whereas others favor mobilization of the lipids and a return of the liver to normal. Choline and similar methyl donors are well known as dietary lipotropic agents. Inositol is also effective under certain conditions in both experimental animals and human beings. Inositol has an added effect even when the diet contains a good supply of methyl donors.

Although little is known of the mode of action of lipotropic agents, at least two (choline, inositol) are essential constituents of phospholipids, and it is likely that their effectiveness as lipotropic agents is related to this. Since all other vitamins finally become structural units of all protoplasm also, it is inconsistent to separate the lipotropic activities of choline and inositol from their activities as vitamins.

Inositol and Nucleic Acid Metabolism If inositol is added, certain yeast strains are able to grow on a synthetic minimal nutrient medium in the presence of uracil. The combination of the nucleic acid uracil and inositol can be replaced

TABLE 10.3

Effect of large doses of the water-soluble vitamins on the quantitative electroencephalogram of normal human subjects

Biochemical treatment	Dose mg	No. of trials	MEC	Control %	Control CV*	1 %	1 CV*	2 %	2 CV*	3 %	3 CV*	4 %	4 CV*	5 %	5 CV*	6 %	6 CV*
				Hours after medication													
Placebo	—	10	70.2	100	20	102	22	105	24	102	18	102	19	102	21	102	20
Niacin	500	10	60.3	100	18	103	15	101	22	95	22	104	20	110	19	99	30
Niacinamide	100	10	69.3	100	24	102	27	104	26	110	33	99	29	114	24	100	35
Roniacol	100	10	96.5	100	29	100	29	90	38	103	37	102	36	102	28	96	39
Riboflavin	50	5	77.8	100	15	88	22	81	22	88	18	101	14	93	20	91	19
Pyridoxine	50	10	47.9	100	25	115	36	115	33	106	41	101	52*	112	34	110	35
Thiamin	100	8	75.0	100	12	93	17	101	18*	101	17	99	20	105	21	99	21
Ascorbic acid	1000	10	50.9	100	28	86	63	118	34	111	37	97	57*	112*	44	91	65
Ascorbic acid	3000	11	70.9	100	20	88	31	90	30	86	33	93	20	89	30	86	25
Placebo	—	20	66.2	100	21	105	24	103	27	103	27	108	26	101	26	108	20

MEC=mean energy content.
*C.V.=coefficient of variation.
__Significant difference from control at the 1 in 20 level of confidence.
Source: C. Pfeiffer, L. Goldstein, H. Murphree and R. Nichols. A critical survey of possible biochemical stimulants. *Psychopharmacology*. 1968.

by cytosine, uridine or uridylic acid. Inositol appears to participate in a biochemical process which permits the transformation of uracil, probably to uridine or cytosine. These nucleic acids are important in the forming of ribonucleic acid (RNA), which may be used to store recent memory traces in the brain.

Inositol as a Structural Component of Cells When cells of certain yeasts were deprived of inositol, the majority of the cell population died rapidly consequent to loss of metabolic activities, nucleotide coenzymes and the cytochrome system.

The investigators postulated that inositol functions as a structural component of the yeast cell. Inositol appears to play a similar role in *neurospora*, for in the presence of its antagonist, isomytilitol, this organism exhibits decreased ability to carry out the synthesis of riboflavin, vitamin B-6, niacin, p-aminobenzoic acid (PABA) and folic acid.

Ghosh observed that inositol deficiency in yeast *saccharomyces carlsbergensis* leads to abnormal cell walls and cells that contain more glucan. These changes were accompanied by an inability of daughter cells to separate from parent cells, and, as a result, large cell aggregates were formed. Other investigators have found that inositol deficiency in the same yeast inhibited the fermentation and oxidation activity, and lowered the level of nucleotide coenzymes and cytochrome.

Inositol probably acts indirectly in stimulating synthesis of biotin in the intestine. This postulate is strengthened by the finding of Lindley and Cunha that inositol alleviated to a large extent the biotin deficiency symptoms when the pig is fed a purified diet. Cunha reported a loss of body hair in rats reared on a natural diet composed chiefly of corn and soybean meal which could be prevented and cured by inositol. The hair loss started in the dorsal part of the head and proceeded along the sides to the tail region and then downward to the hind legs. When inositol was given the hair returned inversely, proceeding from the tail portions forward. Of interest is the finding that the hair loss did not occur until a pyridoxine and folic acid preparation was added to the control ration. The addition of these two factors caused a decrease in growth and the development of the alopecia. This may have been due to some imbalance of the vitamins.

In other tests sulfonamides brought out a special need for inositol which indicates a further interrelation with folic acid or PABA. One group found that survival of rat litters was greater on diets supplemented with inositol and PABA, and milk secretion in the mothers was more abundant.

Inositol in Man A specific need for inositol in man has not been demonstrated, nor have specific deficiency symptoms. However, its wide distribution in the body indicates an important role.

Inositol can be made by some animals, and is present in all tissues with the highest levels in the heart and brain.

TABLE 10.4

Presence of inositol in some animals

Mcg/gm

	Organ	*Free inositol*	*Combined inositol*
Ox	**Brain**	**1300**	—
	Muscle	**50**	—
Sheep	**Brain**	**1750**	—
	Heart	**1550**	—
Rabbit	**Muscle**	**1500**	—
Dog	**Heart**	**1600**	—
Rat	**Muscle**	**130**	**210**
	Liver	**250**	**520**
	Heart	**340**	**450**
	Brain	**560**	**670**
	Kidney	**880**	**1230**

Hartree has found that boar seminal plasma contains 650 mg of inositol per 100 ml. This is more than ½ percent. The single ejaculate of the boar also contains 8 mg of zinc. Human semen contains 0.1 percent inositol.

Abrahamson administered a preparation containing inositol, choline, methionine, liver extract and vitamin B-12 to eighty-six elderly patients with hyper-high serum cholesterol and found significant reduction in the cholesterol levels and an improvement in the health of the patients. Sherber and Levites used a mixture of inositol and choline in sixteen patients with high serum cholesterol and observed lowering of the levels. Similar results with the same mixture have been obtained by others.

Leinwand and Moore found that the administration of 3 gm of inositol daily to older patients resulted in a reduction of total lipids and cholesterol blood levels. They concluded that inositol might be of value in atherosclerosis. In general, the exact value of inositol in any human illness remains to be proven.

Diuresis, as in diabetes insipidus, results in a loss of inositol from the human body. Even excess water ingestion will cause this loss. The usual experimental dose of inositol is 3 gm, but 50 gm has been given by mouth and 1 gm intravenously without ill effects. Inositol may be a typical example of a compound which is useful in therapeutics but on which, because it is in the common domain and is not patentable, no pharmaceutical company is pushing to get valid data.

We at the Brain Bio Center have studied the effect of inositol on the quantitative brain waves of both patients and normals. These studies show inositol to have a typical anti-anxiety effect similar to that of Librium or meprobamate. Since inositol is a higher alcohol, one might expect such a sedative effect, but the high level of this vitamin in the brain might indicate a more specific, but as yet undisclosed, calming effect. Patients using inositol can frequently stop their usual daily dose of Valium or meprobamate.

Inositol in the Brain The spinal cord nerves, brain and cerebral spinal fluid contain large amounts of inositol. Human cerebrospinal fluid contains 2.7 mg percent, which is about four times the level found in the blood (0.68 mg percent). It is also found in both the aqueous humor and lens of the eye.

In mild hypertension, the use of 1 gm morning and night produces sedation and a gradual lowering of the blood pressure. A well-rounded diet of 2,500 calories contains approximately 1 gm of inositol; a reducing diet of 1,000 calories or less would probably have correspondingly less inositol. If chosen poorly, the reducing diet might be much lower in inositol content.

We have used inositol in schizophrenics, in hypoglycemics and in patients who have a high serum copper and a low serum zinc. While the phosphate ester of inositol impedes absorption of zinc, the pure inositol favors absorption. Inositol is sedative and solves many insomnia and anxiety problems. Inositol may also reduce stress-elevated blood pressure.

In animals, the vitamins which work closely with inositol are pantothenic acid, pyridoxine, PABA, folic acid and the lipotropic factors choline, methionine and betaine.

Inositol is available in 250, 500 and 650 mg tablets from various suppliers. Health food stores stock these various sizes.

Linodyl (and Hexanicotol) Linodyl is the nicotinic acid ester of inositol and is available in Canada but not in the United States. Some patients use this instead of niacin because Linodyl does not produce a red flush. We have studied Linodyl for its effect on the quantitative brain waves and on the excretion of copper. Little or no effect is found, so it is possible that this ester does not provide niacin to the body. The slow-release forms of niacin are better possibilities for the prevention of the niacin flush.

Vitamin B-6

In the early 1930s, biochemical research was preoccupied with the discovery of new vitamins, among them a factor found in animal livers which prevented skin disorders in rats. In 1936, Szent-Györgyi and Birch established this factor as a separate entity, naming it pyridoxine or B-6. Pyridoxine is now the name applied to the various forms of the vitamin, these being pyridoxine, pyridoxal and pyridoxamine. All three forms are converted by the body into their phosphate forms for biochemical use in a variety of metabolic functions.

Studies on laboratory animals have elucidated sundry disorders related to relative B-6 deficiency. Studies involving humans have supported these results and have also revealed various B-6 dependency syndromes. Because B-6 is needed for many bodily functions, its deficiency can cause serious mental and physical illness.

The recommended daily allowance of B-6 for healthy, unstressed individuals is determined in part by the amount of protein ingested. For adult men and women it is 2.0 mg per day, for adolescents 1.4 to 2.0 mg per day and for infants 0.2 to 1.2 mg. The stressed individual may require much more because the kryptopyrrole molecule removes both B-6 and zinc from the body. Since B-6 is an important intermediary in amino acid

TABLE 10.5

Inositol content of various biological materials

(Mgm/gm of fresh tissue)

Vegetable products					
CEREALS					
Wheat germ	**6.9**	**Whole wheat**	**1.9**	**Bread, whole wheat**	**1.0**
Flour, white	**0.8**	**Flour, whole wheat**	**1.1**	**Oats**	**3.2**
Barley	**3.9**	**Corn**	**0.5**		
FRUITS					
Oranges	**2.1**	**Apples**	**0.2**	**Cantaloupe**	**1.2**
Grapefruit juice	**1.0 (per ml)**	**Orange juice**	**1.0-1,700 (per ml)**	**Grapefruit**	**1.5**
				Tomatoes	**0.5**
VEGETABLES					
Peas, green	**1.6**	**Spinach**	**0.30**	**Lettuce**	**0.6**
Carrots	**0.50**	**Potatoes, sweet**	**0.7**		
Cabbage	**1.0**	**Potatoes, white**	**0.3**		
MISCELLANEOUS					
Peanuts, roasted	**1.8**	**Molasses**	**1.5**	**Tea leaves, dry**	**10.0**
Yeast, *Torulopsis utilis*	**2.7**	**Yeast, brewer's**	**0.5**		
Animal products					
MEATS					
Beef, muscle	**2.6**	**Beef, heart**	**16.0**	**Beef, brain**	**6.0**
Beef, liver	**3.4**	**Pork, loin**	**0.4**	**Veal, chop**	**0.3**
FOWL AND FISH					
Chicken, breast	**0.5**	**Oysters**	**0.4**	**Salmon**	**0.2**
Eggs	**0.2**	**Halibut**	**0.2**		
MILK PRODUCTS					
Whole milk, cow	**0.2 (per ml)**	**Whole milk, human**	**0.3 (per ml)**	**Cheese**	**0.2**

metabolism, those individuals whose diets are high in protein should receive additional B-6. The RDA is a basal level recommendation; more B-6 may also be needed by those with inborn errors of metabolism that make them B-6 dependent.

The 2 mg per day needed by the adult may be obtained by drinking a quart of milk or eating a pound of meat or unprocessed wheat. Processing the wheat removes the B-6. Other sources of B-6 are whole grains, organ meats and other meats. Because this vitamin is water-soluble, excesses are excreted via the urine so that toxic levels are never reached. Pyridoxic acid occurs in the urine of patients who take any excess of B-6. This is a harmless excretion product.

Vitamin B-6 in the Body Pyridoxal phosphate is a coenzyme for a large number of enzyme systems and is thus needed in sufficient amount by the body to insure adequate function. B-6 is not only an important coenzyme for the intermediary metabolism of amino acids but is also needed for their synthesis, degradation and absorption in the intestine. In addition, B-6 is involved in the transfer of amines to and from amino acids. The removal of acid groups from amino acids (thereby forming active biogenic amines such as histamine, serotonin, dopamine and adrenalin) and the final oxidation of histamine and other diamines are all dependent on pyridoxal phosphate. It is also essential in the tryptophan-to-niacin pathway where a B-6 deficiency blocks the tryptophan-to-quinone-derivative conversion, thereby causing abnormal urinary excretion of the intermediary metabolites with the tongue-twisting names of xanthurenic acid, kynurenine, and hydroxykenurine.

Because B-6 is an important coenzyme in the biosynthesis of hemoglobin, some anemic patients who do not respond to iron may actually be only B-6 deficient. Pyridoxine also functions in fat metabolism, in that the essential fatty acids have a sparing action and will reduce the B-6 requirement. Other evidence indicates a factor in the blood plasma which regulates the passage of pyridoxal from the red cell. After entrance into the tissues it is converted into pyridoxal phosphate or may be converted into pyridoxic acid in the liver with subsequent urinary excretion. The transport of amino acids into the cellular interior is also dependent on adequate supplies of B-6.

A specific B-6 phosphate reaction in the brain is the removal of the acid group from glutamic acid to form gamma aminobutyric acid (GABA), which is a calming chemical and a possible neural transmitter. Deficiency of B-6 may cause seizures due to the inability of this calming chemical to be formed in adequate amounts. In subconvulsive states B-6 deficiency symptoms may go unrecognized and undiagnosed until serious complications finally arise. Infants born to mothers inadequately supplied with B-6 during pregnancy show signs of deficiency starting at birth; convulsions have been reported in many instances. Studies of pregnant women indicate that they retain more B-6 than nonpregnant women, which suggests that they require supplementary doses to insure that the proper amount is being transferred to the baby.

Some reported studies have demonstrated a relationship between B-6 and Parkinsonism. Dopamine has been shown to be important in the brain areas associated with Parkinsonism. Thus, it is possible that any substance known to increase the dopamine content of the brain will reduce the cardinal symptoms of the disease: stiffness, tremor and impaired motor function. These are relieved by dopa in adequate dosage. The total dopamine content in the brain is formed by B-6-dependent decarboxylation. The addition of B-6 may therefore relieve walking and speech disturbances, loss of motivation and loss of memory. Zinc may also be needed, since in some patients B-6 alone may counter the good effect of dopa.

Infantile convulsions may be one of many symptoms resulting from B-6 deficiency. Diets deficient in B-6 fed to laboratory animals produced convulsions, accumulation of cystathianine in numerous organs, dermatitis (skin lesions), nervous symptoms and blood disorders. Human deficiency symptoms include convulsions, hyperirritability, abnormal auditory acuteness, seborrhea-like skin lesions and decreased growth rate. In 1952, the feeding of a vitamin formula deficient in B-6 caused a large number of infants, two months and younger, to develop convulsions and muscle abnormalities. This condition was promptly relieved with the addition of the vitamin. Since the use of some antituberculosis drugs such as Isoniazid increases B-6 urinary excretion, therefore extra B-6 is required where these are used.

Eclampsia during pregnancy may be a B-6 and zinc deficiency. Substantial evidence indicates that the contraceptive pill increases the need for B-6 as well as other vitamins, so that the wise gynecologist prescribes zinc and B-6 to prevent deficiency. As noted before, excess B-6 breaks down in the body to harmless pyridoxic acid, which is excreted in the urine. This acid tends to remove calcium oxalate gravel in the urinary tract which may cause kidney stones. Thus, the urologist may also dispense starter doses of B-6 to his stone-forming patients.

In many instances, an individual may be B-6-dependent due to some inborn error of metabolism which may be characterized by neurological disturbances and mental retardation. There is no overlap in these syndromes. They include (1) pyridoxine-dependent convulsions, (2) pyridoxine-responsive anemia and (3) a form of homocystinuria. Those individuals diagnosed as having one of these diseases will need to take supplementary doses well above the RDA to prevent deficiency symptoms.

Vitamin B-6 and Dreaming Recently, the Brain Bio Center has isolated a specific schizophrenic syndrome that is responsive to B-6 and zinc. Kryptopyrrole (mauve factor) (KP), a substance found in large quantities in the urine of schizophrenics and some normals, complexes with pyridoxal to remove B-6 from the body. A patient with this mauve factor may require as much as 1,000 mg twice daily of B-6 to rid him of the urinary KP. Treatment with supplementary doses of B-6 and zinc has also succeeded in removing schizophrenic symptoms.

It has been shown that because B-6 is vitally important to many enzyme systems, optimal levels must be maintained to insure proper bodily functions. Its stability to heat and acid renders it quite resistant to food processing and storage conditions, so that the nutrition-conscious individual can receive sufficient amounts of this vitamin from his diet. In some instances supplements may be required, but that is to be determined by individual need. Once established, however, supplementation should be maintained to ensure optimal mental and physical function.

Patients who excrete kryptopyrrole in their urine (pyrolurics) have constantly reported to us that they never recall their dreams or have not been able since childhood to recall dreaming. Others will say gruffly, "Only children dream!" or "Everybody dreams but I'm too busy sleeping to bother with mine."

Then, on B-6 and zinc dietary supplements, patients report that they have dreamt and recalled the event for the first time in their adult lives. After many such reports, we have postulated that dream recall can serve as a yardstick to measure brain B-6 deficiency. Patients even wax enthusiastic and want to relate all the details of their new found phenomenon—the vivid early-morning dream. If the dose of B-6 is too large or mainly taken with the evening meal, then dreams become so vivid that the patient is awakened from sleep all night long. This restless-dream phenomenon is disturbing, so the dose should be reduced. Dr. Pfeiffer has found that he presumably needs 50 mg of B-6 each morning in order to dream normally at night. This is because of his stressful life of writing and seeing patients and directing the Brain Bio Center. If he takes this 50 mg dose of B-6 on vacation, he dreams excessively. The tablet then is halved and sleep with dreams occurs on 25 mg of B-6 per day. (This is still ten times the RDA!)

Since anorexia or nausea is a sign of B-6 deficiency and since this occurs in the morning, frequently one wonders if the dream phenomenon in pyroluric patients does not utilize B-6 in the night hours and thus produce deficiency in the morning. Certainly, on this theory, anorexic patients who cannot eat breakfast should have B-6 as the first medication offered in the morning. With this early morning B-6, patients may have their anorexia disappear in an hour.

Low Vitamin B-6 in Nausea and Vomiting of Pregnancy
The chemical determination of blood levels of vitamin B-6 in man is difficult because this vitamin occurs in five forms in the body. The most important form is pyridoxal (PALP). L. Reinken and H. Gant of Innsbruck, Austria, determined PALP levels in early and late pregnancy and compared these levels to those of women with nausea and vomiting in early pregnancy, those of such women when treated with B-6, and those of normal nonpregnant women. The deficiency of PALP was great in those who had nausea and vomiting.

We postulate that pyroluria patients who start pregnancy deficient in B-6 will have the most nausea. The stress of late pregnancy probably produces kryptopyrrole with an abnormal

TABLE 10.6

Levels of vitamin B-6 in the blood of pregnant and non-pregnant women*

	PTS	*PALP (mg per ml serum)*
Normal early pregnancy	**22**	**8.9**
Normal late pregnancy	**18**	**3.0**
Normal nonpregnant women	**29**	**9.1**
Nausea and vomiting of early pregnancy	**24**	**2.1**
B-6-treated nausea and vomiting of early pregnancy	**24**	**7.0**

*Adapted from L. Reinken and H. Gant. Vitamin B-6 nutrition in women with hyperemesis gravidarum during the first trimester of pregnancy. *Clinica Chimica Acta* 55: 101, 1974.

loss of vitamin B-6. Pregnant patients who develop nausea and vomiting should be treated with both vitamin B-6 and zinc.

References

Vitamin C

Anderson, T. W. et al. Vitamin C and the common cold: double blind trial. *Can. Med. Assoc. J.* 107:503-508, 1972.

Anderson, T. W. Large scale trials of vitamin C in the prevention and treatment of colds. *ACTA Citaminologica et Enzymologica* 28:99-100, 1974.

Barboriak, J. J. The megadose vitamin controversy. *Drug Therapy.* May 1974.

Crandon, J. H. et al. Experimental human scurvy. *New Eng. J. Med.* 223:353, 1940.

Ginter, E. *Science* 179:702-704, 1973.

Guizot, M. *Collection des memories relatifs a l'histoire de France.* Paris: Briere, 1825.

Mason and Rivers. Plasma ascorbic acid levels in pregnancy. *Amer. J. Obs. and Gyn.* 1971.

McCurdy, P. and Dern, R. Some therapeutic implications of ferrous sulfate-ascorbic acid mixtures. *Amer. J. Clin. Nut.* 21:284-288, 1968.

Milne, J. S. Leucocyte ascorbic acid levels and vitamin C intake in older people. *Br. Med. J.* 4:383-386, 1971.

Pauling, L. *Vitamin C and the common cold.* New York: Bantam Books, 1970.

Pfeiffer, C.; Goldstein, H; Murphree, H. and Nichols, R. A critical survey of possible biochemical stimulants. *Psychopharmacology,* 1968.

Rivers, J. and Devine, M. Plasma ascorbic acid concentrations and oral contraceptives. *Amer. J. Clin. Nutr.* 25:684, 1972.

Saroja, N. Effect of estrogens on ascorbic acid in the plasma and blood vessels of guinea pigs. *Contraception* 3:269, 1971.

Schneider, M. J. Vitamin C: how much do we need? *The Sciences* p. 11, January-February, 1975.

Spittle, C. Atherosclerosis and vitamin C. *Lancet,* 1971.

Vanderkamp, H. A biochemical abnormality in schizophrenia involving ascorbic acid. *Inter. J. Neuropsychiatry,* 1966.

Wilson and Loh. Relationship of human ascorbic acid metabolism to ovulation. *Lancet,* 1971.

——————— Common cold and vitamin C. *Lancet,* 1973.

Inositol

Bronner, F. et al. *J. Nutr.* 54:523, 1954.

Cunha, T. J. Inositol: deficiency effects in animals; requirements of animals.

Ghosh, A. et al. *J. Biol. Chem.* 235:2522, 1960.

Hartree, E. F. *Biochem. J.* 66:131, 1952.

Jungalwala, F. B. The metabolism of phosphatidylinositol in rat brain. *Int. J. Biochem.* 4:145-151, 1973.

Leinwand, I. and Moore, D. H. *Am. Heart J.* 38:467, 1949.

Sebrell, W. H. and Harris, R. S., eds. *The vitamins.* Chap. 9. New York: Academic Press, 1971.

Sherber, D. A. and Levites, M. M. *JAMA* 152:682, 1953.

Vitamin B-6

Aly, H. E., Donald, E. A. and Simpson, M. H. W. Oral contraceptives and vitamin B-6 metabolism. *Amer. J. Clin. Nutr.* 24:297-303, 1971.

Appleyard, J. G. and Stanley, D. A. The evaluation of the vitamin B-6 status in children with convulsions. *Med. Lab. Tech.* 29:160-170, 1972.

Central nervous system changes in deficiency of vitamin B-6 and other B-complex vitamins. *Nutrition Reviews* 33:21-22, 1975.

Crisp, H. and Stonehill, E. Relation between aspects of nutritional disturbance and menstrual activity in primary anorexia nervosa. *Brit. Med. J.* 3:149-151, 1971.

Heller, S., Skalkeld, R. M. and Körner, W. F. Vitamin B-6 status in pregnancy. *Amer. J. Clin. Nutr.* 26:1339-1348, 1973.

Hsu, T. H.; Bianchine, J. R.; Preziosi, T. J. and Messiha, F. S. Effect of pyridoxine on levodopa metabolism in normal and Parkinsonian subjects. *PSEBM* 143:577-581, 1973.

Klieger, J. A.; Altshuler, C. H.; Krakow, G. and Hollister, C. Abnormal pyridoxine metabolism in toxemia of pregnancy. *Annals of the New York Academy of Sciences* 166:288-296, 1969.

Mars, H. Levodope, carbidopa and pyridoxine in Parkinson's disease. *Arch. Neurol.* 30:443-447, 1974.

Miller, L. T.; Benson, E. M.; Edwards, M.A. and Young, J. Vitamin B-6 metabolism in women using oral contraceptives. *Amer. J. Clin. Nutr.* 27:797-805, 1974.

Pfeiffer, C. C. Observations on the therapy of the schizophrenias. Unpublished data, 1974.

Pfeiffer, R. and Ebadi, M. On mechanisms of nullification of CNS effects of l-dopa by pyridoxine in Parkinsonian patients. *J. Neurochem.* 19:2175-2181, 1972.

Reinken, I. and Gant, H. Vitamin B-6 nutrition in women with hyperemesis gravidarum during the first trimester of pregnancy. *Clinica Chimica Acta* 55:101, 1974.

Rose, D. P.; Strong, R.; Adams, P. W. and Harding, P. E. Experimental vitamin B-6 deficiency and effect of estrogen-containing oral contraceptives on tryptophan metabolism and vitamin B-6 requirements. *Clin. Sci.* 42:465-477, 1972.

Rosenberg, S. J. and Bennett, J. M. Pyridoxine responsive anemia. *New York State Journal of Medicine* 96:1430-1433, 1969.

Sauberlich, H. E.; Canham, J. E.; Baker, E. M.; Raica, N. and Herman, Y. F. Biochemical assessment of the nutritional status of vitamin B-6 in the human. *Amer. J. Clin. Nutr.* 25:629-642, 1972.

Schlesinger, K. and Schreiber, R. A. Interaction of drugs and pyridoxine deficiency on central nervous system excitability. *Annals of the New York Academy of Sciences* 166:281-287, 1969.

Sebrell, W. H. and Harris, R. S., eds. *The vitamins.* vol. II. New York: Academic Press, 1971.

Sourkes, T. L. *Biochemistry of mental disease.* New York: Harper & Row, 1962.

Szent-Györgyi, P. Developments leading to the metabolic role of vitamin B-6. *Amer. J. Clin. Nutr.* 24:1250-1256, 1971.

CHAPTER 11

B-12 and Folic Acid

We must continue to emphasize the importance of sufficient nutrients to the brain as well as to the body. The proper biochemical balance must be maintained for each individual. The correct dose of any given nutrient is *enough*—enough to produce maximal productivity or a feeling of well-being. We find that deficiency of vitamin B-12 and folic acid, like most nutrient deficiencies, is manifested in mental as well as physical signs of deficiency. Folic acid and vitamin B-12 have both proven beneficial in the treatment of mental disorders.

Vitamin B-12

Historical background In 1926 Drs. Minot and Murphy found that patients who ate liver had a remission in their pernicious anemia, a debilitating disease which previously had resulted in more than ten thousand deaths each year in the United States alone. Oral liver therapy became a standard remedy in treatment. Some patients ate 1 to 2 pounds of liver per day to control their anemia. For their discovery Murphy and Minot received the Nobel Prize in 1934.

Scientists worked to find out why liver was effective. Castle named the effective substance in liver "the extrinsic factor" and hypothesized that its absorption required the presence in the body of another substance, the intrinsic factor. He maintained that patients with pernicious anemia lacked the intrinsic factor but were able to absorb some extrinsic factor by simple diffusion from the large amounts of liver consumed. The intrinsic factor occurred in the gastric juices and these patients usually had diminished gastric secretion, as shown by the complete lack of acid in their gastric juices. In the 1930s the active substance was isolated from liver and subsequently was injected into patients with pernicious anemia. Then, in 1948, Rickes and his coworkers in the United States and Smith and Parker in England isolated a few micrograms of a red crystalline compound from liver which produced remission of pernicious anemia and was also effective in certain closely related anemias. This substance was named vitamin B-12. Its structure was established in 1955, and it was demonstrated to be the same as Castle's extrinsic food factor.

The cause of pernicious anemia is now known to be a lack of intrinsic factor, as Castle had suggested. The disease is treated with vitamin B-12 injections and oral doses of folic acid. Because vitamin B-12 (cyanocobalamin) is not effective orally, the anti-pernicious-anemia effect of liver seen by Minot and Murphy was probably due in part to the folic acid also present in the liver.

Physiological function Vitamin B-12, chemically a most complex vitamin, contains an atom of cobalt in its center. The structure of this vitamin is similar to that of hemoglobin (with iron at its center) and to that of chlorophyll (the green pigment responsible for photosynthesis in plants) with a central magnesium atom. The several forms of B-12 are called cobalamins. All are active, but hydroxycobalamin is the most active. Cyanocobalamin is most generally available for subcutaneous injection. Cyanocobalamin's red crystals are stable to heat (thus little is lost by cooking), soluble in water and inactivated by light and strong acid or alkaline solutions. The great chemical stability of B-12 seemed unbelievable to the searching chemists since they were looking for an unstable compound. We now know that B-12 can be extracted from sewage and used for animal feed.

The extrinsic factor (B-12) is absorbed through the small intestine with the aid of the intrinsic factor (IF) in the presence of calcium ions. The amount of the vitamin absorbed is regulated by the IF to about 2.5 to 3 mcg per day. When dietary intake is low, most of the extrinsic factor (60 to 80 percent) will be absorbed, but when ample vitamin B-12 is consumed its absorption is decreased to about 5 to 10 percent. Absorption is also greater when B-12 is provided in several meals rather than in one. Vitamin B-12 is transported throughout the body by serum proteins in the blood and is stored in many, if not all, body tissues—especially the liver, kidney, stomach, muscle and brain. The liver is the main storage site and in good nutritional states contains 2 to 5 mg, enough to last three to five years.

Vitamin B-12 is essential for the functioning of all cells, and it performs many diverse and important activities in the organism. It is vital for the growth of various animal species such as pigs, chicks and rats and for egg laying and hatching. In most of its roles, its biochemical action is intertwined with that of folic acid.

B-12 participates in the rapid regeneration of bone marrow and other tissue. One important role is the synthesis of RNA and DNA, our genetic material. When vitamin B-12 is lacking, the bone marrow is unable to produce mature red blood cells; the cells, instead of maturing and dividing, increase in size and are fewer in number. Thus, the red blood cell's normal capacity to carry hemoglobin is impaired and the hemoglobin's normal oxygen-transport function is reduced. The abnormal enlarged cells are called megaloblasts, and the condition is denoted as megaloblastic anemia; pernicious anemia is then a megaloblastic anemia. Maturation of these red cells also requires folic acid.

Vitamin B-12 is important in protein, fat and carbohydrate metabolism. It is required for the synthesis and transfer of single-carbon units such as the methyl group; in this way it aids in the synthesis of methionine (an amino acid or protein building block) and choline, which are both important lipotropic substances. Lipotropic factors have an affinity for lipids, particularly fats and oils, and they prevent or correct the development of fatty livers. Under certain conditions, vitamin B-12 protects against certain types of liver injury by toxic agents.

Among its other functions, vitamin B-12 increases tissue deposition of vitamin A by improving either carotene absorption or its conversion to vitamin A. B-12 also plays a part in reproduction and lactation. It also helps reduce the possibility of bruising and of developing black eyes. Furthermore, it has been claimed that this vitamin combats hangover, alcoholism, diabetes mellitus, osteoarthritis, osteoporosis, multiple sclerosis, spastic paraplegia (leg paralysis), atrophy of the brain's cerebellum, polyneuritis and certain psychoses.

The cobalamins play a role in the physiology of nervous tissue, but their exact function has not yet been elucidated. However, it seems that this vitamin is somehow needed for the functional integrity of myelinated nerve fibers in the central and peripheral nervous systems. Spinal cord lesions, optic degeneration and psychiatric disturbances are well-known results of vitamin B-12 deficiency.

Requirements, Deficiency and Therapeutic Uses The human species cannot synthesize useable vitamin B-12 and therefore must obtain it from food. An intake of 0.6 to 1.2 mcg is sufficient for normal blood formation and good health, but it will not replenish liver stores. This amount is more than enough, however, for improvement of the blood abnormality in pernicious anemia. The RDA is 5 to 9 mcg for adults, 8 mcg in pregnancy, 6 mcg during lactation and 1 to 2 mcg for infants, with a gradual increase during childhood and adolescence. Man's normal dietary intake is 3 to 30 mcg daily, with a probable average of 5 mcg. We receive B-12 almost exclusively from animal products, the major sources being meat, poultry, fish, eggs, brewer's yeast and dairy products (excluding butter). Seafoods such as clams, oysters and shrimps are especially rich sources.

Vitamin B-12 deficiency, which may result in pernicious anemia, is usually caused by a defect of absorption—i.e., lack of the intrinsic factor or small bowel malabsorption of vitamin B-12. Megaloblastic anemia from vitamin B-12 can also develop three to five years after surgical removal of the part of the stomach that produces the IF or the part of the ileum in the small intestine where the vitamin is absorbed. The occurrence of deficiency in this case can be prevented by vitamin B-12 injections. Megaloblastic anemias resulting from inadequate absorption of vitamin B-12 and folic acid may also be symptomatic of malabsorption syndromes such as sprue.

Because the daily requirement is so small, dietary lack as a cause of vitamin B-12 deficiency is rare, but it does occur among vegetarians who consume no animal products. These people do not, however, always show the characteristic anemia. A fact which had perplexed nutritionists is the observation that although some vegetarians in Britain develop B-12 deficiency this condition is rare in India. The answer was found to lie in differences in food purity which turned out to be a blessing for Indian vegetarians. India, where food standards are low and insects abound, differs from England, where food standards are high and insects are few. Vegetarians in India inadvertently consumed dried bits of insects in their fruits, vegetables and grains, and insects contain vitamin B-12. Another dietary factor which may contribute to B-12 deficiency in some people is the consumption of refined sugar which drains the body's store of vitamins and minerals.

The most common findings in vitamin B-12 deficiency are motor and mental difficulties. Symptoms are many: rapid heart beat, cardiac pain, shortness of breath, edema (swelling) of the face, general jaundice and intense brown discoloration around the small joints, weakness and fatigue as a consequence of the anemia (when present), inflammation of the tongue, loss of hair, lack of appetite, loss of weight, disturbed digestion, diarrhea, and neurological disturbances such as peripheral neuritis, spinal cord changes, intermittent numbness and tinglings in arms and legs, diminished tendon reflexes, unsteady gait, weakness of fine movements of hands, intolerance to noise or light, optic atrophy, auditory hallucinations, impaired memory and ability to learn and concentrate, confusion with paranoid delusions, mental depression, and psychoses. As mentioned, anemia is not always present in B-12 deficiency, and lesions of the nervous system may occur before the anemia is evident and may progress even after the anemia has been corrected. Conversely, neurological symptoms are not always seen in pernicious anemia patients. About 80 percent of pernicious anemia patients show some neurological involvement, and about 60 percent have personality changes. "Schizophrenia" with onset in middle or old age is usually B-12 deficiency.

Pernicious anemia is a fatal disease unless the deficiency is corrected; complete therapeutic remission is obtained with proper treatment. Vitamin B-12 injections will arrest the neurological disturbance, but folic acid is needed in conjunction with B-12 to cure the anemia. As little as 1 mcg of vitamin B-12 is needed, but 15 to 30 mcg are usually given until the anemia is corrected, after which maintenance therapy is continued monthly.

As previously mentioned, emotional disturbances, psychoses and neurological abnormalities are frequently observed in vitamin B-12 deficiency states. Indeed, it has now become obvious that avitaminosis B-12 is the root of much mental illness. Psychiatric disturbance due to this deficiency is well documented. Dr. J. G. Handerson, a consultant psychiatrist to the University of Aberdeen, believes that "a vitamin B-12 deficiency may be a possible diagnosis in the majority of psychiatric patients." Manifestations of the deficiency may include disturbances of perception, thinking, emotions, drive and memory; the clinical syndromes range from mild to severe. Spinal cord symptoms or megaloblastic anemia are seldom present, and therefore exact diagnosis is often difficult.

Dr. Victor Herbert of Mount Sinai Hospital in New York blames a lack of vitamin B-12 for the hospitalization of many patients in mental institutions. H. H. Wieck, et al. found B-12 deficiency in 58 percent of 138 cases of functional psychoses and organic brain syndrome. Rescue with vitamin B-12 has been suggested for many old people labeled as having "senile dementia."

Aside from its use in the treatment of pernicious anemia and B-12-deficiency psychoses, vitamin B-12 has been found beneficial for many who do not display overt signs of deficiency. They may or may not have low blood levels of the vitamin. It has been administered for relief of muscle fatigue and for extra energy. The improvement in general well-being and energy reserves lasts about five days initially and may be sustained for several weeks after treatment is discontinued. Injections of vitamin B-12 cause no local reactions, and the vitamin is nontoxic.

Why should extra B-12 be helpful? We know that a normal blood serum level of the vitamin is not a guarantee that the brain and nervous system are receiving adequate amounts. Linus Pauling has pointed out the possibility that some genetically defective enzyme systems may function better if the levels of the vitamins involved in these systems are increased above the accepted norm. Roger Williams has long insisted on biochemical individuality. More may be needed by some. The correct dose is *enough!* Whatever its mechanism, vitamin B-12 has helped many, whether anemic, psychotic or just plain tuckered-out; it is a most important vitamin and has not in the past received due recognition for its relationship to mental health.

Some internists will not give patients a weekly B-12 injection for fatigue which we know disappears with red vitamin injections. They state that B-12 is only good for pernicious anemia, which is so rare that the marketing of B-12 would not be commercially feasible for this purpose alone. Actually B-12 is almost the only vitamin that should be given by injection. The wise use of B-12 injections with folic acid has helped many fatigued patients.

A monumental work by Drs. Ellis and Nasser published in *The British Journal of Nutrition,* should be read by all doubting internists. The article is entitled "A Pilot Study of B-12 in the Treatment of Tiredness."

Twenty-eight tired subjects were recruited from the practices of local physicians and hospital staff. Under double-blind test conditions they were given hydroxycobalamin (B-12) or a matching placebo by injection twice a week. Fourteen patients were given B-12 for two weeks and fourteen were given a placebo for two weeks. Then, unknown to the doctors or subjects, a crossover was effected for two additional weeks.

Symptoms were assessed by a daily rating scale which included appetite, mood, energy, sleep and general feeling of well-being. The subject responses achieved great statistical significance (P=0.006) (one possibility in 160 that this would occur by chance) in respect to general well-being. "Happiness" received a value of P=0.032 (1 chance in 33). In subjects who received B-12 in the first period, no differences were found between responses in the first two-week period and the second two-week period, which suggests that the effect of the B-12 injections lasted as long as four weeks after injection. The authors hope to try oral doses of B-12 to see if this route is also effective in fighting abnormal fatigue.

The above study was done with injectable hydroxycobalamin (Alpha Redisol MSD) which has twice the effect of cyanocobalamin. Although the Alpha Redisol is more expensive than generic B-12, we find the product to be preferable in the seriously ill patient.

Folic Acid

Historical Background During the 1930s and 1940s, many scientists noted that water-soluble factors were required by many animal species and microorganisms. Some were especially needed for normal growth and protection against anemia. These factors were given various names in accordance with the animal species studied. In 1941, a substance was isolated from spinach and named folic acid by Mitchell and his associates. The name comes from *folium*, the Latin word for "leaf," because folic acid is found most abundantly in bright green leaves, or foliage. Through the identification of the structure and the synthesis of folic acid by Angier and his coworkers in 1945, it was established that folic acid and all the other various factors mentioned above were, in fact, the same substance. Also in that year, Dr. Tom Spies demonstrated that folic acid was effective in the treatment of megaloblastic anemias of pregnancy and also of tropical sprue.

Physiological Function Folic acid (folacin, folate, pteroylglutamic acid) has three chemical components: a pteridine grouping; PABA, a B-complex vitamin; and glutamic acid, an amino acid. Folic acid is bright yellow in color, slightly soluble in water, easily oxidized in an acid medium and easily destroyed by sunlight and heat. Much of the folic acid in foods can be lost by storage at room temperature and by normal cooking.

Dogs, rabbits, and rats can synthesize folic acid, but chicks, monkeys and humans must obtain it from dietary sources. Folic acid is mostly stored in the liver; its conversion to folinic acid, the biologically active form, probably is made with the aid of ascorbic acid. Folinic acid is a coenzyme for many enzyme systems. Much of folates' activity is interrelated with that of vitamin B-12; therefore, most of the functions about to be mentioned will already be familiar.

One of folic acid's most crucial roles is in the synthesis of nucleoproteins, such as DNA and RNA, and thus folate is needed, along with vitamin B-12, for the production of normal red blood cells in the bone marrow. Deficiency leads to megaloblastic anemia. Folate also performs an important function in the biosynthesis and transfer of single carbon units such as the methyl group. These processes result in the making of methylated compounds such as choline and other lipotropic substances previously discussed. The transfer of a methyl group is also essential to one of the components of DNA.

Folate is essential to the functioning of our brains, in that it is selectively concentrated in the spinal fluid and extracellular fluids. Folate is necessary for the synthesis of purines, which are the constituents of nucleic acids, the components of the cellular nucleoproteins DNA and RNA. Methionine, the synthesis of which depends upon folate and B-12, participates in many further transmethylation reactions in the brain and other areas. Folate and other pteridine derivatives also function as coenzymes in the biosynthesis of norepinephrine and serotonin, substances which are believed to be brain neurotransmitters (between-nerve-cell-communicators). Considerable evidence indicates that alterations in norepinephrine levels in the brain, possibly in conjunction with serotonin and dopamine, may play a part in the etiology of manic-depressive disorders. Folic acid appears to be crucial for mental and emotional health, but little is yet known as to the exact mechanism.

Requirements, Deficiency and Administration The recommended allowance of folic acid is 0.4 to 0.5 mg per day for adults, in pregnancy 0.8 mg per day and for nursing mothers 0.5 mg per day. The recommendation during infancy is 0.05 to 0.1 mg daily. The individual's requirement will vary with metabolic rate and cellular turnover, and people with hemolytic anemia or hyperthyroidism need much more.

The several forms of folic acid, or folates, are widespread in nature and are most abundant in foods also rich in other B vitamins and minerals. The best sources include liver, kidney, yeast, and deep-green leafy vegetables (spinach, watercress, kale, parsley, escarole, etc.). Other good food sources are asparagus, broccoli, lentils, lima beans, peanuts, other legumes, mushrooms, whole-grain cereals, lean beef, veal and egg yolks. Notably low in folate are root vegetables, light-green vegetables, corn, rice, dairy products and pork. Eggs are not especially rich in the vitamin, but the folacin of eggs, liver and yeast is better absorbed than that from other sources. Despite folic acid's widespread occurrence in natural raw foods, up to 90 percent of it may be nutritionally unavailable in some foods, and cooking and processing losses are great. From 50 to 95 percent of folate may be destroyed by prolonged cooking, by excess water used in boiling or by the high heat necessary in canning.

The average balanced diet contributes 0.15 to 0.2 mg per day of folic acid, which, you should note, is less than half the recommended allowance of 0.5 mg. Many people suffer from borderline folate deficiency. This deficiency may result from inadequate intake or secondary disease. Congenital inability to absorb folate is rare, but has been found to exist in isolated cases. People who eat no green or leafy vegetables are most susceptible to folate deficiency. The folic acid level is also related to iron intake. An iron-deficiency anemia will result in lowered plasma folate, and correction with oral iron will establish again the proper balance. When carbohydrate foods constitute too large a portion of the diet, folate deficiency may develop because these foods contain only traces of iron and folate.

Surveys have revealed folic acid intake to be one of the most widespread insufficiencies in our diets. It is true that severe anemia and megaloblastic bone marrow changes are not often reported, since these are usually the end result of a severe deficiency state and may never develop. Folate deficiency usually produces irritability, forgetfulness and mental sluggishness. In addition, the deficiency may produce cheilosis, a condition characterized by lesions at the corners of the mouth, which was observed by Dr. G. Rose to be alleviated by folate administration.

Folate deficiency with anemia is most commonly observed in elderly patients with poor diets and various organic diseases, in infants receiving formulas inadequate in folic acid or ascorbic acid, and in pregnant women. The World Health Organization in Geneva reports that from one-third to one-half of expectant mothers suffer folic acid deficiency in the last three months of pregnancy.

A special need for folic acid exists during pregnancy, as is noted by the approximate doubling of the normal adult recommended allowance. The fetus, by drawing from the mother's folate reserves to meet the needs for rapid growth, often depletes the mother's reserves to the point of megaloblastic anemia. Pregnant women are now given daily supplemental folic acid (0.5 to 1.5 mg per day) for protection against folic acid deficiency. Many women with histories of abortion or miscarriage have been able to complete successful childbirth subsequent to folic acid supplementation.

Relative deficiency during old age may also require daily supplementation of the diet with folate.

Folate deficiency has also been observed in mentally retarded children. Deficiency is frequently associated with disease conditions where the requirement for the vitamin is greatly increased, as in Hodgkin's disease and leukemia. Disorders which interfere with the ability to absorb food—tropical sprue, celiac disease or any disorder accompanied by vomiting or diarrhea—may produce deficiency of both folic acid and vitamin B-12. Folic acid is thought to be manufactured to some extent by bacteria in the intestinal tract. Prolonged use of antibiotics kills these bacteria and sometimes leads to a lack of both folate and B-12. In some women, oral contraceptives have produced deficiency of folic acid due to decreased absorption of the vitamin. Excessive alcohol consumption accelerates megaloblastic changes; about 90 percent of alcoholics suffer folic acid deficiencies.

Anticonvulsants (e.g., Dilantin) and phenobarbital can also produce folic acid deficiency. Low serum and cerebrospinal fluid folate levels have repeatedly been found in epileptics receiving anticonvulsant medication. The evidence concerning the effect of folic acid therapy in epileptics is contradictory. Researchers such as Norris and Pratt, Jensen and Olesen, and Horwitz et al. found no effect on seizure frequency in epileptics when their folate deficiency was corrected. Mattson and his associates detected no statistical change in seizure frequency or severity and no improvement in psychological test performance from folic acid therapy in epileptics with low folate levels. The therapy did, however, effect a decrease in serum anticonvulsant and barbiturate concentration and an elevation of folate in the serum, but the folate level did not rise in the spinal fluid; it is believed that anticonvulsants may interfere with the conversion of folic acid to the form which can pass the blood-brain barrier.

However, Hawkins and Meynell reported decreased fit frequency with folic acid treatment. Also Reynolds et al. found marked improvement in the megaloblastic anemia and in the mental state of most of a group of epileptic patients, despite occasional increased frequency and severity of fits. The improvement was in the areas of drive, mood, intellectual speed (both quality and capacity), alertness, concentration, self-confidence, independence and sociability. In two-thirds of the patients who received B-12 concurrently, the improvement of the mental state either was enhanced or, for the first time, became apparent. The so-called deterioration of the epileptic with continued anticonvulsant (Dilantin) therapy is probably B-12 and folate deficiency.

The main side-effect of anticonvulsant medication is apathy and slowing of the mental processes. Anticonvulsant therapy of epilepsy, if prolonged, may lead to paranoid schizophrenia, and there exists a strong temporal relationship between the commencement of anticonvulsant drug therapy and the onset of such psychotic illness. These mental manifestations of therapy are probably due to the patients' lowered folic acid levels. On testing, a significantly higher incidence of low-folate concentrations is found in epileptic patients with psychiatric illness than in those with normal mental states. We have found that schizophrenia produced by Dilantin-induced folate deficiency is usually of the low blood histamine type (histapenia) and that it is characterized by paranoia and hallucinations.

Reynolds et al., and also others, have suggested that folate deficiency may lead to neuropsychiatric disorders. Indeed, all evidence indicates that prolonged folate deficiency, whether drug-induced or not, may cause neurological changes and mental deterioration.

In the discussion of folate function, we mentioned several vital roles in the nervous system, but the actual detailed effects of deficiency are not well understood. Low levels of serum folic acid (more than of vitamin B-12) have been found in psychiatric illness, and megaloblastic anemia is not uncommon in these patients. Hunter reported that 37 of 75 patients admitted to mental hospitals had subnormal folate levels; 13 of these were consuming barbiturates, anticonvulsants or alcohol. Two out of 150 had B-12 deficiency syndrome which cleared with appropriate therapy. Folate deficiency has also been reported in geriatric patients with mental disorders; their most common mental symptoms were apathy, withdrawal, lack of motivation and depression. The World Health Organization has recommended that the aged, pregnant women, and those on the contraceptive pill should receive extra folic acid.

A relationship does exist, then, between folate lack and mental illness. Some leads are available, but the mechanisms are not yet understood. Further research may uncover the complex roles played by folic acid and vitamin B-12 in our mental health.

Again, we must stress the close relationship between folic acid and vitamin B-12. In pernicious anemia, caused by lack of vitamin B-12 in the body, the patient is often also deficient in folic acid. Similarly, in the megaloblastic anemia caused by folic acid deficiency, the patient usually suffers a concomitant deficiency in vitamin B-12.

Almost without exception, both these vitamins are always given together, and extreme care must be exercised if only one is administered. Treatment of pernicious anemia with vitamin

B-12 alone increases the rate at which folic acid is utilized by the body and may lead to a deficiency of folate. Conversely, folic acid therapy alone will produce a remission in the anemia of pernicious anemia, but vitamin B-12 is needed to cure the neurologic symptoms of the disease.

Since a high folic acid intake eliminates the anemia of pernicious anemia, which is the most effective means of detecting the disease, accurate diagnosis will be difficult if the patient is already supplementing his diet with this vitamin. The patient may then incur irreversible nerve and spinal cord damage.

Although new techniques have made possible the diagnosis of pernicious anemia despite folic acid supplementation, this danger has prompted the FDA to limit over-the-counter preparations of folic acid to 0.1 mg per tablet. Since this amount is insufficient to correct an anemia, an effort is now being made to increase the maximum amount allowable without prescription to 0.4 mg per tablet. Even this dose, however, is not usually large enough to thoroughly reverse the megaloblastic bone marrow pattern of pernicious anemia and obscure diagnosis.

How high can one go with folic acid intake and still be safe? Some say hundreds of milligrams per day are not harmful. Folic acid in oral doses greater than 5 mg per day is apt to produce muscle restlessness, myoclonic (muscle) jerking, and occasionally seizures (convulsions). Epileptics on anticonvulsants such as Dilantin need extra folic acid, but the effective administration of folate is difficult because seizures may be aggravated. The slow and careful substitution of Valium for Dilantin may be useful in that Valium is not an anti-folate drug. Certainly the reduction in size of the official (prescription) folic tablet from 5 mg to 1 mg has provided a tablet of a more suitable size for use by epileptics with folate deficiency. Again, folate use without adequate B-12 can be harmful.

Since folic acid and vitamin B-12 are so interrelated in their biochemical actions, and a deficiency usually encompasses both of these B vitamins, it is wise to start B-12 therapy first and then add the folic acid at the level of 1 to 2 mg per day for the schizophrenic and 1 mg per day for the epileptic. We have not found a need for doses above 5 mg per day. Nor have we found a need for any route of administration of folic acid other than by mouth.

Vitamin B-12 and Folic Acid in the Schizophrenias After finding that serum folate levels were low in histapenic (low blood histamine) patients, we used folic acid, logically, to raise blood histamine level. This does occur, and with the rise in blood histamine the patient's hallucinations and paranoia are lessened. Thus folic acid therapy (1 to 2 mg orally per day) may provide dramatic improvement in the histapenic patient. This improvement may continue for several months, when a plateau will occur unless the patient also gets an adequate supply of vitamin B-12. This B-12 dose can be as little as 1 mg given subcutaneously each month, but some may require 1 mg twice weekly. The histapenic patient also responds to large doses of niacin. The niacin dosage can frequently be brought to a more normal range if B-12 and folate are given simultaneously with the niacin. Because zinc is needed to store histamine in the tissues, zinc must be given in the needed dose for each individual.

It follows that patients who are high in blood histamine (histadelics) should have Dilantin regularly to produce an antifolate effect and thus lower their histamine level. When used knowledgeably with calcium, methionine and the trace metal nutrients (zinc and manganese), this is effective therapy for histadelic patients (see page 102, *The Schizophrenias: Yours and Mine*, Pfeiffer et al. Pyramid Books, 1970).

It also follows that some patients who are low in histamine can have their histamine driven higher with folic acid and B-12 therapy, to the point where they may have a high-histamine depression. This has occurred in several of our patients, but as long as regular blood samples are taken and the condition is recognized, no real difficulties are encountered.

Many patients ask, "Shouldn't I receive the vitamins, especially the B vitamins, all together, not singly in high doses?" For the normal human adult this may, in general, be true. It is a good idea to obtain an adequate intake of all vitamins together; many interrelate in the body, and too much of one, relative to another, can upset a proper balance. This is true, as we have seen, of folic acid and B-12; it is probably also the case with respect to calcium, magnesium and phosphorus—minerals essential to normal skeletal growth and maintenance.

This belief in "all vitamins together," does not always hold, however. It is prudent to receive an adequate intake of the B vitamins together, as would be provided by appropriate food sources and a B-complex supplement or ten tablets of brewer's yeast. Nevertheless, many individuals, including half of the schizophrenics (those with low blood histamine) have a special need for extra folic acid and B-12. We also know that such vitamins as C, B-3 and B-6 must be given in adequate doses to certain patients to correct their specific biochemical abnormalities. In each instance, a biochemical imbalance affecting mental capacities is corrected by the use of a large dose of a specific vitamin or vitamins (such as folate, B-12, B-3 and B-6).

References

Ellis and Nasser. A pilot study of B-12 in the treatment of tiredness. *Brit. J. Nutr.* 30:277, 1973.

Hawkins, C. F. and Meynell, M. J. Macrocytosis and macrocytic anemia caused by anticonvulsant drugs. *Quart. J. Med.* 27:45-63, 1958.

Herbert, V. The diagnosis and treatment of folic acid deficiency. *Med. Clin. N. Amer.* 46:1365-1378, 1962.

Horwitz, S. J. et al. Relation of abnormal folate metabolism to neuropathy developing during anticonvulsant drug therapy. *Lancet* 1:563-565, 1968.

Kane, F. Jr. and Lipton, M. Folic acid and mental illness. *South. Med. J.* 63:603, 1970.

Kruger, M. Folic acid requirements during pregnancy. *JAMA* 218, 5:747, 1971.

Lanzkowsky, P. Congenital malabsorption of folate. *Amer. J. Med.* p. 580, May 1970.

Mattson, R.; Gallagher, B.; Reynolds, E. and Glass, D. Folate therapy in epilepsy. *Arch. Neurol.* 29:78, 1973.

Omer, A.; Finlayson, N.; Shearman, D.; Samson, R. and Girdwood, R. Plasma and erythrocyte folate in iron deficiency and folate deficiency. *Blood* 35, 6:821, 1970.

Pritchard, J., Scott, D. and Whalley, P. Folic acid requirements in pregnancy-induced megaloblastic anemia. *JAMA* 208, 7:1163, 1969.

Reynolds, E., Preece, J. and Johnson, A. Folate metabolism in epileptic and psychiatric patients. *J. Neurol. Neurosurg. Psychiat.* 34:726, 1971.

Robinson, C. *Fundamentals of normal nutrition.* New York: Macmillan, 1973.

Rose, J. Folic acid as cause of angular cheilosis. *Lancet* 2:453, 1971.

Sullivan, L. Vitamin B-12 metabolism and megaloblastic anemia. *Semin. Hematol. 7,* 1:6, 1970.

Trager, J. *The bellybook.* New York: Grossman, 1972.

Wieck, H., Pribilla, W. and Heerklotz, B. Psychoses as a manifestation of B-12 deficiency. *Deutsch. Med. Wschr.* 94:1473, 1969.

CHAPTER 12

The Remainder of the B-Complex Vitamins

Understanding of the relationship between diet and psychiatric disorders is in its infancy. The state of the science might be likened to the understanding of the relationship between vitamins and physical illness that existed a few hundred years ago when James Lind found that lemon juice cured scurvy. But we do know that good nutrition, especially with respect to the B vitamins, is a requisite for mental health. Deficiency or even a borderline deficiency can seriously impair mental function, often before any bodily changes appear.

Dr. Michael Jefferson, a British neurologist (along with other scientists), has noted the special importance of the B vitamins to the proper functioning of the nervous system. He finds B vitamin deficiencies to be responsible for many complaints of middle age. Almost all the B vitamins function as enzymes in carbohydrate metabolism, which is the keystone for proper function of nerve cells and tissues. The B-complex vitamins are needed by the brain, yet many people do not receive adequate supplies.

Present findings do not classify the remainder of the essential B vitamins as important in the schizophrenias, unlike niacin (B-3), pyridoxine (B-6), cyanocobalamin (B-12), folic acid, inositol and choline. These remaining B vitamins (thiamin, riboflavin, pantothenic acid, biotin, and PABA) are, however, still vital to health. Further studies may find them more important than those currently used.

Thiamin (B-1)

Thiamin was the first member of the B complex to be chemically identified. The severe deficiency disease, beriberi, was first suspected to be dietary by Japanese scientists who were faced with an outbreak of pandemic proportions in this rice-eating country. Several investigators in various parts of the world demonstrated that the disease was directly related to consumption of a diet consisting entirely of polished rice and that it could be cured through use of a factor in the rice's bran coating (removed during polishing) that prevented the polyneuritis (multiple nerve degeneration) or inflammation of beriberi. Since the basic chemical was an amine (a nitrogen-containing substance), it was named vital-amine, and later vitamin, to indicate a necessary dietary substance. But not until a later time was "vitamin B" identified chemically. Crystalline vitamin B-1 was isolated from rice bran by Jansen and Donath in Holland in 1926. In 1936 Dr. Robert Williams synthesized vitamin B-1, thereby demonstrating its structure. He named this vitamin thiamin (often spelled thiamine) because both sulfur and nitrogen were present.

In the human organism, thiamin performs several functions, one of the most important of which is related to carbohydrate metabolism. It is involved to a lesser extent in the metabolism of fats and amino acids. Thiamin aids digestion and elimination by helping to maintain muscle tone in the digestive tract, is necessary for normal growth and good appetite, and is essential to a healthy nervous system.

Humans need approximately half a milligram of thiamin per thousand calories consumed; athletes and laborers therefore need more than the usual amounts. Diets high in fats and proteins require somewhat less; however, a minimum allowance of at least 1.0 mg is recommended for all adults. The allowance for pregnant and lactating women is increased by 0.1 and 0.5 mg, respectively, beyond the normal requirements for women. Infants and children should receive from 0.2 to 1.1 mg per day. The amount needed increases with the age of the child.

From what sources can we receive our needed thiamin? Whole-grain cereals originally are rich in thiamin, but most of the vitamin is lost in the polishing of rice and the refining of flour. (These grains undergo these processes in order to curtail pest attraction and prevent spoilage.) Nevertheless, Americans obtain about a third of their thiamin from enriched-grain cereal foods; the remainder comes from poultry, fish, meats (lean pork and liver are especially high), legumes, egg yolks and milk. Brewer's yeast and wheat germ, with their concentration of B-complex vitamins, are also good sources and should be used more frequently by Americans. Vegetables and fruits may also make a significant contribution to vitamin B-1 intake if large quantities are consumed and not overcooked.

A potential difficulty in obtaining sufficient thiamin is the vitamin's ready solubility in water and its destruction by heating in a neutral or alkaline (basic) reaction. All B vitamins are soluble in water to varying degrees, but B-1 is the most vulnerable to heat. Cooking results in thiamin depletion of most foods. Thiamin losses from cooking in water such foods as rice, meats and vegetables may approach 50 percent if the liquid is discarded. Thiamin losses can be minimized for meat if the cooking juices are consumed and for vegetables if excess water and overcooking are avoided.

When the dietary intake of thiamin is in excess of tissue needs, the vitamin will be excreted in the urine; if the amount ingested is low, urinary excretion decreases to make the vitamin available to the body's tissues. The storage in the body of thiamin is not very great, and tissues are rapidly depleted during a deficiency. Eating sugar, smoking and drinking alcohol further deplete thiamin.

Thiamin deficiencies have been observed most notably in rice-eating areas where the outer layers containing most of the nutrients have been removed from the grain by polishing. Since rice is the staple food of half the world, vitamin B-1 deficiencies are widespread. In Japan, the danger is compounded by the use of raw fish (which contains the enzyme thiaminase) as a dietary staple; unless thiaminase is inactivated by cooking, it destroys the thiamin in the remainder of a mixed meal. This might explain the low tolerance of alcohol common to the Japanese. Known as *kakke* in Japan, beriberi disabled so many Japanese who ate raw fish and polished rice during World War II that the Japanese government would only allow brown rice to be distributed. But many of the citizens hulled their rice to obtain the traditionally preferred, nutritionally deficient, white rice.

We now know that the potential danger of white rice can be lessened by the process of parboiling. In the 1940s, Gordon Harwell, a former produce broker in Texas, and Eric Huzenlaub, an English food chemist, developed a process whereby the nutrients of the outer layers of rice are diffused and sealed into the kernel's starchy protein center. When the hull and bran are later removed, about 80 percent of the natural B vitamins present in rough rice or paddy are retained. The "converted" rice resulting from the parboiling keeps well, retains its nutrients during cooking, and is much less attractive to weevils and other pests than natural paddy. Perhaps if the Japanese had had access to this process, much of their wartime deficiency of thiamin could have been avoided.

Beriberi is the most severe form of vitamin B-1 deficiency. Adult beriberi, resulting from a prolonged thiamin deficit, is fatal if not corrected. The predominant symptoms are debility, severe weight loss, plugged hair follicles, gastrointestinal disturbances, nervous disturbances, weak and sore muscles, paralysis of the lower and sometimes upper limbs, enlarged liver, and swollen and weak heart with palpitations, difficult breathing and possibly cardiac failure. "Wet" beriberi is mainly characterized by edema (water-swelling of the tissues) and cardiac failure; "dry" beriberi is distinguished by weakness, emaciation and multiple neuritic symptoms. Infants in the Far East may also develop beriberi as a result of the deficiency of thiamin in their mothers' milk. In the treatment of beriberi, B-complex vitamins are prescribed, rather than thiamin alone, usually in conjunction with a diet high in protein and calories.

Beriberi is rare in the United States except among our

alcoholics. The occurrence of the disease in the chronic drinker is the result of multiple factors. We know extra thiamin is required for alcohol metabolism. Yet, the alcoholic receives little of the vitamin from his limited food intake, and furthermore, the alcohol in his blood blocks the absorption of what little thiamin he might receive. Thus, the alcoholic is one who is particularly susceptible to severe vitamin B-1 deficiency. "Wrist drop" and "foot drop" with a flapping gait are characteristic of chronic alcoholism.

Thiamin deficiency can also occur subsequent to gastrointestinal disturbances which are accompanied by persistent vomiting or diarrhea, or following surgery or diseases characterized by fever when the dietary intake has been limited.

Varying degrees of vitamin B-1 deficiency occur. Many Americans do not obtain enough thiamin and may suffer from mild thiamin deficiency. The 1965 USDA food-intake studies indicated that although almost all men got more than the RDA of thiamin, many adolescent girls and many women over sixty-five got only about 85 percent of the RDA.

The symptoms of mild thiamin deficiency are vague and can be attributed to other problems, so that diagnosis is often difficult. Most commonly, the individual experiences fatigue, insomnia, headaches, numbness, neuritis, aching, burning sensation in hands and feet, indigestion, constipation, diarrhea and loss of appetite, weight and strength. Mental symptoms include apathy, confusion, emotional instability, irritability, depression and fear of impending disaster. Often the mental changes are prominent after only a few days of deprivation and are not accompanied by the symptoms or signs of neuritis. Dr. Joseph Brozek of the University of Minnesota has noted significant behavioral decrement in the sensory area with thiamin deprivation. Deterioration of manual speed and coordination, complex body-reaction time, toe-reaction time, motor speed, eye-hand coordination, manual steadiness and body sway were reversed with adequate thiamin resupplementation.

Although neurologic and mental symptoms are commonly seen with thiamin deficiencies, the schizophrenic is usually adequately supplied with vitamin B-1. Exceptions can occur with persons on pep pills and crash diets. We have not seen any benefit in the schizophrenic when megadoses of 500 mg are given twice a day. Large doses intravenously or intramuscularly should never be given because the quaternary nitrogen in thiamin has a curare action on the motor nerve endings. This may result in muscle weakness and paralysis of respiration.

The more severe manifestations of thiamin deficiency are not commonly seen in the United States today because even converted rice is enriched with additional thiamin, riboflavin, niacin and iron. This process gives it a content of these vitamins even greater than that of whole brown rice. However, enrichment does not replace other needed nutrients lost in polishing, and the short-grain white rice preferred by most Americans and used as a staple by many of our poor people is still not always enriched. In the Orient, where rice is still polished and rarely enriched, the disabling disease beriberi remains widespread. Unfortunately, as was indicated by the Japanese hulling their nutritionally superior rice to make it white, it is often easier to enrich and fortify foods, as has been done in the United States, than to attempt to change common eating habits. Even enrichment has its limitations, however, and we believe it is possible to alter eating habits through continued education.

Riboflavin (B-2)

Riboflavin, an orange-yellow fluorescent biochemical, was discovered in 1879. Because this fluorescent pigment or "flavin" was first found in milk, it was designated as "lactoflavin." By 1928, it was evident that vitamin B, which prevented the polyneuritis of beriberi, was more than just one vitamin. The antiberiberi fraction destroyed by heat became known as vitamin B-1 or thiamin. A heat-resistant factor which promoted growth but did not fight polyneuritis was designated as vitamin B-2. Vitamin B-2 was synthesized in 1935 by Kuhn and his coworkers in Germany and later was named riboflavin by Henry W. Sebrell, Jr. of Columbia University.

Riboflavin (B-2) is essential to normal growth and tissue maintenance. B-2 goes into the formation of some enzymes and assists in the metabolism of amino acids, fatty acids and carbohydrates, the three energy-generating food constituents.

The recommended daily allowance of riboflavin is 0.8 to 2.6 mg for adults. During pregnancy and lactation, 1.8 and 2.0 mg daily, respectively, are recommended. Infants should receive 0.4 to 0.6 mg and children to ten years, 0.6 to 1.2 mg per day. The individual need will be increased by hyperthyroidism, fevers, stress of injury or surgery, and malabsorption. People in those parts of the world where the diet consists mostly of starches have the ability to synthesize riboflavin in their gastrointestinal tracts, but the bacteria that accomplish this synthesis are inhibited by fat and protein.

The most important source of B-2 is milk, which supplies almost half of our intake of this vitamin. Significant contributions are also made by organ meats and by dairy products other than butter. In addition, eggs, some other meats, poultry, fish, yeast, wheat germ, green leafy vegetables, legumes and nuts supply important amounts. Cereals and flours do not naturally contain much riboflavin, but through being enriched, they make significant contributions of riboflavin to the diet.

The yellow riboflavin crystals are resistant to heat, acids and oxidizing agents, and are only sparingly soluble in water, but they are quickly decomposed by sunlight, ultraviolet rays and alkaline solutions. Much of the riboflavin in milk is lost in even one hour of exposure to direct sunlight in a glass container. Three and one-half hours of contact with the sun's rays will destroy as much as 70 percent. At maximum, however, 10 to 20 percent of milk's initial riboflavin is lost by pasteurization, irradiation for vitamin D and evaporation or drying. Opaque plastic containers and waxed paper cartons have increasingly replaced glass milk bottles.

Even bread is vulnerable to riboflavin losses through light exposure. Not much riboflavin is lost in the cooking of meat, and because the vitamin is only slightly soluble in water, little is lost in common vegetable cooking procedures. However, if baking soda is used in cooking to preserve the green color, vitamin B-2 will be destroyed.

The body stores riboflavin to some extent, but beyond a certain point of intake the vitamin is excreted in the urine. Thus, riboflavin is nontoxic in large quantities. A marked lowering of the intake of vitamin B-2 correspondingly cuts down urinary excretion If intake falls too low for too long, deficiency can result; riboflavin lack is one of the most common deficiencies repeatedly observed in nutritional surveys. In a 1968-1969 study of American preschool children, 21 percent were found to have substandard levels of riboflavin in their diets. From 1968 to 1970, the U.S. Department of Health, Education, and Welfare (HEW) conducted a ten-state nutrition survey; the resulting preliminary report to the Congress revealed that 17 percent of Americans below the poverty level were low in riboflavin, twice the rate of deficiency in middle-class Americans.

Signs of B-2 deficiency are cheilosis and inflammation of the tongue and cornea. Other symptoms are a purple-red colored tongue; dermatitis around the nose, forehead and ears; eye fatigue, oversensitivity to light, blurred vision, and bloodshot eyes. The ocular manifestations are often among the earliest warnings of riboflavin deficiency. The signs of the deficiency may, however, have other causes.

Although B-2 deficiency can produce trembling, dizziness, insomnia and mental sluggishness, this vitamin is not believed to be as important in mental health as the B vitamins pyridoxine, cyanocobalamin, folic acid, niacin, thiamin and pantothenic acid. No specific need for excess riboflavin has been found in stress or in any mental disease. Riboflavin in doses of 10 mg is quite adequate, and this dose produces a highly fluorescent yellow urine. (This yellow coloration can be used as a tracer to make certain that a patient is taking his prescribed medications.)

Pantothenic Acid (Calcium Pantothenate)

Pantothenic acid was isolated and synthesized in 1940 by the chemist Roger Williams of Texas. Its key role in metabolism is suggested by its occurrence in all living cells, and thus its name was derived from the Greek word for "everywhere," *panthos.*

In 1950, pantothenic acid was found by Lipmann and his associates to be a constituent of coenzyme A, a substance discovered just four years previously to be involved in the transfer of acetyl groups (CH_3CO-) in the body. Coenzyme A is the main form in which pantothenic acid functions in the body. Via this route, pantothenic acid is essential for energy metabolism, for fat and cholesterol synthesis, for antibody formation and for the building of acetylcholine in the nervous system. This vitamin has been found to restore abnormally gray hair to its original color in test rats, but the same has not been found for humans. (Yet some claim pantothenic acid deficiency may result in premature graying of hair.) We have found zinc and sulfur deficiency to be more important in the graying of hair.

The human requirement for pantothenic acid is not known, but a dose of 5 to 10 mg daily is considered sufficient for adults and children; more is probably needed after an injury, after antibiotic therapy or during the stress of severe illness. Since pantothenic acid is synthesized in all animal and plant cells, it is available to us in all foods, but the largest quantities of this vitamin are found in meat, poultry, fish, whole-grain cereals and legumes. We also obtain some pantothenic acid from fruits, vegetables and milk. Little of the vitamin is lost with ordinary cooking procedures, except in acid and alkaline solutions. However, the milling of flour removes about 50 percent of the original pantothenic acid and the dry processing of foods also results in substantial losses.

In addition to its widespread availability in the diet, this vitamin can be synthesized in the body by intestinal bacteria. However, the average American diet easily provides adequate pantothenic acid, and deficiency is not usually found. Even the demonstration of human pantothenic acid deficiency with experimental diets low in the vitamin is difficult.

Under normal everyday conditions, deficiency is seen only in conjunction with severe multiple B-complex deficiencies. The deficit identifies itself through loss of appetite, indigestion, abdominal pain, respiratory infections, peripheral neuritis with cramping pains in the arms and legs, burning sensations in the feet, and adrenal insufficiency. The brain is one of the areas of highest pantothenic acid concentration in the body. As with almost all the B vitamins, mental symptoms accompany the deficiency—in this case, insomnia, fatigue, sullenness and mental depression. Pantothenic acid deficiency may be related to the nervous disease and psychosis seen in some alcoholics. However, when diets are deficient in pantothenic acid, this deficiency is accompanied by others. Therefore, it is probably not legitimate to attribute the alcoholic's neuropathy solely to any single deficit.

We at the Brain Bio Center have studied pantothenic acid extensively, in doses as high as 500 mg per day in patients and even in single large doses, for the effect on the quantitative brain wave. No specific effect on the brain has been found. Large doses make the teeth and joints more sensitive, so that normals find that minor erosions in the teeth become painful and the arthritic patient reports that his painful joints are much more sensitive. (This the arthritic does not need!) Our usual dose in the histapenic patient is 30 mg per day taken in the morning. This dose causes a rapid rise in the blood histamine level.

Biotin

In the 1920s a factor essential for the growth of microorganisms such as yeast and intestinal bacteria was described and named bios. In the 1930s, Dr. Helen Parsons and coworkers discovered that rats fed a diet containing raw egg whites developed loss of fur, rapid weight loss, paralysis of the hind legs, blue coloration of the surface of the body, (due to inadequate oxygen in the blood), and death. These signs did not appear when cooked egg white was substituted for raw. The factor which prevents this sequence of signs was later isolated from egg yolk and established as being identical to the microorganism growth factor bios. This vitamin, which was given the name biotin, was synthesized and its structure determined in 1943.

How is it that raw egg white creates a biotin deficiency? Egg white contains a glycoprotein, avidin, that binds biotin, thereby preventing the vitamin's absorption from the intestinal tract. Heat inactivates the binding ability of avidin, and thus cooking egg white will counter avidin's effect on biotin without affecting the biotin itself, which is very stable to heat (and also to light and to acids).

Biotin, like thiamin, is a sulfur-containing vitamin which acts as a coenzyme of a number of enzymes responsible for many reactions in the body. It is required in the food-energy cycles, in the synthesis of fatty acids and amino acids and in the manufacture of glycogen, our means of storing energy in the liver. It is also essential for the introduction of carbon dioxide in the formation of purines, constituents of DNA and RNA.

The requirement for this vitamin in man has not been established, but it is estimated at about 150 mcg per day in adults. The average diet provides about 150 to 300 mcg daily.

Small quantities of biotin are found in many foods; good food sources include egg yolk, organ meats, yeast, legumes and nuts. Cereal grains, muscle meats and milk contain very small amounts. Biotin is also synthesized by intestinal bacteria, in amounts considerably greater than the diet supplies.

Absorption of the vitamin from the intestine does take place, but much is excreted in the urine. Minute amounts of biotin are stored in the body, mainly in the liver, kidney, brain and the adrenal glands, the same metabolically active tissues in which we find the largest concentrations of pantothenic acid.

Deficiency of biotin is difficult to produce experimentally. When artificially induced by extreme measures in humans, the symptoms of biotin deficiency are similar to those of thiamin lack. They include scaly dermatitis, loss of appetite, nausea, pallor of both skin and mucuous membranes, muscle pains, lassitude and increased sensory sensitivity. The individual will usually show a lowered hemoglobin level, a raised blood cholesterol level and a greatly decreased urinary excretion of biotin. No natural biotin deficiency has been observed in humans, although two kinds of dermatitis in infants respond to biotin therapy. Deficiency does occur, however, as a result of two different circumstances: consuming many raw egg whites for a prolonged time (an amount constituting approximately 30 percent of one's dietary calories) or taking too many antibiotics (which dramatically reduces the number of intestinal bacteria).

We have studied large doses of biotin in both normals and patients. Extra biotin increases the kryptopyrrole excretion in pyroluric patients, and Donald Irvine has found that sterilization of the gut with antibiotics will eliminate the KP excretion. In pyroluria we may be dealing with an overproduction of biotin or with an abnormal form of biotin, since we know that the synthesis of hemoglobin involves the use of biotin as a coenzyme. This is an important research problem in stress-induced psychoses.

PABA (Para-aminobenzoic Acid)

PABA's major importance is as a component of folic acid, a vital B vitamin, but PABA is sometimes classified as a separate B-complex vitamin. It has been noted as the anti-gray-hair factor in animals, and large doses have been tried in man in the hope of darkening gray hair. However, excess PABA is excreted promptly in the urine, and to date gray hair has not been darkened in humans in this way.

This vitamin is one of the best ultraviolet screens when applied to the skin, and is therefore widely used in many sunscreen lotions. Supplementation of the diet with PABA may perhaps lessen the susceptibility to sunburn in those persons easily affected. We find, however, that B-6 by mouth is better than PABA for this purpose.

Some nutritionists have reported that PABA plus pantothenic acid will result in a repigmentation of the patchy dead-white areas of the skin in the condition known as vitiligo. This may be possible, particularly if the patient also ingests good amounts of zinc, manganese and vitamin B-6.

With regard to its possible effects in mental disease, we have tried large doses of the vitamin in man without any definite effect on the quantitative brain waves. Dr. J. E. Carron of Arnold, Missouri, has used large doses (2 gm per day) in problem schizophrenic patients and has reported good results. If this continues to help we may have in PABA a scavenger amine which picks up excess methyl and acetyl groups so that more important amines will not be methylated to form hallucinogens. (We have often thought that ethanol amine would make an effective, harmless scavenger amine.)

References

Brozek, J. Soviet studies on nutrition and higher nervous system activity. *Annals of the New York Academy of Science* 93:687, 1962.

Bruno, M. There's psychotherapy in the vitamins B. *Prevention* p. 75, April 1973.

———— Psychotic symptoms can result from deficiency. *Drug Trade News* p. 52, 3 June 1957.

Irvine, D. G. et al. *Nature* 224:812, 1969.

Parsons, H. T. *J. Biol. Chem.* 90:351, 1931.

Robinson, C. *Fundamentals of normal nutrition.* New York: Macmillan, 1973.

Trager, J. *The bellybook.* New York: Grossman, 1972.

Williams, R. J. *Nutrition in a nutshell.* New York: Doubleday, 1962.

CHAPTER 13

Rutin and Bioflavonoids

The flavonoids are non-nitrogenous biochemicals which are widely distributed in nature as the pigments in flowers, fruits and vegetables. Dr. Szent-Györgyi and his colleagues in the late 1930s isolated from citrus peel a material called citrin (vitamin P) which later proved to be the flavone hesperidin. We now know a whole series of bioflavonoids which may prevent excess capillary fragility. This has been difficult to prove in man, but animal studies indicate that such an effect might be possible.

Bioflavonoids have antioxidant activity and protect both vitamin C and adrenalin from oxidation by copper-containing enzymes. The bioflavonoids can actually chelate copper. Ambrose and De Eds in 1947 proposed this chelation reaction as the major vitamin-like action, namely a preservation of vitamin C and also of the life of adrenalin so that capillary permeability is lessened.

Rutin is one of the bioflavonoids. It is obtained as a by-product of the milling of buckwheat. Rutin, as a bioflavonoid, prolongs the action of adrenalin in animal studies and also appears to have an adrenalin-like effect on capillaries. This action is not sufficient to alter the course of the symptoms of the common cold but may be a factor in easy bruising, which occurs frequently in menopausal women and in rheumatoid arthritis patients. We use rutin and other bioflavonoids, with uneven success, in an attempt to control bruising.

We have studied rutin in oral doses of 50 mg to ascertain the effect on the quantitative brain wave. This method is sensitive enough to disclose the sedative effect of two aspirin tablets or two Miltowns, and both are quite comparable. Rutin, tested by this method, shows a definite effect which is a mixture of sedative and stimulant. With this in mind, we have used rutin in depressed and other patients. An oral dose of 50 mg given each morning would appear to be effective.

We also have data that indicate that rutin in doses of 60 mg by mouth in man will raise the blood histamine and lower the serum copper. The six-hour urinary excretion of three metals studied in twenty-one trials gave zinc 181 ± 93 mcg (normal 150), copper 9.4 ± 5.7 mcg (normal 3.0) and iron 19.1 ± 11 (normal 20). These data show that rutin removes zinc and copper, but not iron, from the body. Rutin might be used to remove copper if a dietary supplement of zinc were given.

Rutin and the bioflavonoids are additional examples of biochemicals (in the common domain) which lack any commercial sponsor. The regulatory bureaucracy has criticized any suggested new uses, and the granting bureaucracy has shown little interest in studying a compound which has some adrenalin effect for its possible usefulness as a brain stimulant or an antiasthmatic compound.

References

Pearson, William N. Flavonoids in human nutrition and medicine. *JAMA* 164, 1957.

CHAPTER 14

Deanol: A Biochemical Stimulant

A vitamin may occur in several different forms which the body can use to make an ultimately active product. These forms are termed vitamers. Two vitamers of the vitamin choline are ethanol amine and DMAE (2-di-methylaminoethanol). Both of these substances can be converted to choline in the body. They are important since choline is highly water soluble and does not pass membranal barriers easily. Such a barrier protects the brain from water-soluble substances which might be poisonous. Unlike choline, ethanol amine and DMAE readily pass through the blood-brain barrier. Pfeiffer et al. introduced DMAE in 1957 as a biochemical stimulant under the trade name Deaner (generic name deanol). The compound has found use as an anti-anxiety agent and as a substitute for drug stimulants in the treatment of hyperactive children.

Deanol has been slow in gaining clinical acceptance for several reasons.

1. Deanol does not have the immediate effect of a strong drug but rather the slow effect of a biochemical, so that the maximal beneficial effect may not be seen until after several weeks of therapy.
2. Side-effects will occur unless the deanol dose is reduced by

one-half as soon as maximal beneficial effects are found.

3. About 25 percent of patients do not respond to deanol therapy, and 10 percent of children may have increased emotional outbursts with deanol.

4. Psychometric tests are not sufficiently accurate to measure the slow improvement produced by a biochemical anti-depressant.

5. We lack a simple biochemical test which might tell us which patients will respond.

Animal studies of deanol have produced the following positive results:

1. Increased speed of learning of both avoidance conditioning and maze running;
2. Brain stimulation, as measured by various tests, in all animals tested;
3. More rapid passage to the brain than choline;
4. Increases of up to 60 percent in brain acetylcholine (Ach)—the working neurotransmitter of the brain;
5. Blocking of amphetamine toxicity in mice;
6. Increases in tolerance to alcohol and barbiturates in mice.

There have now been six double-blind studies of the effect of deanol in behavioral disorders in children. Of these, only one study showed no significant effect. In addition there have been numerous studies showing 45 to 70 percent behavioral improvement in children. The occasional young patient may surprise the parents by speaking for the first time when the parents have despaired because of lack of speech in a three- to five-year-old child.

Because acetylcholine-like stimulation of the brain benefits patients with many obscure diseases such as Huntington's chorea, tardive dyskinesia, l-dopa-induced dyskinesia, mania and blepharospasm, the use of deanol is now being tried in these various disorders. The doses used are large, namely 500 to 1,000 mg orally per day. In each instance we have found a decrease in the symptoms of the disease state. Obviously more confirmatory studies are needed.

Deanol has several advantages over Ritalin or the amphetamines in hyperactivity or learning disorders of children. They produce lack of appetite, insomnia and weight loss in a hyperactive child who already may have feeding problems. Both may wear off before noon, so that a second dose may need to be given at school, whereas a single morning dose of deanol usually lasts all day. Both drugs present a risk of abuse, while deanol does not because of its slow biochemical effect.

Deanol is effective in preventing the mind-racing and hypomania of paranoid schizophrenia. Many of our paranoid patients find effective relaxation when using 100 mg of deanol each morning.

Studies are now in progress on the use of deanol and its esters in elderly patients to produce greater alertness and better memory. The wise physician will first take care of primary nutritional imbalances such as copper excess and zinc deficiency and then carefully add metabolic stimulants such as deanol and perhaps thyroid, depending on the patient's symptoms.

References

Goldberg, A. M. and Silbergelb, E. K. Neurological aspects of lead-induced hyperactivity. Transactions of the American Society for Neurochemistry, 5th Annual Meeting, 5, no. 1:185, 1974.

Janowsky, D. S.; El-Yousef, M. K.; Davis, J. M.; Hubbard, B. and Sekerke, H. J. Cholinergic reversal of manic symptoms. *Lancet* 1:1236-1237, 1972.

Lewis, J. A. and Young, R. Deanol in learning disorders. *J. of Clinical Pharmacology and Therapeutics* 15:210, 1974.

Miller, E.: Deanol in the treatment of levodopa-induced dyskinesias. *Neurology* 24:116-119, 1974.

——— Dimethylaminoethanol in the treatment of blepharospasm. *New England J. of Medicine* 289:697, 1973.

Pfeiffer, C. C.; Jenney, E. H.; Gallagher, W.; Smith, R. P.; Beran, W.; Killam, K. F.; Killam, E. K. and Blackmore, W. Stimulant effect of 2-dimethylaminoethanol, possible precursor of brain acetylcholine. *Science* 126:610-611, 1957.

Walker, J. E.; Hoehn, M.; Sears, E. and Lewis, J. Dimethylaminoethanol in Huntington's chorea. *Lancet* 1:1512, 1973.

CHAPTER 15

The Fat-soluble Vitamins—A, D, E and K

Vitamin A

Night blindness, one symptom of vitamin A deficiency, was described in the Eber's papyrus in Egypt, a document thirty-five hundred years old; ox liver or the liver of black cocks was prescribed as a preventive. Hippocrates, the Greek physician, and the medicine men of Ruanda, Africa, also treated night blindness with ox liver.

In 1887, endemic night blindness was noted among Orthodox Russian Catholics fasting during Lent. Nursing children of fasting mothers developed keratomalacia, or degeneration of the cornea, now known to be a vitamin A deficiency.

In cases of night blindness Newfoundland fishermen have a home remedy, which is to eat codfish liver. This promptly restores their night vision.

Although liver is known to be an effective cure, not all varieties are innocuous. If individuals living in the Arctic eat polar bear liver they get hypervitaminosis A because of the liver's exceptionally high A content. Excess dietary intake of vitamin A may cause complete hair loss, skin peeling, severe headache, drowsiness and vomiting. In the sixteenth century, a

Dutch crew searching for a northeast passage to India ate large amounts of polar bear liver, resulting in severe skin loss.

An eye disease, xerophthalmia, was known in 1865 to be a product of malnutrition. It had previously been observed by slave traders bringing slaves from Africa to the New World. The decrease in secretions from the eyelids and the subsequent drying of the cornea caused blindness. Xerophthalmia was also observed in infants in Japan in 1904. It was again seen in Denmark in 1917, at which time there was a severe scarcity of food fats, most of the butterfat having been exported because of the war. Children subsisting on margarine and pork fat developed xerophthalmia and eventual blindness because of vitamin A deficiency.

The Two Forms of Vitamin A

Despite these early treatments of what are now known to be vitamin A deficiencies, the chemical characteristics of pure vitamin A were not known until they were discovered in 1922 by workers doing studies on cod liver oil. Feeding experiments had indicated that in vegetables with yellow pigments, carotenes (first isolated from carrots and hence the name), were structurally related to vitamin A and were converted to that substance in the living organism. By 1930, the chemical structure of the principal and most potent carotene, the beta form, was described by the researchers who had discovered vitamin A. With this knowledge, the way was paved for the identification of numerous syndromes indicative of vitamin A excess or deficiency.

The human body receives its requirement of vitamin A in two ways: by direct intake of vitamin A, or by eating foods containing beta-carotene, which is changed in the body into vitamin A. The carotenes are synthesized by plants, algae and certain bacteria with photosynthetic ability. In general, those vegetables with a stronger yellow or red pigment contain a larger amount of beta-carotene. Since the carotenes are precursors of vitamin A, they are often called provitamin A. Although beta-carotene predominates in nature, the other forms of carotene do exist in edible plant products. Alpha-carotene is found in palm oil and in mountain ash berries. Cryptoxanthene is a beta-carotene found in citrus fruits, green vegetables and fish liver—a slight chemical difference exists between that found in fresh-water and that found in salt-water fish.

Vitamin A and the carotenes are transported in the blood in a fat-protein complex. Vitamin E is known to prevent the oxidation of fats and is needed for adequate A uptake. Mobilizing vitamin A from the liver stores depends upon adequate protein nutrition and possibly on sufficient dietary zinc. In animal studies using weanling rats given identical amounts of vitamin A but fed a diet either deficient in or adequate in zinc, it was found that the blood plasma concentration of A was significantly lower in the zinc-deficient animals. This suggests that the animals deficient in zinc were not satisfactorily mobilizing vitamin A. When the animals were then fed a diet deficient in A and zinc, both the zinc and vitamin A concentrations in the liver declined and the animals exhibited symptoms of deficiency of zinc and vitamin A. When two groups were fed either vitamin A, or zinc plus vitamin A, the group given only the vitamin had a higher concentration of liver A than the others. The implication is that without plentiful dietary zinc, vitamin A accumulates in the liver due to inadequate mobilization from liver to plasma.

Liver reserves and blood levels of vitamin A vary widely and are generally higher for men than for women. But the blood level of vitamin A remains high even when liver storage is exhausted, so that serum levels are markedly affected only in extreme hypervitaminosis A or extreme hypovitaminosis A. In general, the American diet supplies the body with equal amounts of vitamin A and beta-carotene. Individuals in developing countries may ingest more beta-carotene and less A, owing to their predominantly vegetarian diet.

Carotene stored in body fat gives fat its color, which, therefore, varies with the diet. Vitamin A and beta-carotene combine with bile salts in the small intestine, pass into the blood and travel via the lymphatic system to the liver for storage. Inside the liver, hydrolysis by a liver enzyme produces retinol, or free vitamin A, which then works at the cellular level.

When a diet is low in fat little bile reaches the intestines, and both carotene and vitamin A may be lost in the feces (stool), thereby increasing the need for this vitamin. The use of mineral oil as a laxative will result in excessive loss of all fat-soluble vitamins via the feces. This vitamin loss, plus the occurrence of lipid tumors in the intestinal loops, has made mineral oil obsolete as a laxative.

Natural Sources of Vitamin A The primary sources of Vitamin A are fish and animal livers. The principal commercial sources are cod and shark liver oil. Vitamin A is also present in other animal products—egg yolk, butter, margarine, milk, cream and milk products. Since vitamin A occurs in foods of animal origin, it is fortunate for vegetarians that carotene, primarily beta-carotene, is synthesized in plants and can be converted to vitamin A in the body. The richest sources are apricots (fresh and dried), yellow, red and green vegetables, carrots, beets, beet greens, spinach, sweet potatoes, tomatoes, peaches, oranges, bananas and cantaloupe. It has been reported that even in the United States more than 26 percent of the households consume diets insufficient in A, primarily because some Americans may not drink enough milk or eat enough dairy products, eggs, fruits and vegetables.

Normal Physiological Function The function of vitamin A in the visual cycle was elucidated by Dr. George Wald, who was awarded the Nobel prize in medicine in 1967 for his findings on the biochemical role of vitamin A. The retina, with its nerve cells called rods (which are sensitive to low-intensity light) and other nerve cells called cones (which are receptive to high-intensity light and to colors), forms visual pigments by combining vitamin A aldehyde with opsin, a protein, to produce the retina visual pigments in rods (rhodopsin). The photosensitivity of the rods permits accurate measurement of vitamin A deficiency. Thus, vitamin A is essential for the visual apparatus to perceive light of variable intensities and colors.

Vitamin A affects the development of teeth in children. With deficiency, the enamel-forming cells become abnormal and the crystal structure becomes incomplete and weak. The integrity of epithelial cells depends on vitamin A, and deficiency affects the tissues of the skin, mouth, gastrointestinal tract and genitourinary tract. The process of epithelial change from vitamin A deficiency is called metaplasia; it evokes restoration of the basal cells, which proliferate to alter the nature of the epithelial surface. The mucous membrane cells of these epithelial organs grow but die more quickly; the layer of dead cells prevents mucoid secretion in the epithelium and the manufacture of corticosterone as well as other adrenocortical steroids.

In laboratory animals, vitamin A overcomes the inhibitory effect of steroids such as cortisone on wound healing (normal gain in tensile strength). Since cortisone-treated rats are unable to convert carotene to vitamin A adequately, carotene accumulates in the body.

Do You Have Xanthosis? Xanthosis, a yellow discoloration of the skin due to the excessive accumulation of carotene in the body and the deposition of superfluous carotenoid pigment in the epidermis, often occurs in anorexia nervosa, in diabetes and in cases of low thyroid function. People who make and eat beet or carrot cocktails (usually in a blender) also may exhibit yellow skin, since carrots and beets are high in carotene. The yellow discoloration is most evident in the palm of the hand. We have observed yellow palms in patients who eat spinach at each meal. It is interesting to note that chickens in European markets often look pale blue because European chicken feeds lack corn. American corn-fed chickens have yellow skin, especially since synthetic B-carotene is now added to most commercial chicken feed to make the egg yolk a deep yellow and the skin of the dressed chicken yellowish. We suspect that the meat from such chickens is high in carotene; we have observed yellow palms in hypoglycemic patients who subsist on a high-protein diet and eat the cheap American chicken as their main source of protein.

Vitamin A is commonly used in the treatment of skin problems, especially difficult cases of acne. Retinoic acid (Tretinoin), is a novel treatment for acne; it causes a more intense redness and skin peeling than other medications. The peeling, rather than the vitamin A, may be the effective portion of the treatment.

Vitamin A combined with calcium carbonate has been used successfully to prevent severe sunburn in susceptible individuals. (Pyridoxine and zinc also help.) Rats pretreated with vitamin A can withstand cold stress and the stress of steroid administration better than those deficient in A; and, when all other essential nutrients except A are present in the diet of laboratory animals, the growth of these animals is stunted compared to that of controls.

It is now known that vitamin A and carotene absorption are contingent upon adequate fat and protein uptake. Once in the body, vitamin A is essential for normal growth and dental health, for adequate appetite and digestion and for prevention of infections. The fat-solubility of vitamin A renders it toxic if taken in large quantities. The MDR (minimum daily requirement) is 1,500-4,500 IU (international units) for children and 5,000 IU for adults. Older patients and those on a fat-restricted diet may need 25,000 to 50,000 IU per day. In all patients with diseases in which absorption, storage or mobilization of A is impaired, increased amounts are required. Since normal individuals store the vitamin in their livers, adequate daily consumption is not needed, but is still recommended.

Deficiency and Intoxication In 1969, the United States National Nutrition Survey presented evidence before the Select Committee on Nutrition and Human Needs in the United States Senate that there was substantial vitamin A deficiency in the population. Thirteen percent of the population sampled at the time had serum vitamin A levels of 20 mcg percent, a clear deficiency level. Thirty-three percent of children under six years were deficient in vitamin A. The Food and Drug Directorate of Canada conducted a survey of vitamin A content of the livers of patients and discovered that 8 percent of one sampling had no stores of vitamin A at all. In India, Africa and other developing areas where fat intake is exceedingly low, vitamin A deficiency may be severe, even in the presence of carotene intake. Many are oblivious to the subclinical deficiency that may exist, although clinical deficiency is easily detectable.

Among the first signs of vitamin A deficiency is nyctolopia, night blindness. Characteristically, the patient has normal vision in daylight but has poor vision in dim light from failure of the visual mechanism. The World Health Organization cites vitamin A deficiency as one important cause of blindness in children of developing countries. Xerophthalmia, a manifestation of a greater degree of deficiency, is characterized by burning, itching, inflamed eyelids, and mucus in the corners of the eye and in the cornea. Literally, it means "dry eyes"; the lacrimal duct glands fail to secrete, producing inflammation of the conjuntiva and the cornea. Keratomalacia, a progression of xeropthalmia, produces severe degeneration and perforation of the cornea, resulting in permanent blindness. People working in extremely bright or dim light, such as typists, seamstresses or miners, need more vitamin A because such extremes cause more of the vitamin to be used up.

Faulty bone formation emerges from the delayed lesions of vitamin A deficiency. Intracellularly, it has been suggested by Lucy that vitamin A is involved in the electron transfer chain of membrane-bound enzymes, there being ten enzymes which are affected by vitamin A deficiency. Deficiency also initiates formation of thick bones caused by a disturbed reabsorption of old bone. Cases of dry, scaly, pruritic skin with a lower resistance to infection have also been reported with vitamin A deficiency. There is an increase in keratin which produces plugging of the hair follicles and a sandpapery roughness to the skin, principally on the backs of the arms and legs. Alteration of sebaceous (secretory) glands occurs and secretion may decrease. Hair lacks sheen and luster, dandruff accumulates on the scalp, and nails become brittle when vitamin A is lacking.

Chernov has reported a sharp drop in serum A in severely injured patients. The results of a study of randomly selected injured patients suggest that high doses of vitamin A reduce the risk of gastrointestinal ulceration in severely stressed patients. The severely injured patients entered a state of nitrogen loss and exhibited a high degree of protein deficiency; the sudden drop in vitamin A was directly related to a corresponding drop in serum protein. Chernov believes that the sudden depletion of serum A adversely affects mucous cells, initiating autolysis (tissue self-digestion) and failure to multiply normally. Malabsorption in the intestinal tract accentuates vitamin A and carotene deficiency which can be corrected with large oral doses.

Mental changes, lack of motor coordination, weakness and nerve degeneration have all been attributed to vitamin A deficiency. This is under some dispute, however, and evidence for the direct involvement of A in the metabolism of the peripheral and central nervous system is lacking. In the laboratory, rats with vitamin A deficiency develop neurological lesions characterized by inability to right themselves if placed on their backs. Zinc added to this diet accentuates the deficiency.

Poisoning with Vitamin A Most individuals consuming adequate vegetable and animal products will rarely contract vitamin A deficiency, but many individuals, especially those using A for therapeutic reasons, may inadvertently take too much. Intoxication with vitamin A has been reported in doses as low as 50,000 IU per day. The symptoms are red discoloration of the gums, craving for food, itchy skin, muscle stiffness, bursitis, headaches from increased intracranial pressure and lack of appetite. Pseudotumor cerebri, or vitamin A-induced benign increased intracranial pressure, may occur in individuals taking high doses for dermatologic reasons. Fisher has reported cases of hypercalcemia due to hypervitaminosis A with ingestion of 150,000 IU daily to mitigate acne, even though no hyperactivity of the parathyroid glands was present. Body size is a factor in toxic symptoms; in a group of oarsmen using "vitamins" to build muscles, only the coxswain developed signs of vitamin A overdosage. (The coxswain is chosen for small size and a loud voice!)

Acute hypervitaminosis A has been diagnosed in some adults. It is characterized by spontaneous onset and remission and may occur in an otherwise normal individual who has consumed a large amount of vitamin A over a short period. The syndrome consists of nausea, vomiting, skin peeling, intense headaches, vertigo, irritability, drowsiness, seizures and, eventually, coma. A six-year-old girl suffering from chronic hypervitaminosis A developed hepatic (liver) dysfunction and hypertension associated with clinical and structural evidence of liver damage.

Dr. Robboy and his coworkers have found a significant elevation of beta-carotene and its chemical relatives in the blood of eight patients with anorexia nervosa. The level was 90 mcg percent, compared to 23 mcg percent for controls and 4.4 mcg percent for cancer patients who had no appetite. Since this is an enormous difference and since anorexia occurs with hypervitaminosis A, the possibility of a block in the use of plasma vitamin A needs study in these patients. These patients are usually claimed by the psychologist or psychiatrist as belonging so firmly in his domain, that any metabolic lead should be carefully explored.

In the North Atlantic off Norway, a Dutch crew caught a 6½-foot halibut. One crewman ate two-thirds of a pound of the liver containing approximately 30 million units of vitamin A; he developed severe frontal headaches, nausea, vomiting, abnormal gait and red and swollen skin, with severe loss of the top layers of the skin.

The general tolerance for vitamin A is uniform, and there seems little risk of the development of vitamin A intoxication with prudent administration. As noted before, carotene excess, often seen in vegetarians, produces yellow skin (especially palms) but no serious toxic reaction; the condition is called carotenemia. One must remember that the fat-solubility of vitamin A may cause toxicity. Awareness of the symptoms of both toxicity and deficiency, as described above, may prevent difficulties. If toxicity symptoms should occur, prompt cessation of vitamin A intake will provide relief.

Vitamin A and the Schizophrenias It is noteworthy that the schizophrenic under stress may begin to show skin alteration, as manifested by acne and increased oiliness of the face and scalp from excess sebaceous gland excretion. Vitamin A levels decrease under stress along with the loss of zinc. An increase in vitamin A intake to 25,000 to 50,000 IU daily, in association with an increase in intake of zinc and vitamins B-6, B-2 and E, usually relieves the acne and decreases excessive oiliness.

Vitamin A is implicated in steroidogenesis in the adrenal glands. No definite recommendation can be made concerning the possible implication of vitamin A in the schizophrenic process. Although there appear to be neurological sequelae (locomotor ataxia) in severe vitamin A intoxication, and some old literature has suggested a relationship of vitamin A deficiency to mental changes, there is as yet no definite proof that vitamin A is directly related to mental disease. More study is needed, particularly on the use of adequate B-6, vitamin A and zinc.

Vitamin A is an essential body nutrient and should be consumed in adequate amounts each day. The requirement will vary with the individual, depending on the amount of fat, protein, zinc and vitamin E ingested daily. Most individuals are amply supplied with vitamin A, but if any of the previously mentioned deficiency or toxicity states should arise, proper treatment can prevent any serious complications.

Vitamin D

Relatively few individuals concern themselves with vitamin D, probably because they assume that the "vitamin A and D fortified" label on most milk cartons means that they are supplied with their dietary allowance. For most individuals the 400 IU added to milk may suffice, but even this small amount may be toxic for others. Toxicity is rare, but deficiency is commonly seen in premature infants or children having minimal exposure to the sun. This fat-soluble vitamin can be manufactured in vivo (in the body), but because of variable environmental and dietary conditions serious deficiency syndromes can occur and should be carefully anticipated so that effective treatment can ensue.

Cod liver oil has been recommended for prevention of bent legs (rickets) since the Middle Ages, but only in the present century has it been used with consistency. In 1919, McCollum et al. reported that cod liver oil from which vitamin A had been removed still retained its antirachitic (rickets-preventing) properties. Eleven years later the same scientists discovered the vital substance in cod liver oil—vitamin D. There are ten forms of this substance, but only two are nutritionally valuable. Provitamin D-2 (ergosterol) is found in yeasts and certain plants, and is changed into ergocalciferol (vitamin D-2) in the presence of ultraviolet light. The other provitamin D, D-3 or cholecalciferol, is considered by some to be a hormone because it can be made by the skin upon exposure to ultraviolet sunlight. Adequate exposure to the sun's rays insures sufficient vitamin D, but unlike sun-drenched lifeguards, many inner-city black children in northern climates have minimal exposure to smoggy sunlight and are among the most susceptible to deficiency.

The various pure vitamin forms of D are white, odorless, fat-soluble crystals. Although most natural food sources lack vitamin D, miniscule amounts are present in egg yolk, liver and fish—3½ ounces of sardines, herring or salmon provide the daily requirement. Fortified milk is among the best food sources of vitamin D. As with the other fat-soluble vitamins, vitamin D, whether ingested or manufactured, is absorbed in the intestine with the aid of bile salts. It is then carried to the liver to be transformed into 25-hydrovitamin D-3; it then travels to the kidneys via a protein carrier in the blood and is manufactured into the useable product. Dr. Anthony Norman attributes the dangerously low levels of calcium in kidney disease to the inability to metabolize the liver form of vitamin D to its biologically active form. With a supplement of 100 IU of vitamin D to his patients' diets, he obtained a significant improvement in internal absorption and an elevation of blood calcium level.

Among the normal physiological functions of vitamin D is its ability to regulate the absorption of calcium and phosphorous from the intestinal tract—it is believed that vitamin D renders the intestinal mucosa more permeable to these minerals. Due to its regulation of calcium uptake, vitamin D is also important to the calcification of bones and teeth. Delayed dentition or malformation of teeth can result from inadequate ingestion of vitamin D.

Hypovitaminosis D, as previously mentioned, causes inadequate absorption of calcium and phosphorous from the intestinal tract and faulty mineralization of bone and tooth structures resulting in skeletal malformation. Rickets, rarely observable in the United States because of milk fortification, may occur among children living in northern regions less exposed to the sun, or among individuals with darker skin and an inadequate ability to manufacture vitamin D. Premature infants are particularly susceptible since their greater need for growth and calcification imposes additional demands for vitamin D. Rickets is characterized by bowed legs, restlessness, irritability and lowered inorganic phosphorous. The high incidence of rickets prompted milk fortification.

Another deficiency disease is tetany, a syndrome marked by sharp flexion of the wrists and ankle joints, cramps and convulsions. Tetany is due to abnormal calcium-phosphorous metabolism caused by insufficient dietary intake or failure of absorption of vitamin D. Calcium salts, to control the spasms, and concentrated vitamin D comprise the remedy.

Osteomalacia is a deficiency syndrome in which bone calcification fails to parallel metabolic processes. Lack of vitamin D and inadequate calcium are its causes. It is prevalent in the Far East where many pregnant and lactating women remain indoors for much of the time and subsist on a cereal diet.

Hypervitaminosis D may be seen in individuals ingesting 1,800 IU or more. Toxicity symptoms are: nausea, vomiting, diarrhea, weight loss, excessive urination and uncontrolled nocturnal urination. As hypervitaminosis D becomes more severe, kidney damage and calcification of arteries and soft tissues may occur. Too much vitamin D deposits calcium and phosphorus released from the body's bony tissues in the walls of blood vessels, in the heart, in kidney tubules, and in bronchial passages. Adequate vitamin C may prevent the occurrence of these symptoms.

For infants who are constitutionally hyperreactive to vitamin D, the amount of this vitamin currently supplied by fortified dry and fluid milk often proves toxic. According to Dr. M. Seelig, a pharmacologist of the New York Medical College, this hyperreactivity to vitamin D may account for many infantile medical complications. H. B. Taussig suggests that a genetic trait allowing better utilization of vitamin D may cause this. Infantile hypercalcemia has developed in children on doses of vitamin D which are considered prophylactic. This excessive absorption of calcium in response to vitamin D also seems to indicate an infantile hyperreactivity to the vitamin.

Vitamin D requirements are not uniform, and what may

be appropriate for one individual may be toxic for another. Vitamin D-fortified milk has proven effective in eradicating rickets, but lower fortification levels of D in the United States than in England has resulted in fewer reported cases here of infantile hypercalcemia. Continued fortification will serve to maintain our low incidence of rickets, and awareness of hyperreactivity can prevent serious infantile disease. Pediatricians can advise parents at each visit.

The toxicity of vitamin D has clearly been encountered in the treatment of rheumatoid arthritis. Large doses have been used in the past, with the result that patients had calcium deposited in all of their main arteries. Deposition in the arteries of the kidney results in renal shutdown, elevated blood pressure and, sometimes, death. Large doses of vitamin D should not be used, for they may lead to disease which can be fatal!

Vitamin E (Alpha-tocopherol)

In 1922, Evans and Bishop in California discovered a new chemical substance now known as vitamin E. The absence of this substance led to irreparable damage to the germinal epithelium in male rats and to an inability in female rats to carry their young to term. It was designated the antisterility factor.

The word tocopherol was coined by combining two Greek words, *tokos,* meaning "childbirth," and *phero,* meaning "I bring" and the suffix -ol which indicates that a substance has properties of an alcohol. There are now four known tocopherols —alpha, beta, gamma and delta—all of which have physiological activity in the human being and the laboratory animal. The alpha form is the most active and is the one that is generally being referred to when the term "vitamin E" is used.

Since most of the early work done on vitamin E was connected with sterility, its action was at first believed to be limited to the reproductive mechanism. But vitamin E treatment in women who have a known history of spontaneous abortion has not, to date, been proven beneficial. Thus, in this respect, the vitamin's effectiveness seems to be limited to laboratory animals.

The currently accepted theory on vitamin E's function in the body is that it is an antioxidant—a substance which unites with oxygen to protect other chemicals from being destroyed or modified by exposure to oxygen. Support for this hypothesis comes from the ability of synthetic antioxidants unrelated to vitamin E to substitute for the vitamin in preventing certain deficiency symptoms. Researchers have also indicated that vitamin E inhibits the autoxidation of unsaturated lipids in vitro (in the test tube), but results have not yet been substantiated in vivo. J. Lucy disagrees with the antioxidant theory and feels that vitamin E interacts primarily with polyunsaturated phospholipids and fulfills a physiochemical role in the stabilization of cell membranes. Uncontrolled peroxidation (complete oxidation) of lipids leads to widespread damage to intracellular membranes, enzymes and certain metabolites. Vitamin E supposedly has the ability to unite with oxygen to protect the red blood cells from blood-destroying agents which would otherwise cause the cells to rupture.

The tocopherols are the main antioxidants present in unsaturated fats that protect the fats from becoming rancid. No harm results from taking polyunsaturated fats in natural substances—wheat germ, safflower oil, sunflower oil or soybeans—but if large doses of unsaturated fats are taken, vitamin E should also be taken to protect against oxidation. Ozone and nitric oxides oxidize the unsaturated fats, and vitamin E protects against such occurrences.

Although diets high in polyunsaturated fats (margarine, vegetable oils, fish) will increase the body's requirement for vitamin E, any of the polyunsaturated fats naturally contain the vitamin and may, accordingly, supply the body's needs. For example, margarine has thirteen times more E than butter; thus, when we ingest polyunsaturated fats we may need additional vitamin E, but we receive more vitamin E; so, theoretically, natural foods are already balanced.

Since the discovery of vitamin E, scientists have been searching for a human disease clearly indicative of vitamin E deficiency. Animal studies have indicated the existence of numerous effects of vitamin E deficiency; in most species, a severe vitamin E deficiency causes muscle wasting or dystrophy. Cattle deprived of vitamin E may die from a cardiac ailment; horses display increased fertility and endurance on vitamin E; guinea pigs, rabbits, sheep, goats, hamsters and calves develop muscular dystrophy (degeneration of skeletal muscle) in the absence of this vitamin.

In humans, the only known deficiency is probably a result of poor absorption, or of poor utilization, or of an increased vitamin E requirement peculiar to the individual. Oski and Barness reported in 1967 that babies suffering from hemolytic anemia—a premature destruction of red blood cells—were receiving milk formulas lacking in vitamin E. When a vitamin E supplement was given they promptly improved. In intestinal malabsorption, excessive fatty loss may lead to vitamin E depletion, and correction is made with vitamin E in water-soluble form. Individuals suffering from the relatively rare diseases of cystic fibrosis, celiac disease or sprue have an inability to absorb fat and, consequently, to absorb the fat-dissolved E. Thus, individuals with these or related diseases will be continually deficient in vitamin E. To date, no other deficiency syndromes have been reported, but the search continues for solid indications of the therapeutic usefulness of vitamin E.

Many claim that vitamin E arrests everything from acne to ulcers, with a myriad of illnesses in between; they usually prescribe 200 IU or more as treatment. The MDR has not yet been established, but the National Research Council recommends 5 IU for children and 30 IU for adults. (One international unit is equivalent to 1 mg of alpha-tocopherol in biological activity.)

The best sources of E are the vegetable oils from seeds—such as wheat germ oil, peanut oil and cottonseed oil. Green leafy vegetables, milk and eggs contain significant amounts, as do meats—particularly rabbit and squirrel meat. Alpha-tocopherol, the most active of the tocopherols, is sold as natural or synthetic vitamin E in sealed, opaque, soft gelatin capsules to protect it from light, heat and oxidation. Vitamin E is readily absorbed from the intestinal tract and distributed in fat and skeletal muscles. Since storage is quite effective, depletion in the total absence of dietary intake is very slow.

Little is known of the manner in which vitamin E produces its changes in the body. It appears to have a primary role as a lipid antioxidant, preventing the accumulation of free radicals within cells. Vitamin E is required for the synthesis of coenzyme Q, a factor in the respiratory chain that releases energy from carbohydrates and fats. Vitamin E has been shown to lower the levels of abnormal dienes in the blood and raise the level of antioxidant activity. Thus, the presence of abnormal fractions is reduced by vitamin E. The conjugated dienes presumably lead to the formation of toxic peroxidized fats, which can cause injury to the liver. Rat studies with administered vitamin E and selenium lead to the conclusion that selenium does not appear to influence the absorption or retention of vitamin E and does not affect the plasma level, but that it may modify its distribution in the tissues. Other studies have indicated that vitamin E works with traces of selenium in preventing certain types of liver pathology and red cell hemolysis.

Hemolytic anemia is frequently found in premature infants and infants fed a formula deficient in vitamin E. It is characterized by marked reticulocytosis, pyknocytosis, and shortened red blood cell survival. Unquestionably, this anemia responds to alpha-tocopherol. In addition, red blood cells that hemolyze spontaneously in vitro in a rare genetic disease (acanthocytosis syndrome) have had their hemolytic anemia corrected by vitamin E. When Dr. M. Horwitt put men on a low-vitamin E, high-polyunsaturated-fat diet, the vitamin E concentration in the blood decreased after a year and this was accompanied by an increased fragility of the red blood cells. This decreased red blood cell survival in vitamin E deficiency appears to be due to lipid peroxidation of the red cell membrane.

Vitamin E has been reported to reduce the side-effects from certain pain-relieving drugs such as codeine, morphine and aminopyrine. Vitamin E also apparently is involved with the enzymatic actions which are essential for smooth detoxification of many drugs. A relationship exists with vitamin A, in that adequate amounts of vitamin E allow greater storage of vitamin A. Vitamin E spares, and reduces the requirement for, vitamin A. Goodson and Bolles, upon administering vitamin E or a placebo to subjects suffering from periodontal disease, found a significant decrease in the fluid around the teeth of patients receiving vitamin E.

It has also been reported that intravenous injections of 200 to 400 mg of vitamin E, followed by oral administration of 200 to 300 mg of vitamin E has successfully stopped signs of digitalis intoxication, even while digitalis (a cardiotonic drug) continued to be administered.

Among other reported effects of vitamin E are its salutary effect in preventing the abnormal synthesis of porphoryn. Various metabolites of porphoryn were initially elevated in urinary excretion tests, but fell to normal following vitamin E administration. Because vitamin E deficiency seems to increase the susceptibility to porphyria, the vitamin must in some way be involved in the regulation of the inducible enzyme causing the porphyria. This has an implication in mental illness, since mental illness is related to abnormal porphoryn metabolism and the porphyrias.

In a study of pollution, the exposure of rats to 10 ppm of the oxides of nitrogen for four weeks produced reduction of polyunsaturated fatty acids. One group had vitamin E depletions. Additional exposure to 1 ppm of ozone resulted in death from lung congestion in all animals within twenty-two days, but the vitamin E-depleted group died within 8.2 days on the average, whereas those receiving the vitamin lasted 18.5 days. Vitamin E appeared to protect against the biological effects of these chemical air pollutants.

Vitamin E has also been reported to be effective in eliminating leg muscle cramps, in decreasing breast tenderness and congestion experienced by women premenstrually, and in treating intermittent claudication—a vascular condition in which the blood flow to the limbs is reduced and pain is experienced during walking.

Because, as an antioxidant, vitamin E prevents the oxidation of fatty acids, it has been claimed that it is useful in preventing odor in perspiration without disturbing the natural secretions. This vitamin has also been hailed as having a therapeutic effect on stretch marks, wrinkles and skin blemishes, but dermatologists consulted by Consumers Union have not found any conclusive evidence.

Finally, it has been claimed that vitamin E is effective as

a cure for cardiac diseases. In 1946 Drs. Shute, Shute and Vogelsang in Canada claimed that patients suffering from atherosclerosis, hypertensive, rheumatic and coronary heart disease could be benefited by administration of 200 units or more of vitamin E. Their claims were based on personal experience in treating patients. Since then, controlled blind studies have reported vitamin E ineffective in heart disease. The debate still continues but, as of today, no conclusive new evidence has provided documented proof of vitamin E's beneficial effect on heart disease.

Recently vitamin E has been much advertised. Periodically, new uses are found for the vitamin, new products are put on the market, and more money is spent by people searching for the answer to their problems. Vitamin E is needed by the body, as are all vitamins, and taking a supplementary dose is certainly nontoxic. Before purchasing, the consumer should be familiar with what has or has not been proven for the effectiveness of any given vitamin-containing product.

Vitamin K

The least known of the fat-soluble vitamins is vitamin K, perhaps because reported cases of overdosage or deficiency are rare. Its existence was first suggested by Dr. H. Dam who, in 1935, discovered that a "Koagulations Vitamin" was essential for normal blood clotting and thus prevented fatal hemorrhage in chicks. This quinone-type vitamin consists of a number of related compounds: K-1 (phylloquinone) was first isolated from alfalfa; K-2 is normally found in fish meal but is also produced in the intestine by bacterial synthesis. Both are fat-soluble, resistant to heat, and easily destroyed by irradiation, acids and alkalies.

Vitamin K is regularly produced by bacteria in the lower intestinal tract and requires normal bile for absorption. A large amount is excreted in the feces, but limited stores are maintained in the liver. Variation in intestinal synthesis and in diet has made an estimation of an RDA impossible. Individuals whose diets contain milk and unsaturated fats and are low in refined carbohydrates need not concern themselves with vitamin K deficiency. Yogurt eaters will increase the necessary intestinal bacteria and more vitamin K will be produced.

The newborn infant has a limited supply of vitamin K and, since the intestine may not manufacture the vitamin for the first few days, an adequate supply may be crucial. Human milk only supplies one-fourth as much as cow's milk, so that breast-fed babies sometimes need to be supplemented. The synthetic form of the vitamin may then be prescribed by the pediatrician. The best natural sources of vitamin K are the green leaves of plants (spinach, kale, cabbage and cauliflower) and liver.

The normal physiological function of vitamin K is the formation of prothrombin and other clotting proteins by the liver. High levels of vitamin K indicate good coagulation ability; a deficiency causes an increased tendency to hemorrhage.

The individuals most susceptible to a vitamin K deficiency are premature infants or anoxic (oxygen-deficient) "blue babies," and those born from mothers who are taking anticoagulants. Adults may become deficient because of absorption failure, interference in the intestine due to the continual use of sulfa drugs and other antibiotics, or an inability to form prothrombin in the liver, as in liver disease.

Because premature infants are sensitive to vitamin K deficiency and may hemorrhage profusely, most hospitals administer some vitamin K at birth. Abnormal clotting may occur if large amounts of K-containing vegetables are eaten while a patient is on anticoagulant drugs. The result can be a blood clot in the lung (pulmonary embolism) or elsewhere. Conversely, aspirin can add to the anticoagulants' effect and produce abnormal bleeding.

The body's ability to manufacture its own vitamin K, with the aid of proper diet, means that there is relatively little vitamin K deficiency or overdosage. The supplement given infants by modern hospitals helps prevent early deficiency, and precautions should be taken if anticoagulant drugs are used. Otherwise, we are amply supplied.

References

Vitamin A

Chernov, M. S. *Amer. J. Surgery* 122:674-677, 1971.

Ebrahm, G. Vitamin A deficiency—a continuing health problem in developing countries. *Clin. Ped.*, 1972.

Furman, K. Acute hypervitaminosis A in an adult. *Amer. J. Clin. Nutr.* 26, 1973.

Lucy, J. A. et al. Studies on the mode of action of excess vitamin A. Part I: *Biochem. J.* 79:497-500, 1961. Part II: *Biochem J.* 89:419-425, 1963.

Robboy et al. The hypercarotenemia of anorexia nervosa: a comparison of vitamin A and carotene levels in various forms of menstrual dysfunction and cachexia. *Am. J. Clin. Nutr.* 27, 1974.

Rubin, E.; Florman, A.; Degnan, T. and Draz, T. Hepatis injury in chronic hypervitaminosis A. *Amer. J. Dis. Child* 119:132, 1970.

Tev et al. Chronic vitamin A intoxication. *Med. J. Australia*, 1973.

Zinc: a trace element essential in vitamin A metabolism. *Science*, 1973.

Vitamin D

McCollum, E. V. et al. *J. Biol. Chem.* 53:293, 1922.

Robinson, C. *Fundamentals of normal nutrition.* New York: Macmillan, 1972.

Seelig, M. Are American children still getting excess vitamin D? *Clin. Ped.* 9, No. 4: 380, 1970.

——— Hyper-reactivity to vitamin D. *Medical Counterpoint*, 28 July 1970.

Taussig, H. B. On the evolution of our knowledge of congenital malformations of the heart. *Circulation* 31:768, 1965.

——— Possible injury to the cardiovascular system from vitamin D. *Ann. Intern. Med.* 65:1195, 1966.

Vitamin E

Horwitt, M. K. work mentioned in: E the little known vitamin that sparks vitality. *Family Circle* August 1971.

Oski, F. and Barness, L. Vitamin E deficiency: a previously unrecognized cause of hemolytic anemia in the premature infant. *J. Pediat.* 70:211, 1967.

Robinson, C. *Fundamentals of Normal Nutrition.* New York: Macmillan, 1972.

Shute, E. and Shute, W. *Your heart and vitamin E.* Detroit, Michigan: The Cardiac Society, 1956.

Vitamin E: What's behind all those claims for it? *Consumer Reports*, 6 January 1973.

Vitamin K

Dam, H. *Nature* 135:652, 1935.

——— *Biochem. J.* 29:1275, 1935.

PART THREE

Essential Trace Elements Open New Vistas

INTRODUCTION

The study of the human body's need for trace elements is now at the exciting stage that characterized the study of new vitamins in the early 1930s. Thanks to Dr. A. Prasad, Associate Professor of Medicine at Wayne State School of Medicine, we now know that zinc deficiency occurs in man and we eagerly await the availability of Walter Mertz's "glucose tolerance factor" (GTF), a chromium-containing organic molecule which should lower cholesterol, make insulin more active and perhaps help the hypoglycemic patient.

At a recent conference, Dr. E. J. Underwood of Australia estimated that there are fourteen to fifteen essential trace elements. Since his authoritative book does not include sulfur, the actual number may be sixteen. The biochemical role of these trace elements is sometimes first found in plants and then proven in animals. Finally, studies may be initiated to see if man needs these elements as much as the lower species do.

As life evolved from sea water, the simple enzymes and the building blocks of existence used the materials at hand. The major salts of sea water—namely, sodium, potassium, calcium and magnesium—combined with chloride, phosphate and carbonate to provide the general matrix for cells. The enzymes and vitamins evolved in highly specific and specialized forms to incorporate the trace elements from sea water into the cells. For example, fluorine in tooth enamel is held in a tight complex similar to the mineral apatite. Without fluorine this enamel, and even the bones, become deficient in calcium. With weakened tooth enamel, dental cavities will occur more rapidly.

A second example of a trace element is cobalt. Cobalt is firmly combined in a hemoglobin-type molecule to produce vitamin B-12 (cyanocobalamin). This molecule is chemically very stable and is made by many lower forms of life—yet not by man. Since B-12 is needed by man, it is designated a vitamin. Alone, cobalt is not needed; an excess of cobalt is a heart poison.

Zinc provides us with a third instance of a trace element. Zinc has been incorporated into almost twenty enzymes in the human body. These enzymes may be involved in many important functions, such as burning sugar and phosphorylating (attaching a phosphate group to) vitamin B-6. In zinc deficiency, B-6 will not function because the phosphate group cannot be attached. Many of the functions of B-6 and zinc concern the transformation of amino and nucleic acids, the basic building blocks of proteins and cells.

Many scientists have contributed to the study of trace elements, but the medical pioneer is Dr. Henry A. Schroeder of Brattleboro, Vermont. There, on the Vermont hillside, with clean air from the pine forest, he and his colleagues have made notable achievements. Some of these are:

1. The exact delineation and definition of how to recognize a trace element.

2. The exact delineation and definition of how to recognize a toxic or antagonistic element.

3. A description of the antagonisms between the many types of trace elements and between essential trace elements.

4. The discovery that cadmium produces elevated blood pressure in several species of animals, and the suggestion that cadmium excess and zinc deficiency may be a major factor in early heart disease and hardening of the arteries.

5. The suggestion that a molybdenum deficiency may be a factor in some cases of gouty arthritis.

6. A description of the "body burden" of toxic elements which accumulate in modern man with the aging process in a polluted environment.

7. Interpretation of the findings of nutritionists and biochemists to the all-too-unheeding medical profession. It is to be hoped that orthodox medicine will read more frequently and listen more closely to Henry A. Schroeder, the pathfinder. Dr. Schroeder's recent book, "Trace Elements and Man," should be read by all.

References

Mertz, W. Trace element nutrition in health and disease: contributions and problems of analysis. *Clin. Chem.* 21:468, 1975.

______ Some aspects of nutritional trace element research. *Fed. Proc.* 29: 1482-1488, 1970.

Schroeder, H. A. *The trace elements and man.* Old Greenwich, Connecticut: Devin-Adair, 1973.

CHAPTER 16

Zinc as an Essential Element

During these days when the cloudy viewpoint of the FDA limits the clinical investigation of DMSO (dimethylsulfoxide) because massive doses in the dog produce lens cloudiness, we recall the eye-opening history of an antituberculosis drug named ethambutol (Myambutol Lederle). This drug represents a solid chemotherapeutic advancement but, even more, a genuine triumph for man over animals in the realm of chronic toxicity.

The Question of Testing in Man

In 1960, an international gathering of clinical pharmacologists assembled in the Midwest to discuss the amount and type of animal data needed before trials in man could be started on a new candidate drug. Some were ultraconservative and wanted extensive animal studies, and some wisely stated that almost everything should be carefully tried in man since animal studies can only give guidelines as to biochemical systems which might be blocked or damaged in man.

To test the faith of the liberals, Dr. Paget (then with the Imperial Chemical Industries in Britain) stated that he had made extensive chronic toxicity studies of an effective chemotherapeutic agent against tuberculosis but that, unfortunately, it produced blindness in three different species of animals at the high dosage used in the chronic toxicity studies. Could this be tested in man?

Most looked at him incredulously, but some of us had faith in man's biochemically unique structure and suggested cautious trial in a few patients with slowly increasing dosage—if permission could be obtained from the local drug committee and the patient volunteers.

What helped some of us to keep the faith were faint but distinct memories of a time when we charted eye grounds weekly in patients receiving tryparsamide therapy for their neurosyphilis. Some may also have recalled that extremely large doses of quinine (tonic water) can reduce human vision by action on the retina.

Quite independent of the British study, a division of the American Cyanamid Company, Lederle Laboratories, had developed a drug which they knew to be a chelater of zinc ions and which was also highly effective in tuberculosis. In the dog, chronic toxicity testing disclosed that the drug at high dosage produced a pallor of the *tapetum lucidum* (iridescent layer of choroid of the eye). This is the membrane in the back of the eye that is responsible for the bright reflections (eye shine) from animal eyes when it is activated by automobile headlights. This membrane acts as a photomultiplier to allow animals to see better in the dark. The fluorescent reaction depends on an adequate supply of zinc-containing enzymes, so that the pallor produced by the candidate drug was understandable and on a sound scientific basis. The zinc was chelated and partially removed. Human and other primate eyes do not have a *tapetum lucidum;* therefore, cautious clinical trial in tuberculosis patients was started, and the drug was found to be highly effective.

In the meantime, chronic toxicity testing in the cat disclosed retinal detachment at the high dosage used. The highest level of zinc in the human brain occurs in that extension of the brain which is the retina of the eye. Thus, zinc is also important in the visual process in man.

As a trace metal, zinc is important in biochemical processes of tissues other than the retina. Therefore, great reassurance was supplied by Dr. Buyske and his colleagues at Lederle when they completed their dog and monkey studies which showed that the trapping or chelation of zinc by ethambutol was much greater for the eye than for the pancreas, heart or liver. The clinical trials still went forward cautiously, with careful attention being paid to the vision and ophthalmoscopic (eye) findings in each patient.

With all these warnings from the faithful laboratory animals, imagine the dismay of the clinical investigator when he discovered on morning rounds a tuberculosis patient who appeared to be reading the newspaper upside down! The patient admitted he had not been able to read newspaper print for several days. The drug was discontinued and the patient's vision soon returned to normal. At a later date, reinstitution of ethambutol therapy at a lower dose was not accompanied by any reduction of visual acuity.

The patient's explanation for pretending to have normal vision was simple—and a real moral lesson. He had been hospitalized for more than five years with tuberculosis and had not responded to surgical or standard drug treatments for his tuberculosis. In spite of the best available medical care, he saw himself going out the back door of the hospital as had many of his friends. He, personally, chose to go out the front door—even if he went out blind! This is a logical choice for anyone to make!

Dr. I. D. Bobrowitz of New York City, one of the pioneer clinical investigators of ethambutol, stated in 1966 in the *Annals of the New York Academy of Sciences:*

> There was not a single instance of definite eye toxicity due to ethambutol (i.e., complaints of poor vision, poor color discrimination, decrease in visual fields, and scotomas.) There were many patients on our study in whom there were fluctuations in reading of the Snellen eye chart with a reading loss or improvement. These variations occurred with similar frequency in all regimens, with or without ethambutol.

At the same New York Academy of Sciences Symposium, Drs. Donamae and Yamamoto, of Japan, reported that they had found side-effects in only 22 out of 187 patients treated with ethambutol. The drug was stopped in only 5. In 3 cases the drug was discontinued because of a decrease in visual acuity which later returned to normal.

The drug package insert that accompanies Myambutol gives careful directions for the evaluation of eye changes and the need for constant testing of vision, as with the now historic tryparsamide chemotherapy.

The critical and authoritative *Medical Letter*, in its 31 May 1968 issue, states: "With the doses now recommended, reported ocular effects have generally been minor and reversible, though one consultant has noted some permanent loss of visual acuity due to ethambutol in two patients."

The drug has been acclaimed by Dr. Gordon Meade, Director of Medical Education for the American Thoracic Society, as "An excellent drug . . . that will probably be widely used." The drug is particularly beneficial when used with the previous antituberculosis drugs to prevent the development of drug-resistant strains.

Ethambutol still can produce blindness in many species of lower animals, but thanks to the ability and patience of the pharmacologists, pathologists and clinical investigators at the Lederle Laboratories, the drug has been assayed in man and found to be useful in the treatment of one of man's oldest maladies—tuberculosis.

This human-interest saga reinforces the statement made repeatedly by Bernard B. Brodie that new drugs must be tested in man as well as in animals. We must not let animal studies or governmental committees, either local or national, interfere with the continued fight against crippling diseases. Perhaps this ethambutol report may help to get DMSO out of its present limbo.

Since the whole human populace is borderline-deficient in zinc, these side actions of ethambutol might be lessened if each tuberculous patient were given a dose of zinc and vitamin B-6 at a time interval spaced away from the ethambutol therapy. In the early days, many schizophrenic patients succumbed to tuberculosis and many more had chronic tuberculosis. In one Illinois state hospital the percentage of tuberculous mental patients was 6.5. Early investigators postulated that a toxin from the tubercle bacillus might cause schizophrenic symptoms, since the patient who got well from his tuberculosis also got well from his schizophrenia.

Perhaps the good nutrition therapy of the past, including foods containing zinc, may be the common denominator in the treatment of both diseases. With soil depletion of zinc and other essential elements, the old-fashioned nutrient-and-rest therapy for tuberculosis might not be effective today. Fortunately, we now have specific antituberculosis drugs.

Discovery of Zinc as an Essential Element The Wisconsin group of biochemists who carefully determined in 1928 that copper was needed, concluded from animal experiments by 1934 that zinc was an essential element also. They concluded that man needed zinc, but E. J. Underwood of the Institute of Agriculture University of Western Australia, in 1962 stated in *Trace Elements in Human and Animal Nutrition* that zinc deficiency had never been observed in man. However, a skin disease of pigs, reported in 1955 by Tucker and Salmon, was found to be a zinc deficiency, and at about that time animal feeds were supplemented, since O'Dell and Savage had shown that chickens also needed extra zinc for maximal growth. Some feeds and dog foods are supplemented to the extent of 200 ppm of zinc as soluble salts. This extra zinc has increased feed efficiency up to 25 percent in swine and poultry and is one of the reasons for the comparatively low cost of pork and chicken in the United States.

The American *human* diet contains only one-tenth that of animal feed, namely 15 to 25 ppm of zinc. Soil exhaustion, food processing, careless cooking and the consumption of junk foods all contribute to this low level. Man should get 15 mg of zinc per day, but analyses of well-rounded diets served at cafeterias and hospitals show that only 8 to 11 mg of zinc per day is provided. Institutional diets are even lower in their total available zinc content.

Lack of Zinc in Soils Since zinc, like iodine, sulfur, and selenium, occurs in the soil as water-soluble salts, excessive rainfall can leach the zinc from the soil. Glaciated areas (e.g., many northern sections of the United States) may have soils deficient in zinc. This is well known to agriculturists who advise the addition of zinc to fertilizers. In Florida, where the sandy soil has little in the way of trace elements, zinc is a routine metal in fertilizer. Some land plants accumulate from the soil as much as 16 percent of their ashed weight as zinc. When a crop containing 100 ppm of zinc is removed from a field, the soil will lose 1 ppm of zinc. The average soil contains only 50 ppm of zinc, so theoretically 50 such annual crops would exhaust the soil in fifty years or two generations. Some of the fertile lands of the earth have been tilled for many centuries and their zinc content is totally exhausted. Such soils occur in Egypt, Iran and Iraq, where the first zinc-deficient humans were found.

Dwarfism, Hypogonads and Failure of Sexual Maturity In 1961 Prasad, Prasad and Halsted published a detailed clinical study of eleven Iranian male dwarfs who, in addition to iron deficiency, had, by modern tests, zinc deficiency. The symptoms were dwarfism at the age of twenty years, infantile sex organs and lack of mental acuity. The iron deficiency was corrected without improvement. Later, in a controlled study on seventeen male dwarfs, the control group of eight on a normal diet required 224 days for normal sexual activity, while the nine fed the normal diet plus 100 mg of zinc sulfate each day developed normal sexual function in 59 days—4 times as fast. These twenty-year-old dwarfs grew in height because the growing ends of the long bones had not closed. The hospital diet produced 4.2 cm of increased height, while the same diet plus zinc produced 10.5 cm—more than twice as much.

The normal diet of the Iranian villages from which these patients came consisted in large part of unleavened bread which contains phytate, a compound that prevents the absorption of zinc. (In the cities of Iran leavened [yeast-raised] bread is used.) We now know that the biochemical process of leavening bread destroys the phytate.

What Factors Modify Our Zinc Intake? At present no factor *increases* our zinc intake. In the "olden days," the use of galvanized (zinc-coated) food-processing vessels resulted in some useful zinc contamination. Now stainless steel is used instead. In the case of water pipes, acid well water took off some of the lining of the galvanized pipes and provided zinc (but also some cadmium because the zinc was not pure). Now acid drinking water gives us too much copper.

Many factors *decrease* the effective zinc in food and water in modern society. If the plant, grain, fruit or nut has enough zinc from the soil, then it will have a normal zinc level. In the case of lettuce, we know that farmers can grow great greenery without the requisite zinc and manganese if they just put lime and nitrate on the soil. With *adequate* fertilization and scientific farming, the zinc should be there for the eating!

Scientific farming differs from organic farming in that the available trace elements such as zinc are determined and the fertilizer adjusted to fit soil conditions. Organic farming may (as in Europe) add the manure of animals that have been fed 250 ppm of copper in their food. Manure from animals with this amount of copper can poison the soil of the unsuspecting organic farmer! The easiest type of scientific farming is hydroponics, wherein only diluted minerals—and no soil—are used. Sprouting of seeds for food approaches scientific farming.

Food Processing Removes Zinc Food processing is designed, however, to remove anything from food that will discolor, turn rancid or attract bugs. Bugs cannot grow without zinc, so 80 percent of the zinc is removed from wheat flour in the milling process. Cornstarch has much less zinc than corn meal. Frozen peas have less zinc than backyard peas because the surface layer of trace metals is removed with EDTA to produce a brighter green when the peas are cooked. This can happen to broccoli and spinach too! This bright green may be more appealing but is certainly less nutritious.

In the preparation of foods, the vegetable pot liquor may go down the drain, taking the water-soluble zinc salts with it. (But if not thrown away, the water used to cook vegetables may be high in copper from the copper plumbing or pan bottom, and copper antagonizes zinc in the body!) Red meat is a good source of zinc, but the hamburger may contain the cheaper protein from the soybean which is high in copper and low in zinc. The frankfurter may be loaded with cereal which, with its phytate content, will prevent the absorption of any zinc which wanders in with the meat. The oyster is commendably high in zinc, and 100 gm of Atlantic oysters will provide 120 mg of zinc —enough for a whole week if the body could only store zinc. However, along with the zinc in the oyster there occurs copper in large amounts and cadmium in great excess if the oyster is grown in contaminated waters. This makes the oyster less desirable as a source of zinc. Under the best circumstances, the level of zinc in any modern diet may be minimal, contaminated or downright missing. Hence the need for zinc supplements.

Levels of Zinc in Man All told, Bartlett's *Familiar Quotations* list 101 separate items on gold. Silver merits 39 items and *zinc is not even listed.* Yet, to the body, zinc is more precious than gold. This is "Truth purer than the purest gold."

While rodents and nocturnal animals have higher levels of zinc in the back of the eye (retina), man in general has higher tissue levels of zinc than animals. If we except the retina and pineal gland in the brain, the highest level of zinc in the brain is in the hippocampus, where histamine is also present.

Several studies have been made on trace metals in the brain. Harrison et al. in 1968 studied copper, zinc, iron and magnesium distribution in the human brain. They found copper to be highest in the caudate nucleus, zinc and magnesium highest in the hippocampus and iron highest in the globus pallidus. Ibata and Otauka, in 1969, using histochemical techniques, found zinc to be present mainly in the terminal vesicles of the nerve endings of the hippocampal formation of rabbits and rats. The zinc was distributed as follows: hippocampus, 95 ± 38 mcg per gm; caudate, 81 ± 21; putamen, 75 ± 13; globus pallidus, 69 ± 16; corpus callosum, 49 ± 30; thalamus, 58 ± 9. Thus, of the parts of the brain tested, the hippocampus has the highest zinc level.

Since zinc occurs with histamine in both basophils and mast cells, one can speculate that the terminal vesicles of the mossy fibers of the hippocampus may be histaminergic—that is, a nerve impulse may be generated when histamine is released.

Histamine: Neurotransmitter Stored with Zinc Histamine is a biochemical which normally occurs in all soft tissues of the body. It is made by the removal of the acid group from the amino acid histidine. This amino acid can apparently be made in the bodies of adults but perhaps not in those of children. Histidine is usually not listed with the essential amino acids. Both histamine and histidine will chelate, or nab onto, trace elements such as copper and zinc. Perhaps because of this, histidine is available as a food supplement and is occasionally used in the treatment of arthritis. We know that one factor in arthritis is a tissue overload of copper, iron or other heavy metals—thus, the chelating action of extra histidine is beneficial in that these metals are removed from the body.

Swedish scientists have studied histaminergic nerves for many years, and others have noted that histamine will increase stomach acid secretion and salivary secretion. Histamine may therefore be a humoral agent which will be released in the brain and cause the transmission of neuronal impulses. Dr. Michaelson of Cincinnati was the first to use the ultracentrifuge to separate the rat brain into particles of various sizes to test for the presence of histamine in the small vesicles which carry the neurotransmitters in the brain cells. He found histamine in this vesicle fraction, and his work has been confirmed by Kataoka and De Robertis of Buenos Aires and also by Snyder and Taylor of Baltimore.

All of these workers have studied the subcellular localization of histamine in rat brain, using the same separation methods that have been used to demonstrate the presence in synaptic vesicles of the other brain transmitters acetylcholine, norepinephrine, dopamine and serotonin. When the mitochondrial and microsomal-20 fractions are disrupted, a high concentration of histamine is found in these vesicle subfractions. The presence of histamine in small nerve endings and in synaptic vesicles of rat brain cortex suggests a transmitter role for histamine as well as for the other biogenic amines. In other words, histamine is a neurotransmitter in some as yet unspecified portion of the brain.

Several workers have studied the hippocampal mossy fibers for their zinc content; others have studied these same areas of the brain for histamine content. These studies are doubly important in that these may be histaminergic fibers, and the hippocampus is an important structure in regard to integration of thoughts, memory and emotions. If the histamine, of the histaminergic nerve fibers, is stored with zinc, as histamine appears to be in both the mast cell and the basophil, then a functional role of histamine storage could be ascribed to the zinc in the terminal vesicles of the mossy fibers.

The use of zinc in the storage of the neurotransmitter histamine of the hippocampus has been suggested in 1971 by Niklowitz. Haug et al., in the same year, found that the depletion of zinc in the hippocampus after degeneration of the mossy fibers is compatible with the concept of a neurotransmitter role for zinc. McLardy, in 1973, found a decrease in the cells of the hippocampus in both schizophrenics and alcoholics. Any deficiency in mossy fiber cells, or of zinc or histamine in the cells, might result in schizophrenic behavior.

Other Signs of Zinc Deficiency While the original studies on zinc deficiency in males disclosed infantile sex organs, dwarfism and anemia, we know that many more signs and symptoms of zinc deficiency can be detected by the informed clinical observer.

Skin The skin may show striae (stretch marks) over the hips, thighs, abdomen, breasts and shoulder girdle. Young ladies present themselves with mental difficulties and with striae of the skin to such an extent that they cannot wear a bikini. Young men who have tried to exercise away their disperceptions by weight lifting present themselves with striae in the skin of the shoulder girdle. As one lad put it, "I was in a YMCA class in weight lifting and I was the only one out of twenty-five who developed stretch marks. I could feel my skin breaking as I lifted the weights." His initial blood serum level of zinc was 60 mcg percent, compared to a normal of 100 mcg percent. Hair and nails do not grow well and the brittle nails may have white spots or be generally, opaquely white in zinc deficiency. The hair will be brittle and lack pigment, and may change to a deeper color with zinc therapy. We have seen carrot-red hair turn to auburn and dead-white hair turn to rich brown. The facial skin may have acanthosis, a severe form of acne; the skin lesions frequently clear with zinc and vitamin B-6 therapy.

Sex and Endocrine Problems The zinc-deficient girl may not have a regularly established menstrual cycle until age fourteen to seventeen, or the menses may start at thirteen, only to skip for months or even a year. If treated with birth control pills (to regularize the cycle) the patient will have a rise in serum copper which may precipitate depression and intensify disperceptions. However, if placed on vitamin B-6 and zinc, these patients usually establish a normal menstrual cycle within two to three months. Since normal ovulation may start first, it is even possible for a young lady who is at risk (if she is not using effective contraceptive measures) to become pregnant before she menstruates.

With impotent young males who are zinc deficient, a return of sex function may take as long as four to five months of daily zinc supplementation. They may sometimes have an abnormal fear of microphallus (small penis), but with zinc and vitamin B-6 the sex organs develop to full size and the beard and axillary hair become more abundant. Masturbation or sex become more gratifying.

Joint Pain Painful knee and hip joints may plague the teen-ager who has zinc deficiency. One such patient had such painful knees that he chose rowing in prep school because he knew he could not run. We know that poultry with zinc or manganese deficiency get hock disease. We know that active children in the eight-to-thirteen-year-old period are subject to interruption of the blood supply of the growing head of long bones (Perthes' and Osgood-Schlatters' diseases). The zinc-deficient patient has cold extremities with poor peripheral circulation. Because of previously acquired needle trauma, these patients may dread having to give a blood sample. Frequently we must warm the hand and arm before blood can be obtained. They may faint with blood sampling. As they become less zinc-deficient, blood taking is no longer an ordeal; furthermore, they no longer faint. With poor circulation and this tendency to faint, the zinc-deficient patient is a poor risk for dental anesthesia and other operations. Care should be taken to recognize the zinc-deficient patient and correct the deficiency before elective operations. Not only will the patient be prone to shock, but bleeding can be abnormal and wound healing will be delayed.

Retarded Wound Healing Drs. Walter Pories and William Strain have pioneered in the careful study of wound healing in zinc-deficient patients. Most surgeons give salt, glucose and sterile water to their patients in the postoperative period; some surgeons realize that the alcoholic needs more magnesium and vitamins; some surgeons use Ringer's solution which contains the chlorides of sodium, potassium, calcium and magnesium. Some surgeons prepare their patients for operation by assessing nutrient status and give them preoperatively what their patient lacks. Drs. Pories and Strain use zinc salts preoperatively and postoperatively to promote wound healing and to correct zinc deficiency.

Stress of any kind depletes the body of zinc—so much so that the burned patient ends up with body tissue zinc at such low levels that normal healing is retarded. Some of these patients have serum zinc levels of 30 mcg percent (one-third of normal)! Most burn centers now use dietary zinc supplements in all their patients, many of whom are young and need all the zinc they can get for normal growth. Burns are so painful that the stress causes great losses of zinc via the urinary pathway and also in the exuding of fluid from the burned area.

Loss of Taste Several side actions of chelating agents should have suggested that one of the vital trace metals was involved in the sense of taste. When penicillamine was introduced for the treatment of Wilson's disease (excess copper) the side-effect of loss of taste occurred as the excess copper was removed from the body. But chelating agents (and penicillamine is no exception) are seldom specific for a given metal. With penicillamine, copper and zinc are both removed and the zinc must be replaced or side actions such as loss of taste occur.

After publishing his finding that copper, nickel and zinc were involved in loss of taste, Dr. Robert I. Henkin finally settled on zinc deficiency as the main factor in hypogeusia (loss of taste). Older patients, particularly those with cancer, are particularly prone to this annoying symptom. When the mother has loss of taste, she oversalts all the food served to the family. When loss of smell and taste occur, the usual early recognition that food is burning or the house is on fire must depend on other members of the family or other senses such as the visual detection of smoke or flame.

Dr. Henkin and his colleagues (for no good reason in our opinion) are against correcting the loss of taste with the most common salt, zinc sulfate. Numerous studies have shown that zinc sulfate is as well absorbed as other zinc salts, and chelated zinc has no special virtues. Dr. Henkin has not recognized that many patients with loss of taste are also deficient in vitamin B-6 (pyridoxine). (Zinc will not work without other nutrients, including vitamin B-6.) In our clinical experience, patients with loss of taste should be given B-6 for the first two days. Otherwise, zinc alone can increase hallucinatory experiences and/or depression. Patients with loss of taste are usually severely depressed, and for a good reason: the food they eat tastes like so much sawdust.

Birth Defects The nauseated pregnant woman is usually deficient in both vitamin B-6 and zinc. Both are needed for growing tissues of any kind, and the fetus in the uterus makes extraordinary demands on the mother's supplies. Vitamin B-6 has been used for nausea and vomiting of pregnancy with uneven success. We have had many pregnant patients who had difficulty with previous pregnancies go through a pregnancy on a zinc and B-6 nutrient program with no difficulties.

Several workers, notably Dr. Lucille Hurley of the University of California, have shown that zinc deficiency in pregnant rats will result in many stillborn pups and that those born may have one of a number of birth defects. Dr. Caldwell and his colleagues in Detroit have shown that the rats born of zinc-deficient mothers are mentally retarded and do not learn as well as rats born to zinc-supplemented mothers. Our colleagues visiting Iran and Egypt are told that 30 percent of the young children are slow learners. These areas of the world no longer have available zinc in much of the soil.

TABLE 16.1

Clinical disorders and possible zinc deficiency

Syndrome	*Associated B-6 deficiency*	*Scientist*	*Place*
Dwarfism	+	**A. Prasad**	**Iran**
Poor growth	+	**Hambidge**	**U.S.A.**
Hypogonadism	+	**Prasad**	**Iran**
Hypogonadism	+	**Caggiano et al.**	**U.S.A.**
Wound healing	?	**W. Pories**	**U.S.A.**
Loss of taste and smell	?	**R. I. Henkin**	**U.S.A.**
Cadmium poisoning	?	**H. A. Schroeder**	**U.S.A.**
Cirrhosis of liver	+	**Sullivan et al.**	**U.S.A.**
Parenteral nutrition	+	**M. E. Shils**	**U.S.A.**
Poor circulation	?	**J. H. Henzel**	**U.S.A.**
Childhood hyperactivity	+	**Allan Cott**	**U.S.A.**
Epilepsy	+	**A. Barbeau**	**Canada**
Diabetes	+	**E. J. Underwood**	**Australia**
Enlarged prostate	?	**I. M. Bush et al.**	**U.S.A.**
High cholesterol	?	**H. G. Petering**	**U.S.A.**
Effects of oral contraceptives	+	**R. Alfin-Stater**	**England**
Psoriasis	?	**Voorhees et al.**	**U.S.A.**
Cutaneous striae	+	**Pfeiffer et al.**	**U.S.A.**
Pregnancy, nausea	+	**Pfeiffer et al.**	**U.S.A.**
Kwashiorkor	?	**S. Kumar and K. S. Jaya-Rao**	**India**
Acanthosis	+	**Hallbook**	**Sweden**
Acrodermatitis enteropathica	+	**E. J. Moynahan**	**England**
Acne	+	**Pfeiffer et al.**	**U.S.A.**
Sickle cell disease	?	**S. Dash et al.**	**U.S.A.**
Lack of ovulation	+	**Pfeiffer et al.**	**U.S.A.**
Impotency & amenorrhea	+	**Pfeiffer et al.**	**U.S.A.**

Coarse hairs—eyebrows	**?**	**F. M. Dementzis**	**Greece**
Body and breath odor	**?**	**F. M. Dementzis**	**Greece**
Pyroluria, white spots in nails, lack of dream recall, disperceptions, hallucinations, or depression	**+**	**Pfeiffer et al.**	**U.S.A.**
Retinal detachment	**+**	**Pfeiffer (postulated)**	**U.S.A.**
Reye's syndrome	**?**	**Pfeiffer (postulated)**	**U.S.A.**

Male Growth Lag Have you ever attended an eighth-grade dance and seen tall girls dancing with boys who only came up to the girls' shoulders? In contrast, at the junior prom or twelfth-grade dance, you see girls only coming up to the boys' shoulders. Why do the boys lag in growth behind the girls? One does not see this disparity in growth between the two sexes in the animal kingdom, where most pet foods are over-adequate in their supply of zinc. Gaines dog food, for instance, has a zinc content which is a hundred times the recommended level. Male pups do not lag behind the females in growth as they become sexually mature.

The sex organs of boys are loaded with zinc in their mature or functioning state. During puberty, as the prostate, seminal vesicles and testes develop, the body's borderline zinc supply is taxed severely to provide all the zinc needed for the male sex glands to function. To compensate, the voracious appetite of the growing male teen-ager finally overcomes this hypothetical, but probably real, zinc deficiency in the four-year period from eighth to twelfth grade.

Since junk foods and soft drinks contain no zinc, the growing teen-ager who consumes them needs, more than ever, his whole grains, eggs, milk, vegetables and meat. We know from the Iranian male dwarfs that short stature and hypogonadism can result from zinc deficiency. Parents should make sure that this does not happen to their son, since failure to develop sexually can lead to many neuroses.

Summary In summary, then, the situations in which zinc deficiency or copper excess may occur are:

1. During pregnancy, when growth and development require zinc.
2. During the first year, when the newborn has excess copper and needs zinc to balance the copper.
3. During rapid growth, the child requires adequate zinc.
4. From the twelfth year, zinc is required for normal pubertal development of the male, and deficiency may cause a growth lag. The pubertal development of the female may require less zinc.
5. During the teen-age years, at the time when zinc is lowest and copper is high, premenstrual tension occurs. This is an endocrine effect which might be corrected with additional dietary zinc.
6. From fifteen to twenty years, stress of any kind causes loss of zinc, and in some people stress causes the excretion in the urine of kryptopyrrole, which takes with it both zinc and vitamin B-6.
7. In adult life, chronic zinc and B-6 deficiency may predispose cells to cancerous change. Wounds and burns require zinc to heal. Hypertensives are high in copper and low in zinc.
8. In older patients who suffer from confusion resulting in senile behavior, the confusion may be caused by excess copper.

Stretch Marks in the Skin (Striae) Clinicians have known that the stretched skin of the abdomen of the pregnant woman may break under the surface layer and leave scars. This also happens in some obese individuals. Surprisingly, many women go through several pregnancies without any stretch marks. This indicates that nutritional or familial factors may be involved. We see many young people with stretch marks in the skin owing to normal growth at puberty. The skin of the breasts, abdomen, thighs and hips is frequently scarred with these subcutaneous breaks. These breaks in the connective tissue also occur in diabetics and in persons who have excess cortisone secretion.

The two major components of connective tissue are collagen fibers and elastic fibers. The collagen fiber is formed by fibroblasts in the healing of wounds; the elastin is formed outside the cell in a manner similar to the manufacture of our modern polymers. Elastin is built rapidly and perfectly during normal growth, and the elastic fiber lives as long as the individual. Elastin comes from four molecules of lysine in a process furthered by lysyl oxidase—a copper-containing enzyme. This enzyme requires pyridoxal phosphate (vitamin B-6) to make either collagen or elastin fibrils (very small muscle fibers found in striated muscles). Vitamin C is also necessary in this process to stabilize the easily oxidized chemical groups of a metallo enzyme (enzyme containing a metal, such as a copper-containing enzyme). Both zinc and copper are needed for effective cross-linking of the elastin chains to make the perfect elastic tissue. When imperfect, any overstretching will cause long tears which appear as striae or stretchmarks.

Copper-deficient animals lack pigment in their hair and die of ruptured elastin in their main arteries. Zinc-deficient animals have hock disease—imperfect formation of cartilages—and cannot make B-6 phosphate. Animals deficient in B-6 would also lack skin and hair pigment, since B-6 phosphate is needed in the formation of both elastin and collagen. The biochemical cause of the stretch marks in teen-agers with pyroluria is thus understandable, because both vitamin B-6 and zinc are lost from the body in abnormal amounts.

Fingernail White Spots: Possible Zinc Deficiency Many children and teen-agers and a few adults have white spots in the fingernails. These occur more frequently in the nails of the index and little finger of the dominant hand—i.e., the right hand for right-handed individuals. Trauma is thus a factor, but not the primary cause, since patients with numerous white nail spots will also have such spots in the toenails. White banding may occur in the nails of both hands.

Attention was called to these spots or paired bands by

R. C. Muerhcke in 1956. He ascribed the phenomenon to a serum albumin level lower than 2.2 gm per 100 ml. His largest group of patients suffered from nephrosis, and those in a second group had hepatic cirrhosis. All had low serum albumin levels. Two patients responded to cortisone therapy with disappearance of the white banding, and several patients responded to albumin-replacement therapy. We now find that spots or paired bands will occur in patients with zinc and pyridoxine deficiency that is metabolically induced by the abnormal excretion of kryptopyrrole derivatives which combine chemically with pyridoxal phosphate and then complex with zinc. These patients have normal serum protein levels but are zinc and pyridoxine deficient. The major portion (70 percent) of the serum zinc is bound to albumin and our observations are therefore in accord with Muerhcke's findings, since patients with albuminuria also have a significant zincuria and patients with hepatic cirrhosis have a very low serum zinc level.

Our suggestion is that the metabolic white banding of finger and toenails is primarily the result of zinc deficiency. This deficiency can be caused by zinc loss due to albuminuria as well as in other ways. We further find that with therapy, only small white spots resolve; large white spots must grow out with the fingernail, a process taking five to six months. The banding of the nails may result from the menstrual cycle in the female. Copper level is high and zinc is low one week before the menstrual period when women are more liable to depressive disorders.

Religious days of fasting may cause white spots that can be traced to the food abstinence in orthodox Jews, some of whom, like some of the rest of the populace, are borderline deficient in zinc.

An acute psychotic episode may be accompanied by the broad white banding. Fasting with inadequate intake of zinc may accompany the psychosis.

The minimal daily requirement for zinc is 15 mg, but analysis of various diets shows an average of only 11 mg. Zinc deficiency may be aggravated by the ingestion of excess copper, as in drinking water or in vitamins plus minerals, many of which contain 2 mg of copper in each tablet. The situation can also be aggravated by increased estrogen ingestion—for example, in contraceptive pills. Pfeiffer and Iliev reported in 1972 that estrogens raise ceruloplasmin and serum copper and lower serum zinc.

Fingernail furrows known since 1846 as Beau's lines are crosswise depressions in the nail produced by a fever lasting a week or more. These furrows grow out with the nail so that the approximate date of the severe fever can be estimated by the slow forward march of the furrow, which takes one month to appear. The growth of the adult fingernail is 0.104 to 0.108 mm per day. The entire nail is replaced in 5½ to six months, but women with long nails may provide the doctor with almost a year of nail growth to inspect. (Once polish is removed!)

Women's nails are more brittle than men's. When men go on estrogens their nails become brittle within six months. The birth control pill makes women's nails more brittle. Brittle or thin nails are not helped by gelatin therapy. Nails are made stronger by zinc and sulfur supplements to the diet. The zinc can be in the form of zinc gluconate tablets, and the sulfur is most conveniently given as eggs (yolks). The diet should, of course, contain adequate protein.

Dermatologists have named these white spots *leukonychia*. Some internists have stated (without giving evidence) that these spots are deposits of calcium. The more frequent occurrence of these spots in teen-agers than in atherosclerotic patients is evidence against the calcium hypothesis. Actual analysis shows no increase in calcium, but the zinc level rises, as does the copper level.

The types of white spots are summarized below (see Figure 16.1).

1. Frequent small white spots in the nails of people living in historically glaciated countries. (Glaciers leached iodine, sulphate, selenium and zinc from the soil.)
2. Fasting or "Yom Kippur" white spots. (The whole populace is so borderline deficient in zinc that one to two days of fasting may produce white spots.)
3. Menstrual white bands. (Serum zinc is low at the menstrual

period, while serum copper is high. This results in rhythmic monthly banding, since six months are required for the nail to be replaced.)

4. Weekly or fortnightly bands produced by dietary binges.

5. White bands seen in backpackers, perhaps because of zinc lost in sweat and also because of their frequent avoidance of red meat in their backpacked diet.

6. Influenza white spots, with a furrow in the nail if the patient had a high fever at the time of the influenza. (If the patient is not zinc deficient, only the furrow occurs. Pecarek and Biesel have shown that most types of virus infections deplete the body of zinc.)

7. "We ran out of zinc" white spots. (Teen-aged patients will develop white spots if they fail to take their zinc dietary supplement over a weekend or if they run out of zinc before the next visit to the physician.)

8. A homogeneous white opacity in the entire nail, instead of white spots. (When adequate zinc and vitamin B-6 are given, sections of the nail corresponding to the months in which this therapy took place have a normal pink appearance.)

9. After treatment with zinc, the opaque part of the nail grows out and is replaced by normal healthy pink nail.

Miller Laboratories of West Chicago, Illinois, markets a Zn-Plus which contains 5 mg of zinc combined with soy protein and torula yeast. For most people this dose of zinc would be too low, and the company has not proven that better absorption of zinc occurs with their product. Several studies have shown that zinc as the sulfate is adequately absorbed. The other PDR (1974) preparations of zinc are too low to be useful.

Plus Products have a Formula 85 which contains 15 mg of zinc as the gluconate plus unstated amounts of manganese and magnesium in a mixture of bone meal and dolomite. The price is competitive with that of zinc gluconate tablets.

For use by children, most pharmacists, on a doctor's order, will make up a 10 percent solution of zinc sulfate which can be used three drops morning and night. This dose provides 5 mg of zinc in soluble form, which for a child would approximate half of the needed daily intake.

Zinc is like many other trace metals: the body will ordi-

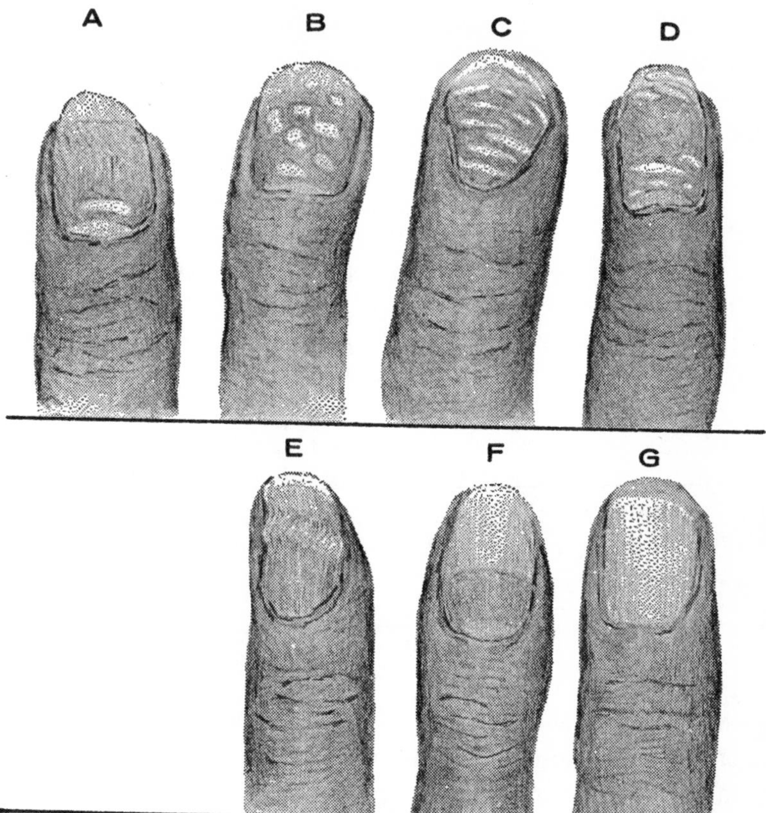

Types of white spots on fingernails (leukonichia) seen in zinc-deficient patients

A. Isolated white spot originating from a period of fasting or altered diet. Yom Kippur fasting, or a day of anorexia can cause such a white spot. A back-packing trip (which usually does not include fresh red meat as a source of zinc) can also produce a white spot. A hospital stay of 5 days also caused a white spot indicating the low level of zinc in that hospital's diet.

B. Multiple white spots in the finger and toe nails of an eleven-year-old child whose serum zinc level was low and whose behavior was inappropriate.

C. Monthly white bands or menstrual white spots in a female pyroluric patient. Copper is high and zinc is low premenstrually when many women feel depressed.

D. White spots in the nail of a female pyroluric patient who ran out of zinc and vitamin B-6 after a 2½ month period of treatment. The center band of normal-appearing nail represents the period of zinc therapy.

E. Opaquely white nail of an older pyroluric patient who also had hypertension and elevated serum copper. The hypertension responds to zinc and vitamin B-6 therapy and the nail becomes normal pink in color.

F. Opaquely white nail after 3 months of zinc B-6 therapy.

G. White spot in a depression in the nail (Beau's Groove) caused by a virus infection with a high fever. Virus infections cause a loss of zinc via the urinary pathway and the altered metabolic rate of a fever results in the transverse groove.

narily take from the intestines only the daily needed amount; the rest will not be absorbed. An exception might be metallic zinc in an oily base, since an Iranian youth became oversleepy when he ingested zinc and peanut butter.

What Doses of Zinc Are Safe? In the latest edition of the *U.S. Pharmacopoeia* zinc sulfate is listed as a substance to be used orally as an emetic. For a while a midwestern company that markets zinc sulfate $7H_2O$ in pellets of 220 mg could not ship its product to the many surgeons interested in wound healing without a label reading, "Dissolve 4 tablets in water and use as an emetic"! This peculiarity of bureaucracy is a hint as to the safety factors of the soluble salts of zinc. If too much is taken, then vomiting will occur. The patient who slowly takes increasing amounts of zinc will probably develop diarrhea before he has nausea and vomiting. Either of these symptoms requires a decrease in dosage.

As with most trace metal salts, only a certain percentage of the swallowed zinc dose will be absorbed from the stomach and intestine. An excess may lead to nausea and diarrhea. In the case of iron, we are only modestly protected and children can easily be poisoned by eating a bottle of candy-coated iron salt tablets. The same may be true of soluble zinc salts if they are ever (God forbid!) supplied in the form of candy-coated pills. Even the dose forms presently available should be kept out of the hands of children.

As Dr. Murphy reported in the *Journal of the American Medical Association* in 1970, a lad of sixteen living in Tehran, Iran, read in *Time* magazine for 19 November 1965 that zinc was good for wound healing. He had a minor wound, and he had just purchased 12 gm of elemental zinc to use as a rocket fuel. He therefore mixed the zinc with peanut butter, spread it on his bread, and ate it all to speed his recovery. The next day he had difficulty awakening and staying awake at breakfast. He also fell asleep in school. The sleepiness increased over the next four days and on the fifth day he was taken to the U.S. Air Force hospital in Tehran for treatment.

On the morning of admission he was difficult to arouse, but when awakened he consumed a normal breakfast and then returned to sleep while sitting on a stool. He was dizzy, staggered as he walked, and wrote illegibly. He had no nausea and denied any diarrhea. Reflexes and speech were normal, and he successfully completed simple psychological tests. Many laboratory tests were done, and the only abnormalities were slightly high activities of serum lipase and amylase. He recovered the next day and a follow-up a month later disclosed no abnormality. On the eighth and fifteenth days after dosing, his serum zinc level was not abnormally high.

We know that ingestion of alcohol with fat will delay absorption of the mixture, so the slow release of zinc from the peanut butter might be expected. It is surprising that this rash act did not result in greater harm. As a matter of fact, if this procedure could ever be proven safe, many insomniacs would consider zinc and peanut butter a real blessing. The elemental zinc must have been of high purity; otherwise the lad would have ended up with cadmium or lead poisoning. Both of these substances are more poisonous than zinc.

The most recent scientific study on the safety of zinc in man was done by Czerwinski et al. in Oklahoma in 1974. To sixteen geriatric patients these doctors administered 220 mg zinc sulfate three times a day, which is a large dose for patients in their sixties. Diarrhea occurred in six of the sixteen patients. In four weeks plasma zinc rose from a normal average of 100 mcg percent to 150 mcg percent and remained at this high level for the twenty-four week duration of the study. Some behavioral tests indicated that several of the zinc-treated patients might have benefited. The urinary, blood, kidney and liver tests did not differ from the findings in the fourteen patients who, as controls, received placebo capsules. From this and other studies we can state that this large dose of zinc as the sulfate is probably very safe.

Most patients do not need 220 mg doses, particularly when zinc is given with B-6 and E vitamins. The one exception may be those patients with psoriasis. Vorhees et al. found in 1969 that these patients need more than the usual zinc dietary supplement.

The elevation of serum zinc from a normal of 100 mcg percent to 150 mcg percent might seem dangerous. If more B-6 were given the rise might have been less. However, we have many patients who are deficient in B-6 and live for months with serum zinc levels of 150 to 300 mcg percent. These levels fall to the 100 to 150 mcg percent range when adequate B-6 is given. These patients may have an increase in their abnormal mental symptoms if zinc dietary supplementation is started before the B-6 deficiency has been treated. In epileptics, seizures may increase unless the B-6 therapy is started first.

In summary, we have treated over 1,700 patients with zinc dietary supplements, using various salts, and have not seen a serious side-effect attributable to the zinc alone. The use of a double dietary supplement such as zinc and manganese in a ratio of twenty to one can raise blood pressure. This is helpful in the hypoglycemic, but in the older patient the blood pressure level must be monitored at regular intervals.

Case History: Fran and the Fried Oysters Before listing the food sources of zinc, we must summarize the case history of Fran, a baby adopted at the age of two weeks in August 1955. Although Fran was overactive as a baby, her parents saw no evidence of difficulty until she started school, where she repeated the first grade because of poor learning.

Her behavior and learning problems seemed to be emotional in nature, but psychological counseling did not help. In the sixth grade she was diagnosed by a psychiatrist as having minimal brain dysfunction and later by a clinic as having learning disabilities involving poor visual perception and auditory memory.

At age thirteen her pediatrician, believing her erratic and irritable behavior might be caused by low blood sugar, finally hospitalized her for three weeks and placed her on a high-protein, sugar-free diet plus vitamins. After she had been in the hospital a few days her behavior—which had been extremely antagonistic and uncooperative much of the time—dramatically and suddenly changed. The unprovoked temper tantrums involving ranting and raving, the cruel swear words—all suddenly stopped.

The parents tried to keep her on a sugar-free diet at home. However, for a less-than-cooperative teen-ager this was almost

TABLE 16.2

Dietary supplements of zinc, magnesium and manganese in the physicians' desk reference (PDR)

Manufacturer (sells to pharmacies)		*Pharmacist (sells to the public)*
Meyer Laboratories, 1900 W. Commercial Blvd., Ft. Lauderdale, FL 33309.		*Willner Chemists, 330 Lexington Avenue, New York City, NY 10016.*
Vicon-C		*Zimag-C*
Ascorbic acid	**300 mg**	**is the same as Vicon-C**
Nicotinamide	**100 mg**	
Magnesium sulfate, USP	**70 mg**	
(As 50 mg dried magnesium sulfate)		
Zinc sulfate, USP	**79 mg**	
(As 50 mg dried zinc sulfate)		
Thiamine mononitrate	**20 mg**	
D-calcium pantothenate	**20 mg**	
Riboflavin	**10 mg**	
Pyridoxine	**5 mg**	
Vicon Plus		*Ziman Fortified*
is the same as the above with 4 mg of manganous chloride added.		**is the same as Vicon Plus.**

Supplements

Health food stores now have in stock zinc tablets (as the gluconate) in various sizes. The 15 mg content of zinc is the most popular since this represents the daily needed intake of zinc metal for each adult.

impossible, especially since she seemed to have a craving for candy. They learned, after repeated experiences, that candy or candy wrappers could usually be found in her room after one of her destructive tantrums. However, she still was in much better condition than before they knew about the sugar. She still was immature, had very poor logic, made mostly C's and D's in school. But the tantrums had decreased in frequency and in degree.

Her parents had noticed several years before that after

Fran had eaten fried oysters she was always unusually alert and cooperative—and never had any tantrums. So they all ate fried oysters an awful lot. They kept wondering what could be in the oysters that could have this effect on her. The parents' massive reading program included the book *Orthomolecular Psychiatry,* in one chapter of which Pfeiffer describes a high-histamine-level patient in a way that seemed to fit Fran and recommended a zinc dietary supplement. They also found, in a book on nutrition by Roger Williams, that oysters contained 143 mg percent of zinc and that the next best source of zinc was roast beef, with only 6.4 mg percent zinc. This had to be the answer!

Although the parents had tried megavitamin therapy without any significant improvement, they had again started Fran in August 1973 on a closely supervised megavitamin dosage of mostly vitamin C, niacinamide (2 to 3 gm daily) and B-6. After four months of this therapy, they could not ascertain any significant improvement. Then, on 27 December 1973, they gave her the first dose of zinc. The very next day she was positively improved. Within two weeks after she had started the zinc she had (1) obtained her driver's license (for two years she had had a learner's permit but had not wanted to try for the license); (2) obtained a full-time job from midnight to 8 A.M. (the first job she had ever had); and (3) enrolled in a college for a three-hour-per-day course (she had been out of high school for several weeks and had not previously expressed any desire to attend college). Although after two more weeks she had to drop the college—no time for sleep—they just couldn't believe the change that had taken place in their Fran.

They continued the megavitamins for two months and gave her one Vicon Plus (Meyer Lab multivitamin with 80 mg zinc and 4 mg manganese) in the morning and one chelated zinc (Rich-Life, Inc., 200 mg zinc) in the evening. Then, they stopped the megavitamins completely (except what was in the Vicon Plus) but continued the zinc. There was no discernible change —the very great improvement remained. They continued the zinc for a total of 3½ months (from 27 December), then stopped everything to see what would happen. For two days there was little change, but on the third day Fran had a "blowup"—a real temper tantrum. The next day, another. This one included the ranting alone in her room. It was the first time such ranting had taken place since she had begun receiving the zinc. One week after they stopped the zinc her behavior had deteriorated so much that they felt they had to resume it. They gave her the zinc capsule at 8:30 A.M.; by 6:00 that night she was, once again, a changed person—and continues to be, as the zinc is continued.

Fran still has problems. She is immature, still has poor logic (although this seems to be improving) and few friends. Her parents have a strong feeling that she has lost the sugar compulsion, although they are not yet certain. But after eighteen years of watching Fran try to cope with her frustrations and failures, the parents thank God she is not in prison. No one can imagine how much the parents are enjoying the new Fran. They say, "She has a great sense of humor, is considerate and fun to be around. *There is no doubt whatsoever in our minds that zinc has saved her.*"

TABLE. 16.3

Food sources of zinc

Mg per 100 gm=3 oz

*Vegetables **		*Sea foods*	
Peas	4.0	Atlantic oysters	143
Carrots	2.0	Herrings	100
Beets	0.93	Hard clams	21
Cabbage	0.80	Soft clams	17
Watercress	0.56	*Meats*	
Asparagus	0.32		
Rutabaga	0.30	Pork liver	9.0
Lettuce	0.30	Beef liver	5.5
Potato	0.29	Lamb	5.3
Corn	0.25	Beef	6.4
Tomato	0.24	Chicken thigh	2.8
Sweet potato	0.23	Chicken breast	1.1
Cauliflower	0.23	*Cereals **	
Green beans	0.21		
Turnip greens	0.21	Wheat bran	14.0

Turnips	**0.08**
*Fruits **	
Dates	**0.34**
Banana	**0.28**
Pineapple	**0.26**
Red currants	**0.20**
Lemon	**0.17**
Prune juice	**0.16**
Cherries	**0.15**
Apricots	**0.12**
Orange juice	**0.11**
Grapefruit juice	**0.10**
Cantaloupe	**0.09**
Pears	**0.08**
Peaches	**0.07**
Apple juice	**0.07**
*Nuts **	
Whole nuts	**3.42**
Peanut butter	**2.0**
Whole oatmeal	**14.0**
Wheat germ	**13.3**
Whole corn	**2.5**
Unpolished rice	**1.5**
White rice	**0.5**
Breads	
Whole rye	**1.34**
Whole wheat	**1.04**
White	**0.12**
Dairy products +	
Whole egg	**1.5**
Egg yolk	**1.5**
Egg white	**0.02**
"Egg Beaters"	**0.46**
Cow's milk	**17-66**
Human milk	**2-138**
Human colostrum	**70-900+**

* Actual level in food crops depends on adequate zinc level in the soil. Many soils are deficient. In the case of cereals, the calcium phytate present in the products will prevent the absorption of zinc. Thus, the available zinc may be less. The feeding of copper to chickens and pigs (a practice which is legal at 250 ppm of copper in England and Europe) results in high copper and low zinc levels in the liver. These livers frequently end up in liver sausage which may be inedible because of the high copper content. Foods or drinking water high in copper can negate much of the zinc obtained from food.

+The human infant is born loaded with copper. This can be corrected by an adequate zinc intake. Notice that human colostrum (first breast secretion) is high but variable in zinc content, perhaps for this specific purpose. But note also that the variability of human milk is from *2 to 138* mg percent, while the better-fed cows have a variability in the zinc content of their milk from only *17 to 66* mcg percent. Rather than on milk from a zinc-deficient mother, the baby might thrive better on cow's milk. The obvious answer is to give the mother zinc.

Zinc Responsive Disorders In Farm Animals

For more than fifty years, New Zealand agriculturalists have sought effective means of preventing and treating a fatal disease which afflicts farm animals in this country during the autumn. The disease, caused by a fungus toxin found in certain pasture grasses, produces liver damage and severe facial eczema (abnormal sunburn) in sheep and cattle. It has cost New Zealand farmers millions of dollars in deaths, damage to stock livers and lower production.

Recent studies, based on the observations of Mrs. Gladys M. Reid, a New Zealand dairy farmer, indicate that zinc sulfate is an effective prophylactic for the disease. Mrs. Reid has long been concerned over the numbers of New Zealand breeding stock that develop difficulties late in pregnancy. Extreme muscular weakness, a teetering walk, failure to eat enough and gain weight, eczema on the face and at the base of the tail, failure to lift the tail with subsequent soiling and lethargy precalving are symptoms of what New Zealand farmers term "the sulky cow syndrome." If the animal does not collapse in the last week of pregnancy, she will produce a dead or weak calf after prolonged and stressful labor.

Mrs. Reid found that animals who suffer this condition could be revived by coaxing them to eat hay soaked in molasses and a special proprietary stock meal, both extremely high in zinc.

Mrs. Reid was familiar with the studies of Dr. Jean Apgar of the U.S. Agricultural Research Service which showed that zinc deficient laboratory animals suffer considerable lethargy in advanced pregnancy and have a long and difficult labor. She began administering zinc sulfate to her "sulky cows." Given one teaspoon (about 5 grams) of zinc sulfate "straight down the throat" even the most seriously ill animals ("downer cows") were on their feet within hours, their appetites returned in several days and they gave birth to healthy calves.

Zinc is stored in the liver and Mrs. Reid observed that the collapse of the cow with toxin-induced liver damage occurred at the same time, and in a similar manner, to the collapse of the zinc deficient animal at the birth of the young. In fact, most of the "sulky cows" were professionally diagnosed as suffering from previous liver damage.

Mrs. Reid's observations interested scientists of the Ruakura Agricultural Research Center near Hamilton, New Zealand. In laboratory studies, these scientists found that rats fed synthetic diets deficient in zinc became severely ill and died shortly after administration of the fungus toxin while rats fed synthetic diets supplemented with zinc escaped serious liver damage when the fungus toxin was administered and survived.

In field trials, using sheep and milking cows, large doses of oral zinc sulfate significantly reduced toxin-induced liver damage following administration of the fungus toxin. Scientists conclude that oral zinc sulfate, in large doses, will protect farm animals against the fungus toxin.

In another study, New Zealand veterinarian, Dr. B. F. Rickard, divided a group of 50 yearling calves affected with facial eczema into two mobs. Twenty-five calves were treated with oral zinc sulfate while the remaining calves served as controls. Within 10 days, the treated group showed considerable improvement. The animals' skin lesions were healing well, they gained weight and their coats began to shine. Animals in the control group failed to improve and many died.

These studies confirm Mrs. Reid's observation that zinc sulfate is the key to solving the animal health problem which has long troubled New Zealand farmers.

Mrs. Reid has also found zinc supplementation beneficial for improving the health and disposition of young animals. Weaning is a stressful situation for the little calves. Separated from their mothers, the calves refuse to eat, crowd together and bellow constantly. When she recalled that Dr. Apgar had found zinc to be stress-protective, Mrs. Reid put zinc sulfate in the weanlings' watering troughs. The following day the young animals were peacefully grazing and were spread all over the paddock.

Mrs. Reid further notes that when calves are fed extra zinc they are happy and play. She comments that, "in a large herd, the younger animals are pretty low on the social order. After a few days on zinc sulfate, the calves kick their heels in a frisky fashion. They walk in a purposeful way and their tails are not soiled because they lift their tails high to defecate in a purposeful way."

Mrs. Reid's experiences indicate that the addition of zinc salts to farm watering troughs could contribute greatly to the prevention of disease states and the promotion of optimal health in farm animals.

References

Apgar, J. Effect of zinc repletion late in gestation on parturition in the zinc deficient rat. *Journal of Nutrition* 103: July 1973.

Bush, I. M.; Sadoughi, N.; Shah, M. S. and Berman, E. Zinc: a key urological element. Presented at the meeting of the American Urological Association, Washington, D.C., 1972.

Caldwell, D. F. et al. *Proc. Soc. Exp. Biol. Med.* 133:1417, 1970.

Calhoun, N. R., Smith, J. C. and Becker, K. L. The role of zinc in bone metabolism. *Clinical Orthopedics.* 103:212-234, 1974.

Czerwinski, A. W.; Clark, M. L.; Serafetinides, E. A.; Perrier, C. and Huber, W. Safety and efficacy of zinc sulfate in geriatric patients. *Clinical Pharmacology and Therapeutics.* 15:436-441, 1974.

Dolar, S. G. and Keeney, D. R. Availability of Cu, Zn and Mn in soils. *Journal of Science Fd. Agriculture* 22:273-286, 1972.

Fernandez-Madrid, F., Prasad, A. S. and Oberleas, D. Effect of zinc deficiency on nucleic acids, collagen and non-collagenous protein of the connective tissue. *Journal of Laboratory and Clinical Medicine* 82:951-961, 1973.

Fjerdingstad, E., Danscher, G. and Ferdingstad, E. J. Zinc content in hippocampus and whole brain of normal rats. *Brain Research* 79:338-347, 1974.

Garbarg, M.; Babbin, G.; Feger, G. and Schwarz, J. C. Histaminergic pathway in rat brain evidenced by lesions of the medial forebrain bundle. *Science* 186:833-835, 1974.

Halstead, J. A., Smith, J. C. and Irwin, M. I. A conspectus of research on zinc requirements of man. *Journal of Nutrition* 104:345-378, 1974.

Hardjan, P. M.; Smith, C. G.; Herman, J. B. and Halstead, J. A. Serum zinc concentration in acute myocardial infarction. *Chest* 65:185-187, 1974.

Harrison, W. W., Netsky, M. G. and Brown, M. D. Trace elements in human brain: copper, zinc, iron and magnesium. *Clinica Chimica ACTH* 21:55-60, 1968.

Haug, F. M. et al. Timm's sulfide-silver reaction for zinc during experimental anterograde degeneration of hippocampal mossy fibers. *J. Comparative Neurology* 142:23-31, 1971.

——Depletion of metal in the rat hippocampal mossy fiber system by intravital chelation with dithizone. *Histochemie* 28:211-219, 1971.

Haug, F. M. On the normal histochemistry of trace metals in the brain. Presented at the Trace Elements and Brain Function Symposium, Princeton, New Jersey, 1973.

Henkin, R. J. Zinc in wound healing. *New England Journal of Medicine* 291:675-674, 1974.

Hurley, L. S. The consequences of fetal impoverishment. *Nutrition Today* 3:2, 1968.

Hussey, H. H. Taste and smell deviations: importance of zinc. *JAMA* 228:1669-1670, 1974.

Ibata, Y. and Otsuka, N. Electron microscopic demonstration of zinc in hippocampus formation using Timm's sulfide-silver technique. *J. Histochem. Cytochem.* 17:171-175, 1969.

Kazimierczak, W. and Maslinski, C. Effect of zinc ions on selective and non-selective release in vitro. *Agents and Actions* 4:1, 1974.

McBean, L. D.; Dove, J. T.; Halstead, J. A., and Smith, J. C. Zinc concentrations in human tissues. *Amer. J. Clin. Nutr.* 25:672-676, 1972.

McClain, P. E.; Woley, E. R.; Boecher, G. R.; Anthony, W. L. and Hsu, J. G. Influence of zinc deficiency on synthesis and cross-linking of rat skin collagen. *Biochimica et Biosphysica ACTA* 304:457-465, 1973.

McLardy, T. Hippocampal zinc and structural deficit in brain from schizophrenics and chronic alcoholics. Presented at the Trace Elements and Brain Function Symposium, Princeton, New Jersey, 1973.

Muerhcke, R. C. The fingernails in hypoalbuminuria: a new physical sign. *Br. Med. J.* 195:1327-1328, 1956.

Murphy, J. V. Intoxication following ingestion of elemental zinc. *JAMA* 212:2119-2120, 1970.

Niklowitz, W. J. Interference of Pb and Mg with essential brain tissue Cu, Fe and Zn as main determinant in experimental metal encephalopathy. Presented at the Trace Elements and Brain Function Symposium, Princeton, New Jersey, 1973.

O'Dell, B. L. and Savage, J. E. Effect of phytic acid on zinc availability. *Proc. Soc. Expt. Biol. Med.* 103:304, 1960.

Pecarek, R. S. and Biesel, W. R. *Appl. Microbiol.* 18:482, 1969.

Pfeiffer, C. C. and Iliev, V. A study of zinc deficiency and copper excess in the schizophrenias. *Int. Ref. Neurobiol.* Supp. 1:141-165, 1972.

Pories, W. J.; Henzel, J. H.; Rob, C. G. and Strain, W. H. Acceleration of wound healing with zinc sulfate. *Ann. Surg.* 165:432, 1967.

Pories, W. J. and Strain, W. H. Once upon a trace metal: the zinc story. *Medical Opinion*, 7, 1971.

Prasad, A. S. *Zinc metabolism*. Springfield, Illinois: Charles C. Thomas, 1966.

Reid, G. M. (Personal communications)

Rickard, B. F. Facial eczema: zinc responsiveness in dairy cattle. *New Zealand Veterinary Journal* 23:41-42, 1975.

Rodale, R. The zinc story. *Prevention*, July, 1973.

Schroeder, H. A. Losses of vitamins and trace minerals resulting from processing and preservation of foods. *American Journal of Clinical Nutrition*. 24:562-573, 1971.

Strain, W. H., ed. *Clinical applications of zinc metabolism*. Springfield, Illinois: Charles C. Thomas, 1975.

Towers. Role of Zn^{+2} in protecting against sporedesmin damage. Biochemistry section, Ruakura Agricultural Research Center, August 1975.

Tucker, H. F. and Salmon, W. D. Prakeratosis or zinc deficiency in pigs. *Proc. Soc. Expt. Biol. Med.* 88:613-616, 1955.

Vorhees, J. G.; Chakrabarti, S. G.; Botero, Fernando; Miedler, L. and Harrell, E. R. Zinc therapy and distribution in psoriasis. *Arch. Derm.* 100:669-673, 1969.

CHAPTER 17

Iron

Iron is essential to human body chemistry, since it combines with protein to make hemoglobin, the coloring matter of red blood cells. The body makes efficient use of iron stores by "re-cycling," but when blood is lost through menstruation or hemorhage iron is also lost and must be replaced by adequate dietary intake. If this deficiency is not adjusted, an anemia may result.

The similarity between iron-deficiency anemia and other anemias, particularly pyridoxal-deficiency anemia, presents the possibility of an iron accumulation overload when iron is given in abundance. Doctors who fear incipient iron-deficiency anemia or who misdiagnose another deficiency may prescribe iron supplements for their patients. Current advertising warns consumers of the danger of iron deficiency, with the result that self-medication with products like Geritol, Hadacol, Ironized Yeast and One-a-day Vitamins Plus Iron is not uncommon. This adds up to too much "TV-iron" for some people.

Iron deficiency is more likely to occur in women than in men, and in teen-agers whose rapid growth may require additional iron. In pregnancy and cases of overt blood loss, the risk of deficiency is enough to merit supplements. Iron overload is most likely to occur in older men, as the excess iron accumulates gradually over the years. The individual who has fortified himself with daily doses of "TV iron" for the last thirty years is a likely candidate for iron overload. As with copper, excess iron can have pernicious consequences. Among these are hemachromatosis or siderosis (an iron-excess disease), damage to the liver and pancreas, arthritis and heart damage.

Bread and cereals are usually fortified with iron, but there are much better choices of nutrients to add. Pyridoxine (B-6) and zinc are two such nutrients. A deficiency of these can cause blood disorders which mimic iron deficiency. Based only on hemoglobin levels, some claim that iron deficiency is our most critical nutritional problem. We believe that deficiency in B-6 and zinc is more critical.

Excess tissue iron is more insidious than iron deficiency. It develops gradually over the years, potentially developing into hemosiderosis or hemochromatosis. In those already suffering from hemochromatosis, thalassemia or sickle cell disease, the extra iron can be fatal. Because iron-deficiency anemia may sometimes be confused with other anemias, the best way to diagnose an iron deficiency is by measuring the serum iron level, *not* the hemoglobin. The propensity to equate "iron deficiency" with "anemia" is responsible for much of the present controversy.

Types of Anemia

An anemia is any one of many disorders which involve a reduction in the concentration of hemoglobin (number of red blood cells per unit volume of blood). It results in a decreased ability of the blood to carry oxygen. Symptoms include weakness, pallor, loss of appetite, and the wide array of symptoms which may occur with any disease underlying anemia.

The breakdown of hemoglobin takes place constantly, and iron from this is added to the absorption iron and to the iron released from body reserves which is needed to maintain homeostasis. Iron is withdrawn from the plasma into the bone marrow and synthesized into new hemoglobin with the aid of copper as a catalyst. The life cycle of a red blood cell is about 120 days.

Iron deficiency is often without symptoms other than those associated with anemia of any cause. The establishment of a diagnosis involves measurement of the plasma iron concentration and the iron-binding capacity of the carrier protein, transferrin. It must also be demonstrated that iron stores have been completely depleted. The patient's history must also be scrutinized and a demonstrable blood loss should be sought. This may occur in regular blood donors and those with a history of gastrointestinal bleeding (sometimes due to salicylates such as aspirin, and other drugs). Growing children and women during the reproductive years are most susceptible to blood-loss anemia.

Iron-deficiency anemia rarely constitutes a life-threatening predicament. Patients can walk with only 20 percent of their normal hemoglobin. The first thing which is treated is the cause of the blood loss. Then body iron is replenished, usually by an oral preparation. If the hemoglobin level does not steadily rise (at least 2 gm per 100 ml of blood for every three weeks of therapy), it is possible that the anemia is not caused by iron deficiency.

Pyridoxine-deficiency (or pyridoxal-responsive) anemia may be mistaken for iron-deficiency anemia. Here, however, the serum iron level is often elevated and bone marrow hemosiderin increased. Then, in addition to pernicious anemia (for which there is no cure but which is controlled by periodic doses of folic acid and B-12), there are the significant anemias of blood loss, of protein deficiency, of kidney failure and of liver failure, which must be differentiated from iron deficiency.

Excess Iron

When an excessive amount of iron is ingested frequently over long periods, several pathological conditions of far greater life-threatening potential than those of iron deficiency can arise. An example is the hemosiderosis found in the Northern Veld Bantu tribe of South Africa. These tribesmen used iron pots for preparation of beer and sour porridge. Since these foods are acidic, the iron can leach out into them. Adult Bantu males, who drank large quantities of this beer, had a high incidence of hemosiderosis and scurvy. The scurvy was due to the irreversible oxidation of ascorbic acid by the tissue iron deposits. These men were also susceptible to liver injury and may have shown evidence of liver scarring (cirrhosis).

Hemosiderosis is a disease of the iron metabolism characterized by deposits of iron in the liver. Typical symptoms of cirrhosis may evolve from this. The transferrin (iron-carrying transport protein) becomes saturated with iron and is no longer able to bind all of the absorbed iron. Excess iron may end up in the lungs, pancreas and heart, as well as in the liver. The daily iron intake among Bantu men ranges from 30 mg to 100 mg, so it comes as no surprise that the disease may occur after any prolonged therapy with unneeded iron.

Iron-storage disease may result from a serum iron level permanently elevated by prolonged medicinal iron in the form of oral preparations or injections. Other sources include extensive blood transfusion, presence of other disease, hemolytic anemia, aplastic anemia and early acute hepatitis. All are characterized by high iron levels. A strict vegetarian regime may also produce iron overloading.

The iron-overloading diseases are basically an inability of the digestive tract to screen out unneeded iron. They appear mostly in men over the age of forty, and symptoms include headache, shortness of breath, increasing fatigue, dizziness and loss of weight. The iron becomes deposited in the tissues, and in time the iron deposits give the skin a grey hue. While heredity may contribute to the disposition of some toward the disease, a high intake of iron appears to be the main cause. Persons who drink large quantities of iron-containing red wine, and persons who are addicted to certain iron tonics have a proclivity toward acquisition of the disease.

One organ in which iron deposits may accumulate is the heart. Cardiac iron deposits which are easily visible at autopsy occur in patients with idiopathic hemochromatosis. Another place the iron ends up is the synovial membrane of the rheumatoid joints. Studies have shown a disturbance in iron metabolism among arthritic patients, and although no cause-effect relationship has been shown, it is possible that the synovial membranes are acting as storage depots for excess iron. Dr. K. D. Muirden has hypothesized that regional lymph nodes in rheumatoid arthritis are areas of iron storage.

Iron overload often goes unnoticed due to the fervor associated with the elimination of iron deficiency. Pyridoxine- and zinc-deficiency syndromes may be responsible for the anemia or other condition, and in these cases a daily dose of iron is not the nicest thing you can do for yourself.

Ninety percent of the dietary iron intake remains unabsorbed, never even entering the blood. There is a small daily excretion in the urine and feces, from menstruation, in perspiration and in exfoliation of the skin which requires replacement from dietary sources. Extra dietary iron is required when blood volume expands (as with rapid growth or development of the fetus) or when blood loss occurs.

Sources of Iron

Lean meats, deep-green leafy vegetables, whole-grain cereals or breads, liver, other organ meats, dried fruits, legumes, shellfish and molasses are rich in iron. Iron cookware is another source, although iron skillets are generally the only such items still in use since the advent of aluminum, copper and stainless steel. The daily requirement of iron is probably twice as great in women and adolescents than in men, but pregnancy is the only general condition for which iron supplementation is recommended. Again, the general population would benefit more from more B-6 and zinc supplementation than from more iron.

References

Arora, R.; Lynch, E. C.; Whitly, C. E.; Alfrey, E., Jr. and Clarence, P. The ubiquity and significance of human ferratin. *Texas Rep. Biol. Med.* 28:3, 189-196, 1970.

Brody, K. and Will, G. Iron absorption in rheumatoid arthritis. *Annals of the rheumatoid diseases* 28:5. September 1969.

Crosby, W. H. Intestinal response to the body's requirement for iron. *JAMA* 208:2, 347-351, 14 April 1969.

Goodman, L. S. and Gilman, A. *The pharmacological basis of therapeutics.* New York: Macmillan, 1955.

Muirden, K. D. The anemia of rheumatoid arthritis: the significance of iron deposits in the synovial membrane. *Aust. Ann. Med.* 2:97-104, 1970.

________ Lymph node iron in rheumatoid arthritis. *Annals of Rheumatic Diseases* 29:1, January 1970.

Robinson, C. H. *Fundamentals of normal nutrition.* New York: Macmillan, 1973.

Siimes, M. A., Addiego, J. E., Jr. and Dallman, P. R. Ferratin in serum: diagnosis of iron deficiency and iron overload in infants and children. *Blood* 43:4, April 1974.

CHAPTER 18

Manganese

The high copper level of many schizophrenics can be reduced by dietary intake of zinc and manganese. Manganese is similar to zinc in the way it increases urinary copper excretion; a combination of zinc and manganese is more effective than either alone. High-copper schizophrenics are improved by the zinc-manganese combination in Ziman drops or tablets.

Manganese is one of the essential trace metals, a necessary dietary constituent obtained from nuts, seeds, and whole-grain cereals. It is necessary for bone growth and development, reproduction, lipid metabolism and the moderation of nervous irritability. Manganese is also important in the building and breakdown cycles of protein and nucleic acid (the chief carrier of genetic information). As an activator of such enzymes as arginase (required for the formation of urea) and some peptidases (which cause the hydrolysis of proteins in the intestine), manganese may also contribute to a mother's love and instinctive maternal protection of her child. (Through certain enzymes, manganese affects the glandular secretions underlying maternal instinct.) Manganese is important in the formation of thyroxin, the principle of the thyroid gland.

Required Intake

Every day a healthy person excretes approximately 4 mg of manganese; this amount is then needed in the diet for replacement of the lost manganese. Adequate intake is required for the lipid and glucose metabolism and oxidative phosphorylation (among other intrinsic biochemical processes). On normal lipid metabolism manganese has a beneficial effect, particularly in cases of atherosclerosis.

Manganese Deficiency

Analysis of hair samples has indicated that manganese deficiency may be common among older males. Manganese deficiency may be a cause of atherosclerosis, although no studies have clearly demonstrated a true deficiency of this trace metal in man. Similarly, manganese deficiency is suspected in diabetes. A study by L. G. Kosenko in 1964 implicated manganese deficiency after an examination of 122 diabetics from fifteen to eighty-one years of age. Dr. Kosenko found that the manganese content of whole ashed blood was approximately half that of normal control subjects. In 1968 G. J. Everson and R. E. Shrader reported that manganese deficiency can impair the glucose metabolism so as to lower glucose tolerance (the ability to remove excess sugar from the blood). The deficiency may produce abnormalities in the pancreatic secretion of insulin, the agent which utilizes excess sugar. Thus, a diabetic condition may result.

The enzymes which manganese activates are also necessary for the utilization of vitamin C, choline and other B vitamins (biotin and thiamin). Without the ability to use choline or deanol properly, the body underproduces acetylcholine, a neurotransmitter in the brain. In a body deficient in acetylcholine and properly utilized B vitamins various conditions may result, among them myasthenia gravis (grave loss of muscle strength). This condition may respond to manganese if doses are given at each meal, in addition to a high-protein diet, vitamin E and all the B vitamins. All these nutrients aid in the transmission of impulses between nerve and muscle.

Poisoning

Manganese overloading or poisoning has been reported only in industries where manganese-containing dust may be inhaled. In mining operations in Chile and in the dry battery industry, where workers are exposed to manganese oxide dust, cases of manganese poisoning have been recorded. Symptoms are similar to those of Parkinsonism and include tremor, muscular rigidity, irritability and impotency. Symptoms of chronic manganese poisoning in these industries may also resemble those of schizophrenia. A drug used in treating Parkinson's disease, l-dopa (dihydroxyphenylalanine) has been found useful in treating manganese overload.

Metabolism

Manganese metabolism is somewhat similar to that of iron. Manganese is absorbed slowly from the small intestine, and the unneeded portion is excreted. The absorbed portion is transported through the blood by the protein transmanganin; the manganese quickly leaves the bloodstream and is stored mainly in the kidney. Some is excreted in the urine, most into the bile.

Manganese and Schizophrenia

Manganese chloride was first tested and found effective in treating schizophrenia by Dr. Reiter of Denmark. This finding was confirmed in 1929 by Dr. W. M. English, superintendent of a hospital in Brockville, Ontario. A later study by Hoskins, however, found manganese dioxide ineffective and since then, little attention has focused on the possibility of its therapeutic effects. The finding of high copper levels in the schizophrenias has also been ignored by the medical establishment. Furthermore, there is little dispute over the biochemical fact that zinc and manganese may replace copper and so reduce high copper levels. In evaluating the relative merits of the trace metals, then, we might categorize manganese as one of the "desirables" and copper as one of the "undesirables." This applies particularly to the schizophrenic.

In oral doses, manganese is never harmful, although in patients older than forty it has occasionally elevated blood pressure. The elevated pressure returns to normal when zinc alone is used.

Soil Depletion

Manganese is removed from the soil by current farming and food-processing practices. Soil erosion, leaching and soil exhaustion deplete the amount of manganese available to vegetables. Even normally manganese-rich foods are subject to wide variations. This depletion of the soil may be unsuspected since the foliage of plants may be lush without manganese. This is typified by the growth of lettuce. If lime is applied to solid clay, leafy vegetables grown in the more alkaline soil that is produced will contain much less manganese—simply because of the application of the lime. This finding points up the real need for scientific farming wherein the fertilizer will contain all of the trace elements in which the soil is deficient.

TABLE 18.1

Selected foodstuffs with appreciable amounts of manganese

Mg per 100 gm edible parts

		Cereals			
Corn germ	**10**	**Corn**	**1.0**	**Corn flakes**	**0.04**
Wheat bran	**14**	**Wheat**	**5.0**	**White bread**	**0.25**
Rice bran	**26**	**Rice**	**2.0**	**Rice Krispies**	**1.0**
Oat bran	**10**	**Oats**	**3.0**	**Oatmeal**	**0.30-3.0**
				Buckwheat	**1.3**
		Nuts			
Walnuts	**15**	**Peanuts**	**1.9**	**Pecans**	**1.5**

Chestnuts	3.7				
Spices					
Cloves	30.0	Cardamom	27.0	Ginger	17.6
Fruits					
Strawberries	0.33	Blueberries	0.15-1.9	Pineapple	0.1-3.0
Raspberries	0.12	Apples	0.20	Cherries	0.03-0.78
Bananas	0.2-0.8	Prunes	0.08	Watermelon	0.03
Vegetables					
Lettuce	0.7-0.80	Lima beans	0.5-1.0	Green beans	0.2-2.0
Spinach	0.2-15.0	Parsley	0.90-8.5	Dandelion greens	0.30
Peas	0.11	Onions	0.52-1.0	Carrots	0.06-0.6
Proteins					
Meat	0.03	Clams	0.25	Fresh-water fish	0.06
Whole egg	0.05	White	0.01	Yolk	0.10
Shrimp	0.04	Sea fish	0.02	Snails	1.6
Liver	0.12-0.53				
Miscellaneous					
Yeast	0.53-0.90	Tea leaves	5-71	Coffee beans	2.0
Spaghetti	0.54	Macaroni	0.5	Egg noodles	0.78

Sources: D. Schlettwein-Gsell and S. Mommsen-Straub. *International Journal of Vitamin and Nutrition Research 41*:268, 1971, and A. Gormican. *Journal of the American Dietetic Association 56*:397, 1970.

Leafy vegetables and grains constitute our main sources of dietary manganese. The more alkaline the soil, the less manganese there will be in the leaves. This accounts for the variable range of manganese content. Liming of the soil increases foliage but decreases the manganese content. The germ or bran of the grain contains most manganese, but this is lost in the milling process. Note the drastic losses of manganese in corn: corn germ (10), corn (1) and corn flakes (0.04). Similarly drastic losses in manganese occur in the processing of wheat. Except for the organ meats (such as liver) protein is not a good source of manganese. Fish is low except for shellfish such as clams and snails. The daily requirement of man for manganese is about 4 mg.

References

Cook, D. G. et al. Chronic manganese intoxication. *Arch. Neurol.* 30:59, January 1974.

English, W. M. Report of the treatment with manganese chloride of 181 cases of schizophrenia, 33 of manic depression and 16 of other defects of psychoses at the Ontario Hospital, Brockville, Ontario. November 1929.

Everson, G. J. and Shrader, R. E. *J. of Nutr.* 94:89, 1968.

Hoskins, R. G. *J. Nerv. and Ment. Dis.* 79:59, 1934.

Hurley, L. S. Disproportionate growth in offspring of manganese deficient rats. *J. Nutrition* 74:274.

Kosenko, L. G. *Klin. Med.* 42:113, 1964.

Manganese for muscles and mother love. *Prevention*, p. 115, May 1969.

CHAPTER 19

Sulfur: The Forgotten Essential Element

In his comprehensive and recent book on trace elements in nutrition, E. J. Underwood does not discuss sulfur. (The two references to sulfur in his book are to its interaction with selenium.) Schroeder, in his several comments on sulfur as an essential element, indicates that for ordinary turnover in an adult body which contains a total of 140 gm, the daily requirement is 850 mg. Sulfur content is equalled by a potassium content (also 140 gm), and both sulfur and potassium content exceed that of sodium, which is only 100 gm. Yet we merrily salt our food each day, paying little heed to our sulfur and potassium needs.

The turnover of potassium and sodium is greater than that of sulfur. Both sulfur and potassium are found inside the cells, while sodium is found mainly outside the cells in the extracellular fluid. Every cell in the body contains sulfur, but the cells that contain the most are those of the skin, hair and joints. The horny layer of the skin, keratin, has a high content of sulfur as have the fingernails, toenails and hair. Sheep's wool and hair contain about 5 percent sulfur, and about 13 percent of sheep's wool is made up of the amino acid cystine. Since the curliness of hair depends on the sulfur-to-sulfur bonds of cystine, hair straighteners and curlers are designed to open up the S-to-S bonds and then set them in new arrangements, either straight-chain or curled-chain. If the waving solution is too strong or the hair too fine, the hair can be entirely dissolved instead of curled.

Peculiar odors in biology are usually due to sulfur compounds. The odor of burned hair or wool is no exception; this characteristic odor indicates the high sulfur content of hair.

Dietary Sulfur

Most of man's sulfur must come from food protein which provides four sulfur-containing amino acids—cysteine, cystine, taurine and methionine. The first three can be made in the body as long as adequate amounts of the essential amino acid methionine are contained in man's diet. Elemental sulfur will also allow the building of the first three amino acids by the tissues of the body.

Vegetarians may become deficient in sulfur, particularly if they do not eat eggs. Many adults may be deficient in sulfur because of the misguided warnings against egg eating—our widespread cholesterol phobia. (Two eggs per day raise blood cholesterol by only 2 percent, which is not sufficient to cause atherosclerosis.)

Egg yolk is one of two foods that will darken a silver teaspoon. Since the other is red-hot peppers, most of us will choose the egg yolk as a source of our sulfur. For those who cannot eat eggs in any form (because of sensitivity), the local druggist will, on a physician's order, fill No. 1 capsules with flowers of sulfur. This dose, taken once each day, will provide one-quarter of the daily need, or 200 mg, of pure elemental sulfur. The other 600 mg can be obtained from the sulfur-containing amino acids. Even egg albumen or white of egg is higher in sulfur (1.62 percent) than casein from milk (0.80 percent) and soybean protein (0.38 percent). Muscle protein (as in beef) approaches egg white with 1.27 percent sulfur. Smelly foods such as onions and garlic contain appreciable amounts of sulfur. Indeed, the tear gas from sliced onions is a simple sulfur compound, and any blood-pressure-lowering effect of garlic is related to its "garlic" smell—one that is characteristic of an organic sulfur compound.

Cattle in feed lots lick on modern salt cakes made yellow with elemental sulfur. Chickens and pigs have sulfur added to their feed. Grandmother advocated sulfur and molasses each spring, and homeopathic physicians have continued to prescribe small doses of sulfur for many ailments. In early times some patients travelled to mineral springs or spas to drink regularly of the sulfur water, and even went so far as to bring home a jug of the medicinal waters for the rest of the family.

Sulfur water contains hydrogen sulfide. Ruminant animals such as sheep can make do with sulfur in the form of sulfate because the bacteria of their various stomachs will reduce the sulfate to sulfur. When man takes magnesium sulfate (Epsom salts) or sodium sulfate (horse physic), the sulfate is not absorbed but gathers water from the tissues and goes through the body with cathartic violence. When elemental sulfur was compared to sulfate sulfur in sheep (both at 0.5 percent level in the diet) either form produced better growth and better wool. The general dietary recommendation for sheep is for 0.2 percent elemental sulfur in the diet. The proper amount for man might be as little as 0.01 percent in cereal foods or a 100-mg scored tablet as a dietary supplement.

At present, dietary supplements containing sulfur are not available. One cannot give extra sulfur in the form of one of the amino acids since these often have adverse effects. For instance, methionine produces feelings of unreality. Simple organic sulfur compounds are not cleared for human use and all have a noticeable odor. One possible candidate for sulfur supplementation is the sulfur analogue of acetone called DMSO (dimethyl sulfoxide). This has the advantage of lipid solubility but has the disadvantage of being partially oxidized, so that the body may not be able to use it as a source of sulfur. Since DMSO is under careful clinical investigation, some answers may be forthcoming if the scientists remember to ask the crucial question: does DMSO supply sulfur in a form usable by the body? The great lipid solubility of DMSO might get sulfur to the brain for the regrowth of nerves and treatment of epilepsy by allowing the brain to synthesize the stabilizing amino acid taurine.

Taurine and Epilepsy

Biochemical texts barely mention taurine; after all, it is not an essential sulfur amino acid like methionine. Taurine is a simple chemical with two carbon atoms separating a primary amino group and a sulfuric acid group. These chemical groups at both ends make taurine very water-soluble and thus hard to pass through the lipid membranes of the body. Taurine's function is to perch on cellular membranes, probably in neutralized form, and facilitate the passage of simple things such as the potassium and sodium ions and perhaps calcium or magnesium ions. Since taurine passes the blood-brain barrier very poorly, much of the brain taurine is probably built by the brain tissue.

Andre Barbeau, a dynamic physician at the Clinical Research Institute in Montreal, has studied taurine's role in animal and human epilepsy. The distribution of taurine in the human brain is similar to that of zinc and GABA (gamma-aminobutyric acid), both of which play an important calming role in nerve action. The injection of zinc in trace doses produced stretching and yawning in Barbeau's animals, as did GABA (which is monosodium glutamate with the one acid group removed). Because serum zinc is low and copper high in epileptics, Barbeau theorizes that seizures may occur when the zinc-to-copper ratio falls suddenly in the absence of adequate taurine, which cannot reach the brain easily and must be built in the brain. He believes that oral doses of taurine may help epileptics (but then, the other dietary forms of sulfur have not been tried—these are, of course, elemental sulfur or methionine or cysteine). We have found that elemental sulfur taken by mouth increases man's urinary taurine excretion.

Taurine is a stabilizer of membrane excitability and thus could control the onset of epileptic seizures. Taurine and sulfur could be factors in the control of many disorders, including the known biochemical changes in the aging process. Disorders of the skin and nails might improve with added sulfur in our diet. (In 1899, the *Journal of the American Medical Association* published an article on the use of sulfur in psoriasis.)

Previous Uses of Sulfur in Therapeutics

In the nineteenth century, elemental sulfur was used to treat many disorders because no better remedies were available. If these uses are reviewed with the thought that sulfur deficiency may perhaps occur in man as well as in animals, then some of the old uses of sulfur make good sense.

Psoriasis is a scaly condition of the skin which, in mild cases, occurs on the elbows and knees or behind the belt buckle—i.e., at pressure points. The scales may disappear in summer with sunlight, but return quickly in winter. Large doses of zinc are helpful, and small oral doses of sulfur may also help. The normal formation of melanin pigment requires two amino acids and sulfur plus sunlight. Nutrients which help the skin to tan (pigmenting process) should help psoriasis. These would be adequate protein, vitamin B-6, zinc and sulfur. Patients with psoriasis are more likely than others to get arthritis or joint diseases.

Rheumatoid arthritis patients seem, as a rule, to dislike eggs—at present, our only good source of sulfur. Since yolks turned grandmother's silver spoons black (because of silver sulfide) grandma had special little bone spoons for eating soft-boiled eggs long before the fad of throwing plastic spoons away. In the 1920s, colloidal sulfur was given intravenously or intramuscularly to arthritic patients without adequate control as to the possible benefit. Sulfur in oil was also given in both arthritic and mental patients. The joints are high in sulfate-containing compounds. The most common is chondroitin sulfate of the cartilages. All patients with rheumatoid arthritis would do well to eat at least two eggs per day to provide adequate sulfur for their needs.

The use of sulfur in large doses as a laxative dates back to antiquity. With bacterial action, hydrogen sulfide is formed in the intestine and (as with most intestinal gas) is absorbed. The local hydrogen sulfide is reported to promote peristalsis of the large bowel and facilitate daily bowel movements. Modern studies on sulfur as a laxative have yet to be done. Hydrogen sulfide was thought to be useful in heavy metal poisoning, but here again, modern data are not available. (The sulfur and molasses of grandma's day was probably given for the laxative effect.)

The physician frequently wishes to normalize the flora of the intestine after antibiotic therapy. Acidophilus tablets or buttermilk is sometimes suggested. Certainly egg yolks, with their high sulfur content, or elemental sulfur could be used to normalize the flora or change an unwelcome yeast or fungal flora.

Lack of Sulfur in Soil

The soil in many areas of the world is deficient in sulfur. The glaciated areas are known to have lost sulfur, selenium, iodide and zinc. Commercial fertilizers seldom restore these trace elements to the soil. Plants depend on the soil for sulfur in the form of the sulfate ion. This is taken into the plant, where enzymes convert the sulfate into the many organic sulfur compounds which both plants and animals need. In most instances, the major sources of animal dietary sulfur are the two amino acids, methionine and cysteine. From these the body builds the essential compounds coenzyme A, heparin, glutathione, lipoic acid and biotin. The flora of the world build with sulfur the various penicillins and the characteristic odors of garlic, onion and mustard—not to mention horseradish.

References

Barbeau, A. and Donaldson, J. Zinc, taurine and epilepsy. *Arch. Neurol.* 30:52, 1974.

Martin, W. G. The neglected nutrient sulphur. *The Sulphur Institute Journal* p. 5, Spring 1968.

Math, O. H. and Oldfield, J. E. *Symposium sulfur in nutrition.* Westport, Connecticut: The AVI Publishing Co., 1970.

Schroeder, H. A. *The trace elements and man.* Old Greenwich, Connecticut: Devin-Adair, 1973.

Shohl, A. T. *Sulfur in mineral metabolism.* chap. 8. New York: Reinhold Publishing Co., 1939.

Underwood, E. J. *Trace elements in human and animal nutrition.* 3rd ed. New York: Academic Press, 1971.

Van Gelder, N. M. Antagonism by taurine of cobalt induced epilepsy in cat and mouse. *Brain Research* 47:157, 1972.

CHAPTER 20

Selenium: Stepchild of Sulfur

Selenium, occurring naturally as either a red powder or a gray crystal, is among the most poisonous elements in the universe; and yet, in pure form, it is an essential trace mineral for animals and man. It is a byproduct of copper refining and is used in the manufacture of photoelectric equipment, in paints and in xerography. It is widely but unevenly distributed in the earth's crust. South Dakota's soil is very high while Ohio's is very low.

Selenium-rich soils are thought to result from ancient volcanic eruptions and subsequent leaching to ancient inland seas long since evaporated. Wind and rain may remove selenium from the soil into the sea, thus causing a deficiency in locally grown plants and animal feed. Areas which were glaciated in the ice age have had all of the selenium removed by slow-melting glaciers. This action also removed zinc, sulfur and iodine from the soil. The wheat and corn grown in Ohio are so low in selenium that cattle feed was, at one time, shipped from South Dakota in order to supply adequate selenium. The United States Department of Agriculture now allows the fortification of animal feeds with trace amounts of selenium.

However, too much selenium in the soil—as in South

Dakota—produces toxicity and occasionally death in ruminant animals. Selenium also occurs as a water contaminant around heavily irrigated land. The animal feeds of South Dakota must be diluted with forage grown elsewhere. An adequate dietary intake of selenium for animals is 200 parts per billion (ppb). This level would probably suffice for man also.

Too much selenium, generally absorbed from inorganic salts or from organic compounds in plants, produces toxic symptoms. These include loss of hair, nails and teeth; dermatitis; lassitude and progressive paralysis. Acute poisoning causes fever (103° to 105°), increased respiratory and capillary rate, gastroenteritis, myelitis (inflammation of the spinal cord and bone marrow), anorexia and even death.

Selenium also has some important beneficial effects. It protects against the toxic effects of the pollutant cadmium. Tests on laboratory animals have shown that it also protects against high-mercury tuna fish. In humans, it increases the effectiveness of vitamin E, and it appears to reduce the chances of all types of cancer. Selenium is an antioxidant that helps prevent chromosome breakage in tissue culture. Damaged chromosomes cause not only birth defects but also cancer if the damage to the DNA (found in the cells' nuclei) disturbs the inhibitors that control the cells' tendency to multiply. Studies have shown that in communities where selenium intake is low, the cancer rate is high.

Amount in the Human Blood

Rhead et al. in California have analyzed human blood and found detectable levels in every fraction tested. Hemoglobin has 0.65 ppm, alpha-2 globulins 5.76 ppm, transferrin 3.4 ppm, and ceruloplasm 5.4 ppm. Insulin, which is known to contain much sulfur, has 4.0 ppm of selenium. In these instances selenium may occur as a contaminant of sulfur. In one enzyme, glutathione peroxidase, however, selenium is the only active trace element. The study of the levels of this enzyme in mental disease and also cancer would be most worthwhile.

Males seem to have a higher requirement for selenium

than females. Most infants who die are males. Of the thirty-five thousand infant deaths per year in the United States, about one-quarter are associated with selenium and/or vitamin E deficiency. Almost none of these babies is breast fed, and it is significant that human milk contains up to six times as much selenium as cow's milk and twice as much vitamin E. Also, some children suffering from malnutrition fail to grow when given a recuperative diet unless selenium is added. Australian investigators have suggested that selenium deficiency may be involved in sudden and unexplained crib deaths. Selenium is necessary for protein synthesis; thus, its importance cannot be ignored.

One disadvantage of selenium, however, is its possible tendency to increase dental caries in children up to the age of ten. Trace elements may alter susceptibility to caries by changing the chemical composition of the dental enamel during the period of tooth formation. Heavy consumption of selenium seems to decrease the beneficial effect of fluoride, which helps prevent tooth decay. However, ethical considerations have prevented the carrying out of experiments on human subjects.

Food Sources

Good food sources of selenium include brewer's yeast, garlic, liver and eggs. Foods from animal sources are generally richer in the mineral than those from vegetable sources, so vegetarians should supplement their diet with brewer's yeast tablets to fulfill the requirement. Unfortunately, all foods lose selenium in processing—for example, brown rice has fifteen times the selenium content of white rice, and whole-wheat bread contains twice as much selenium as white bread. It is to be hoped that in future the government will encourage the addition of selenium to staple foods with the goal of preventing deficiency and further reducing the cancer rate in this country.

References

Hadjimarkos, D. M. Selenium in relation to dental caries. *Fd. Cosmet. Toxicol.* 11:1083-1095, 1973.

Harr, J. R. and Muth, O. H. Selenium poisoning in domestic animals and its relationship to man. *Clinical Toxicology* 5(2):175-186, 1972.
Rhead, W. J. et al. Selenium in human plasma: levels in blood proteins and behavior upon dialysis acidification and reduction. *Bioinorganic Chemistry* 3:217-223, 1974.

CHAPTER 21

Calcium and Demineralization

Every school child knows that the mineral calcium is necessary for strong bones and teeth. In fact, 99 percent of the calcium in the body is found in the bones. The other 1 percent is just as vital because it is involved in controlling blood clotting mechanisms, the excitability of nerves and muscles, the function of parathyroid hormone and the action of vitamin D.

Calcium occurs in the blood, the fluid surrounding cells, cell membranes and intracellular organelles. Unfortunately, according to a survey released in 1968 by the USDA, over 30 percent of the human population of this nation is calcium deficient. Calcium is of further interest in mental disease since intravenous injections were used in the early 1930s to produce lucid intervals in some schizophrenics. Those patients who responded may have been the histadelic or high-histamine type, since only one out of five patients responded. Calcium ion is a histamine-releasing agent.

What Is Calcium Deficiency?

Without calcium, muscles cannot contract. Deficiency causes

increased irritability, osteoporosis (softening of the bones), osteomalacia (another type of bone-softening disease) and rickets. According to Leo Lutwak, Professor of Medicine at the School of Medicine, University of California at Los Angeles, "Various surveys have indicated that approximately 30 percent of women over the age of 55 and men over the age of 60 have had sufficient mineral loss to have produced at least one fracture."

The bone-softening disease cannot be detected reliably by X rays until 30 percent or more of the bone mineral has been lost. Unfortunately, in Dr. Lutwak's opinion, his studies suggest that once vertebral fracture has occurred, the progression of softening of the bones cannot be stopped! Other researchers disagree, and some suggest that fluoride in addition to calcium might be more helpful than calcium alone.

Loss of Calcium with Bed Rest or Space Flights

Bed rest is bad for human physiology since calcium is lost from bones and nitrogen is lost from muscles. In the confinement of their spaceship the astronauts in their eight-day space mission lost 200 mg of calcium per day in spite of a daily routine of vigorous exercises. The absence of gravity in space makes walking impossible, so that the bones start to lose calcium from inactivity, and continue to do so. More ingenious elastic apparatus is needed to exercise the big muscles of the legs and back.

Going to bed with a cold or minor misery may impair health because of this calcium and nitrogen loss. With serious illness some bed rest may be necessary at the start, but the resourceful individual will start exercising after the fever breaks or the heart pain stops. Otherwise, the road back from absolute bed rest will be a long and weary one.

For example, on the sixth day after a severe heart attack most individuals can start finger exercises, the next day arm exercises and the tenth day leg exercises while still in bed. Unless this type of exercise program is initiated, always on the advice of the doctor, the bright day will dawn when the doctor says, "Now you may get out of bed," and the patient experiences rubbery knees and even invalidism because of inactivity.

Extra Calcium Tablets Require Extra Zinc

We know from numerous animal studies that extra calcium in the diet decreases zinc absorption. Most animals are on a high-cereal diet which contains considerable phytate. Calcium phytate chelates (nabs onto) zinc ions so that they are lost from the body. Since older patients usually need both zinc and calcium, these should be separated. Even inositol should be separated in time from the zinc and calcium so that maximum absorption of both calcium and zinc are effected.

Hypoglycemics on High-protein Diets Require More Calcium

Drs.Bekha and Linbowiler at the University of Wisconsin have studied young men on a standard calcium intake of 500 mg per day. When the protein intake was 47 gm per day, calcium retention was 31 mg. At 92 gm of protein per day, retention was *minus* 58 mg and—even worse—*minus* 120 mg at 142 gm, with none of the nine subjects in calcium balance. The fecal excretion of calcium was not affected, so the great loss of calcium was all by the urinary pathway. The calcium loss can be overcome by extra calcium in the diet. Older patients on a high-protein diet develop osteoporosis while older vegetarians do not. The acid ash of the protein is responsible for the calcium loss. Obviously, hypoglycemic patients need bone meal or dolomitic calcium tablets twice a day.

Calcium Levels and Psychiatric Depression

Dr. F. F. Flach of Cornell Medical Center has pioneered the study of calcium balance in psychiatric depression. Effective treatment of the depression lowers the blood serum calcium level and increases the retention of calcium by the body. Patients with lack of response to treatment do not show this shift in calcium metabolism. These authors relate the calcium shift to adrenalin-like neuro-humors which might relieve depression.

Dr. John S. Carman has a similar idea involving the urinary excretion of calcium and magnesium. Patients placed on lithium therapy may show a high serum level of both calcium and magnesium. If their depression is lifted by the lithium therapy, the serum blood levels will decrease and urinary excretion of these two elements increase. Carman and his colleagues propose this as a test for the antidepressant response to lithium and other drugs.

What Amounts of Calcium Are Needed in the Body?

The National Academy of Sciences states that men, women and children (aged 1 to 10) need 800 mg of calcium daily. Infants need only 360 to 540 mg, while older boys and girls and pregnant and lactating women need 1200 mg daily. Dr. Lutwak believes 1000 mg of calcium daily in older people may completely prevent osteoporosis.

Regardless of age, whether a person is ingesting adequate calcium or not, the body will lose this mineral every day. Approximately 100 to 200 mg of calcium is filtered from the blood and excreted in the urine. An additional 125 to 180 mg is excreted in the digestive juices, remains unabsorbed and passes out of the body in the feces. Also, a small amount is lost in sweat. Ingesting 380 mg of calcium daily will *not* prevent the bones from wasting away. For example, if a woman at the age of twenty consumed only 380 mg of calcium per day, she would probably have lost two-thirds of the calcium in her body by the age of fifty. As aging occurs, the body's absorption of calcium becomes less efficient. Also, excitement or depressive emotional states can markedly increase calcium loss.

Like most other substances, an excess of calcium may produce undesirable results. If an excess of calcium is added to blood plasma, it prevents coagulation. Nervous and muscular functions can be depressed by overly large quantities of calcium. Children receiving an excess of vitamin D take up too much calcium and may have stomach upsets and retarded growth. However, since a sizeable portion of the population suffers from calcium deficiency, hypercalcemia (excess calcium) is a rare problem by comparison.

Calcium is essential, but its interaction with other vitamins and minerals must not be overlooked. A lack of magnesium can cause calcium deposits in muscles, heart and kidney. This results in kidney stones. The use of enough vitamin B-6 to produce recall of nightly dreams will allow enough pyridoxic acid to form to prevent kidney stones of the calcium oxalate type. Many urologists put their stone-forming patients on some vitamin B-6, but real success depends on a dose adequate to ensure that some goes over into the urine as pyridoxic acid. In hyperparathyroidism, calcium is mobilized from the bones excessively. Patients with this condition may also have kidney stones, but the removal of the enlarged parathyroid gland provides prompt relief.

Calcium in the Histadelic Patient

The Brain Bio Center introduced the use of calcium gluconate 500 mg A.M. and P.M. for the treatment of the histadelic patient (high blood histamine). Calcium ions have a histamine-releasing effect so that when given with Dilantin and methionine the blood histamine level is reduced. In the treatment of 100 histadelic patients with calcium gluconate 1 gm per day only 2 cases of kidney gravel were encountered—in both instances in female patients. Because of this, we usually recommend only one tablet of calcium gluconate per day in smaller histadelic females.

Good Sources of Calcium

Milk is ordinarily the best source of a balanced solution of calcium, magnesium and phosphorus. Two glasses of milk per day should be drunk by every growing individual and every pregnant woman. One 8-ounce glass per day should be drunk by every adult, and if this rule is followed then the adult will not lose the ability to burn lactose or milk sugar. Twenty percent of white adults and 80 percent of black adults cannot digest lactose, mainly because they stopped using milk in early adulthood.

One 8-ounce glass of whole milk supplies 30 percent of the daily calcium requirement. This glass of milk has 160 calories, while skim milk has only 90 calories and contains all of the calcium, magnesium and phosphate of whole milk. The color of skim milk can be improved by stirring in the yolk of an egg, which adds almost 5 percent of the daily need for calcium. The glass of milk also provides 25 percent of the daily need for riboflavin (vitamin B-2). Cheese (made from milk) is another good source of calcium.

Dolomitic calcium and magnesium can be used by the adult who is sensitive to milk. Since the magnesium makes the calcium soluble, the danger of kidney stones which occurs with calcium alone is eliminated. Two 300 mg tablets A.M. and P.M. are sufficient.

Bone meal provides calcium and magnesium and other minerals such as fluoride as they occur in our well-fed animals. Since the fluoride content may not be sufficient to prevent osteoporosis in older people, some should have a daily sodium fluoride tablet in addition.

The eggshell—usually thrown out—is a splendid source of calcium and trace elements. Eggshells can be used to sweeten vinegar and lemon juice by neutralizing the acid, so that sugar is not needed. Salad dressings made from vinegar or lemon juice neutralized with egg shells need no sugar. Eggs allowed to stand for twenty-four hours in either cider or wine vinegar will have a soft shell. The whole egg can then be thrown into the blender to make an eggnog. (So-called white vinegar is only diluted acetic acid and should be avoided.) The eggshells, ordinarily too gritty to eat, can thus be recycled to fill human calcium needs. When eggshells are used to sweeten cider or wine vinegar, the calcium is then in the vinegar as calcium acetate. Since the vinegar is less sour and is now loaded with natural trace elements, it will be more nutritious when used in salads or to make home-made mayonnaise.

Calcium nutrition is a complex matter which must be regarded as a whole rather than discussed in a fragmentary manner. Dr. William Strain of Cleveland has stated that trace element nutriture is like a giant spider web; if one branch of the web is pulled, the whole web of trace elements becomes distorted. Calcium balance, so closely related to magnesium, zinc, iron, selenium and sulfur balance, exemplifies this analogy very well.

References

Adams, R. and Murray, F. *Minerals: Kill or cure?* New York: Larchmont Books, 1974.

Flach, F. F. Calcium metabolism in states of depression. *Brit. J. Psychiat.* 110:588-593, 1964.

Flach, F. F. and Faragalla, F. F. The effects of imipramine and electro-convulsive therapy on the excretion of various minerals in depressed patients. *Brit. J. Psychiat.* 116:437-438, 1970.

Lutwak, L. Continuing need for dietary calcium through life. *Geriatrics* 29, 1974.

Robinson, C. H. *Fundamentals of normal nutrition.* New York: Macmillan, 1973.

Sollmann. *A manual of pharmacology.* Philadelphia: W. B. Saunders, 1957.

Trager, J. *The bellybook.* New York: Grossman, 1972.

CHAPTER 22

Magnesium

Magnesium derives its name from the Greek city Magnesia, where large deposits of magnesium carbonate were found. The first record of the medical use of magnesium dates back to the Italian Renaissance when salts of magnesium were used as a laxative. Today magnesium is used in Epsom salts (magnesium sulfate) and milk of magnesia (suspended magnesium hydroxide) because of its laxative properties.

Magnesium is a mineral essential to most living things and is found in abundance in man. Because of the large quantity in the body, magnesium is termed a bulk or major element rather than a trace element. Humans need magnesium for the production and transfer of energy, muscle contraction, protein synthesis and nerve excitability. Magnesium functions as a cofactor, assisting enzymes in catalyzing many chemical reactions.

Can I Have Too Much Magnesium?

An excess of magnesium can be toxic, but magnesium intoxication is rare, occurring only if the body experiences an unusual decrease in urinary excretion or a great increase in absorption and sometimes after intramuscular injection. Certain types of bone tumors and cancer in women may also raise the magnesium in the plasma to high levels. Hypermagnesia (excess magnesium) can cause depression of the central nervous system (it has been used for anesthesia), and an extreme excess of magnesium can cause death. Magnesium intoxication, however, is almost unknown.

Can I Be Magnesium Deficient?

Magnesium deficiencies are found in chronic alcoholism, cirrhosis of the liver, diabetic acidosis and various other illnesses. Patients who are fed magnesium-free fluids intravenously often become deficient.

Hypomagnesia (lowered blood magnesium) occurs in arteriosclerosis (degeneration of the arteries) and may lead to disturbances of heart rhythm. Dr. Janos Rigo of Semmelweis Medical University, Budapest, found that a high-magnesium diet lowered blood pressure and prevented "precocious aging" of the aorta in rats with experimentally induced hypertension.

Everyone is apt to become magnesium deficient, since the mineral is stripped from many of our foods through processing. Wheat loses almost all magnesium through refining, and refined sugars and fats contain almost no magnesium.

In addition, magnesium can be lost in the cooking process. Water-softening agents remove magnesium (and calcium) from the water, and the boiling of vegetables will further destroy the mineral content. Also, oxalic acid (as in spinach) and phytic acid (as in cereal foods) tie up magnesium by forming salts that the body cannot absorb.

The symptoms of a magnesium deficiency are depression, irritability, muscle tremors and, occasionally, convulsive seizures accompanied by delirium. Adelle Davis in her book *Let's Get Well* states that a daily dose of 450 mg of magnesium, when used to treat thirty epileptic patients, resulted in control of the seizures so that all drugs were discontinued. (Since this appears in her chapter on vitamin B-6, we suspect that magnesium plus adequate B-6 plus a better diet might have been the effective remedy.) Epileptic patients should certainly *not* have their anticonvulsant medications abruptly discontinued or replaced by magnesium oxide tablets. Continued seizures may result, with consequent brain damage. Dr. Pierre Muller, addressing the First International Symposium on Magnesium Deficit in Human Pathology in 1971, stated that data supports the belief that painful uterine contractions at the end of pregnancy are due to a deficiency of magnesium and suggested that a large number of premature interruptions of pregnancy may be related.

Fortunately, our kidneys are efficient in conserving magnesium. Therefore, unless one suffers from a kidney disease or loses an excessive amount of the mineral in sweat or feces, hypomagnesia is not likely to occur.

Where Can I Obtain Magnesium?

The National Academy of Sciences has set the RDA for magnesium at 350 mg for men, 300 for women, and 450 during pregnancy and lactation. Milk, nuts and whole grains are excellent sources of this essential mineral. Magnesium is found in green vegetables, particularly as part of the chorophyll molecule. Seafoods also contain appreciable amounts. The amount of magnesium obtained can be supplemented by taking dolomite, a naturally occurring mixture of calcium and magnesium.

References

Robinson, C. H. *Fundamentals of normal nutrition.* New York: Macmillan, 1973.

Schroeder, H. A., Nason, A. P. and Tipton, I. H. Essential metals in man: magnesium. *J. Chronic Dis.* vol. 21, 1969.

Seelig, M. S. Electrographic patterns of magnesium depletion appearing in alcoholic heart disease. *Annals of the New York Academy of Sciences* vol. 162: 2:906-917. 15 August 1969.

Wacker, E. C. and Vallee, B. L. Magnesium metabolism. *New Eng. J. of Med.* 259:9.

CHAPTER 23

Potassium

Those water pills that give relief from premenstrual tension and relieve water-logged tissues have the side-effect of producing potassium loss as well as salt (sodium) excretion. The daily intake of potassium may be marginal because some patients do not eat adequate amounts of vegetables and fruits which accumulate potash (potassium) from any well-nurtured soil. Symptoms of potassium deficiency are muscle weakness, fatigue, constipation and mental apathy. These symptoms will disappear when dietary changes provide sufficient potassium.

Studies show that the junk-food diet of high fat, refined sugars and oversalted food leads quickly to a state of potassium deficiency. In addition to those on water pills, patients on prednisone, ACTH, or digitalis require extra potassium. Patients with diabetes, high blood pressure or liver disease require a regular dietary supplement of potassium.

Foods particularly rich in potassium are green leafy vegetables, wheat germ, citrus juice, beans, lentils, nuts, dates, prunes and fruits of all kinds. With cooked vegetables, careful conservation of the pot liquor is necessary in order to minimize the water-soluble potassium loss. This pot liquor can be saved to make soups and broths or used immediately if the peas or beans are thickened with instant rice or instant rolled oats. While these prepared foods have lost some potassium, they can nonetheless be restored with the vegetable water. If the vegetable water is used to cook rolled oats, then the potassium content should be even greater.

Pharmaceutical preparations of potassium chloride are Kaochlor liquid, Kay Ciel Elixir, K-Lor, K-Lyte-CL and Slow-K. Most of these are 10 percent flavored potassium chloride. Patients who take daily a full dose of a water pill (thiazide diuretic) may need three tablespoons of 10 percent potassium chloride each day. This dose can be reduced, however, by the careful selection of foods high in potassium. Potassium tablets irritate the stomach and cause pain. Enteric coated potassium can cause deep ulcers in the small intestine.

References

Kosman, M. E. Management of potassium problems during long-term diuretic therapy. *JAMA* 230:5, 4 November 1974.

Schwartz, A. B. and Swartz, C. D. Dosage of potassium chloride elixir to correct thiazide-induced hypokalemia. *JAMA* 230:5, 4 November 1974.

CHAPTER 24

Molybdenum

One of the more difficult names to spell, molybdenum is an essential trace element, important to human life. It is a silvery-gray metal that looks something like lead, is used in ferro-alloys in small proportions (molybdenum steel hack saws) and is mined, almost exclusively, in one large deposit in Colorado.

Life Would Not Be Possible Without Molybdenum

In the nitrogen-fixation process, molybdenum is an essential catalyst, since bacteria-fixing atmospheric nitrogens require its chemical attributes to begin protein synthesis. Where molybdenum is lacking in the soil, the land is barren. When molybdenum-containing fertilizers are added to lawns, this will encourage clover, with its nitrogen-fixing root nodules, to thrive. (If you want an all-clover lawn, then use molybdenum plus some vanadium!)

Molybdenum is essential to all mammals; it is in all of our

tissues. Three important enzymes need molybdenum. Deficiencies are a distinct possibility in man, since our main source of caloric energy—fats and carbohydrates—have molybdenum only in whole grains or wheat germ. We process these grains, of course. Our white flour has lost its molybdenum to the bran (which is fed to chickens and cattle). Our refined sugar has lost its molybdenum to molasses. Only a judicious choice of protein foods and vegetables will ensure adequate amounts of the trace metal in the remaining caloric intake.

Like fluorine, molybdenum appears to prevent dental caries. When U.S. Navy recruits from Ohio were found to be surprisingly free of dental cavities, this was traced to the molybdenum in foods which came from the Ohio soil.

Molybdenum may also be responsible for lack of esophageal cancer in many parts of the world. In the Transkei region of South Africa, where cancer of the esophagus is increasing at an epidemic rate, researchers have found that indigenous vegetation is highly deficient in molybdenum. In the United States, areas deficient in molybdenum also had high rates of cancer of the esophagus. A third condition which might be the upshot of molybdenum deficiency is sexual impotency in older males.

Molybdenum overload or poisoning in humans is very unusual, even when the metal is inhaled as industrial fumes. However, sheep and cattle grazing on molybdenum-rich pasture may develop a copper deficiency. This is evidenced, in black sheep, by lack of pigment in their wool. With alternation of high molybdenum or high copper in the black sheep's diet, one can produce wool which is banded black and white. This demonstrates the dependency of copper metabolism on molybdenum intake, although the exact role of each mineral is an enigma. Conversely, a copper overload may be corrected by administering molybdenum. (Actually, the interaction is tripartite, involving sulfur as well.)

Molybdenum is obtainable in a number of foods. It also can be purchased as drops which can be added to milk or water. A good commercial source of molybdenum is Mol-Iron, which contains both molybdenum and iron.

TABLE 24.1

Food sources of molybdenum

Mcg%

Food	Mcg%
Grain	
Buckwheat	485
Oats	114
Corn	50
Cornflakes	8
Barley	138
Rice	47
Wheat	60
Wheat germ	200
Soybean	—
Bread	
Whole wheat	30
White	21
Rye	50
Prepared foods	
Noodles	45
Macaroni	51
Molasses	18
Nuts	
Coconut	25
Sunflower seeds	103
Miscellaneous	
Butter	10
Eggs	50
Milk	3
Milk powder	14
Honey	—
Cheese	5
Cocoa	50
Coffee	—
Tea	8
Wine	5
Beer	6
Scotch whisky	17
Meal	
Buckwheat	8
Corn	9
Wheat	50
Soybean	182
Fruits	
Apple	Trace
Apricot	14
Banana	3
Cantaloupe	16
Plums	6
Raisins	11
Strawberry	9
Vegetables	
Lima beans	400
Canned beans	350
Lentils	120
Green beans	66
Yams	59
Potato	25
Carrots	8
Celery	2
Lettuce	2
Spinach	26
Endive	4
Watercress	10
Zucchini	12
Eggplant	—
Green peppers	—
Tomato	—
Onions	—

Meats

Chicken	**40**	**Kidney**	**75**
Hearts	**75**	**Fish**	**4**
Liver	**200**	**Shellfish**	**20**

Some mineral waters in Switzerland have high levels of molybdenum (Eglisau—25 to 52 mcg/1 and Bex—26.5 mcg/1). Drinking water only has traces of molybdenum except in the S-charl region of Switzerland (29.0 mcg/1).

Source: D. Schlettwein-Gsell and S. Mommsen-Straub. Ubersichtsartikel spurenelemente in Lebensmitteln X. Molybdan. *International Journal for Vitamin and Nutrition Research* 43:110, 1973.

References

Brody, J. E. Dietary factors linked to cancer of digestive tract. *The New York Times* p. 24, 29 September 1972.

Schroeder, H. A., Balassa, J. J. and Tipton, I. H. Essential trace metals in man: molybdenum. *J. Chron. Dis.* 23:481, 1970.

CHAPTER 25

Vanadium: Little-known Element

One of our earliest ancestors was the *Amphioxas*, a cross between a fish and a worm, a link between vertebrates and invertebrates. This first chordate fish had a spinal cord with a slight bulge on the end which, over the millenia, developed into the human brain. The *Amphioxas* was fortunate in choosing iron as the chief transporter of oxygen in its blood, for, through some evolutionary quirk, a very close relative of the *Amphioxas* was forced to use vanadium for this purpose. Vanadium, more limited in availability than iron, produced an evolutionary regression; the *Amphioxas* became us, while its close relative became the common sea squirt. Instead of red blood cells full of iron, the squirt has green blood cells full of vanadium. And while the larvae of the squirt still have ganglionic bulges on their spinal cords, the mature squirts do not—hence they are brainless.

One may appreciate the presence of iron in one's hemoglobin and pity the poor sea squirt, who somewhere along the line was cut off from a supply of iron and lost his chance to have a brain. But one need not fear vanadium. (Ingesting vanadium will not make your blood green, nor will it shrink your brain and turn you into a sea squirt!) Vanadium is an element that is present throughout the human body. At maximum possible intake from trace amounts in dietary sources and air pollution, vanadium has no known toxicity.

Nutritional studies from four laboratories have shown beyond a doubt that vanadium is an essential trace element for both the rat and the chicken. One study conducted by Hopkins and Mohr in 1970 demonstrated that a vanadium-deficient diet produced a significant loss of feather growth in young chickens. He also showed that a vanadium deficiency decreases the reproduction rate in rats and increases mortality in their offspring. Other independent studies have shown that vanadium is essential to the growth of rats. Vanadium can be assumed to be essential to humans as well, because it is rapidly used by the body and excreted in the urine and it is found in most tissues. All other elements with these same properties, such as zinc, have been found essential. The dietary need for animals is 0.2 ppm. Many animal diets do not reach this level.

Sources of Vanadium

Vanadium is highly concentrated in fats and vegetable oils. At high levels, it helps to lower serum cholesterol, particularly in people of middle age. Vanadium shares with chromium and zinc this cholesterol-lowering ability. Like molybdenum, it is needed by the nitrogen-fixing bacteria of the soil. Another source of vanadium is the burning of coal and certain types of crude oil; there need not be concern for this particular air pollutant. Although vanadium accumulates in the lungs with age, it has little or no toxicity and apparently no adverse effect on longevity.

Nutrients and Evolution

The probable need for vanadium in human nutrition is one more reason to rise to the challenge of maintaining natural, nutrient-rich diets. Little-known elements such as vanadium are certainly not restored to processed foods after they have been stripped away in the food factory, and yet they occur readily in nature and in unprocessed foods.

Trace elements are the nutrients man evolved on, abundant in our diets and those of our ancestors for all but the last twenty of the many millions of years it took life to evolve. In these past twenty years, food processing and high-yield farming techniques have caused depletion in the amounts of these nutrients found in our foods.

And who knows? Long after the human race has disappeared from earth, perhaps sea squirts will evolve a new race of green-blooded, vanadium-rich, intelligent creatures who put too much vanadium back in their processed foods after stripping away all the iron!

References

A new essential trace element—vanadium. *Medical News, JAMA* 222:3:255-256, 16 October 1972.

Hopkins, L. L. and Mohr, H. E. Vanadium as an essential nutrient. *Fed. Proc.* 33:1773, 1973.

Schroeder, H. A. *The trace elements and man.* Old Greenwich, Connecticut: Devin-Adair, 1973.

Schwarz, K. and Milne, D. B. Growth effects of vanadium in the rat. *Science* 174:426-428, 22 October 1971.

CHAPTER 26

Chromium

Chromium-Glucose Tolerance Factor Essential for Burning Blood Sugar

A certain desert rodent, the sand rat, develops sugar diabetes when raised on laboratory food. When the sand rat is returned to the desert, its diabetic condition disappears. What is the key nutrient missing from rat food which the rat finds in its natural forage? Extensive laboratory analyses indicate that it is *chromium*. Chromium bound in an organic form in the glucose tolerance factor (GTF) potentiates the effect of insulin on glucose intake and so suppresses the latent diabetes of the sand rat. The saltbush which is hoarded by the rat in its burrows contains enough GTF to prevent diabetes.

Other trace elements contained in the saltbush and known to have a hypoglycemic effect are manganese, zinc, calcium, potassium and sodium. Manganese, zinc and chromium are the most effective. Chromium is known to be essential to the effectiveness of the insulin hormone.

Dr. Walter Mertz of the Human Nutrition Laboratory in Beltsville, Maryland has spent the last fifteen years studying chromium and its availability to human life. Dr. Mertz has found that with glucose, as in the glucose tolerance test (GTTest), the chromium level of the blood rises with the glucose (blood sugar) level. With this glucose load, significant amounts of chromium are excreted in the urine and lost to the body. The GTTest is stressful, while sugars slowly released from fruits and vegetables would not dissipate the GTF and might even have enough GTF to take care of the contained starches and sugars.

Chromium Deficiency

In Western countries the body content of chromium decreases with age, while in Eastern countries where natural foods are eaten the chromium content is maintained. Many women in Western countries are so deficient in chromium that the white blood cell chromium level may decrease by 50 percent with each pregnancy, resulting first in complete alcohol intolerance and later in glucose intolerance (adult-type diabetes). The two best sources of chromium are brewer's yeast and sugar beet molasses. Because this molasses is less sweet than cane molasses, it is seldom marketed, and that leaves brewer's yeast as the best available source.

Glucose Tolerance Factor

Humans, like rats, need this glucose tolerance factor (GTF). GTF is an organic chromium compound whose exact chemical structure is now being determined. Trivalent chromium is known to be the center of the molecule which also contains two niacin molecules (vitamin B-3) and three amino acids. These amino acids are now known to be glutamic acid and glycine and cysteine. The scientists at Beltsville have tried to put this jigsaw puzzle together. Now that they have crystallized the GTF from commercial brewer's yeast they can subject the crystals to X-ray analysis and so disclose the exact configuration of the two niacins, three amino acids and the trivalent chromium. GTF works with the hormone insulin to maintain the delicate balance between hypoglycemic (low blood sugar) and hyperglycemic (high blood sugar) conditions. Glucose is required for every cellular function. It supplies the energy that is burned every time a muscle contracts or a nerve impulse is transmitted.

The pure GTF is completely nontoxic when given by mouth or even intravenously to the mouse and rat. Yet it is now undergoing chronic toxicity studies to determine whether that which has been separated from brewer's yeast is toxic when administered over a long period of time! That's silly, of course, but that's the way the food and drug laws are written. Because of having to work within these legal restrictions, the pure GTF is not yet available for use in man. In the meantime we must all take six brewer's yeast tablets morning and night if we wish to make sure we get enough of this new vitamin which contains chromium.

A similar vitamin, B-12, contains cobalt rather than chromium. B-12 is the only vitamin which must be given by injection because absorption from the intestines is so poor. GTF is well absorbed by mouth both in man and in animals, so injection will not be necessary. The human dose of pure GTF is now estimated to be 2 to 6 mg per day by mouth. GTF is not entirely new since brewer's yeast and soluble chromium salts have been used to lower the insulin requirement of unstable diabetic children and also to get older patients off insulin and oral insulin substitutes.

GTF is then a trivalent chromium in an organic chemical complex which cannot be easily synthesized in the body but may be synthesized by the normal bacteria of the intestine when enough chromium is contained in the diet. Older people in Western nations are depleted of their GTF and need a good dietary source. Eventually Cr^{+++} will be shifted from rare-trace-metal-nutrient status to full-fledged-vitamin status since adequate synthesis in the human body is questionable.

If you think the GTTest is stressful, imagine what happens to the GTF when glucose 5 percent or 10 percent is given intravenously to nourish the patient in the postoperative period. Pecarek and his colleagues have found that the blood chromium drops precipitously when 60 gm of glucose is given intravenously—for example, 600 ml of 10 percent glucose. If the postoperative patient also has a virus infection, the blood chromium may drop to one-third (from 1.49 to 0.45 ppb). If the patient is then given intravenous glucose, the end results might be disastrous. Our hypoglycemic patients avoid hospitals and put off needed elective operations in justified fear of the intravenous glucose which may be given like the daily bath whether the patient needs it or not!

With Dr. Mertz's discovery we should have the GTF available in the 5 or 10 percent glucose, perhaps with a trace-element nutrient solution containing at least zinc, calcium, magnesium and manganese. The evidence for the need for each of these with GTF in glucose metabolism is scientifically solid—so why wait? Because of the food and drug laws, we must wait until scientific intravenous nutrition is slowly justified—at great expense.

Brewer's Yeast for GTF

Simple measurements of the chromium content of food can be misleading because chromium occurs in several forms with the range of oral absorption between 1 percent and 10 percent. Inorganic chromium is only 1 percent absorbable or less. Eggs have a high chromium concentration, but little of their chromium content is in the organic form biologically available as GTF. Chromium-containing foods with biologically active chromium are brewer's yeast, black pepper, liver, beef, whole-wheat bread, beets, beet sugar molasses, mushrooms and beer. Among these, far and away the highest in chromium content is brewer's yeast. For the patient suspected of impaired glucose tolerance, brewer's yeast tablets are an indispensable supplement to the diet.

Questions to Be Answered

Since the GTF contains two molecules of niacin and since some schizophrenics respond to extra niacin and many schizophrenics have impaired glucose tolerance, we must work harder to correlate one or more of the schizophrenias with deficiency of niacin or of the GTF or both. Do large doses of niacin make trivial dietary amounts of chromium more effective? Will the GTF be effective in the hypoglycemias or only in diabetes? Is any type of mental disorder produced by deficiency in the GTF? All of these questions and more must be answered.

We know that certain vegetables will form the GTF when the soil is supplemented with the chromium ion. Perhaps further supplementation with niacin and chromium might allow more of the GTF to be formed. At least, the riddle is almost solved, and we look forward to the time when pure GTF will be available for use in schizophrenic and hypoglycemic patients and in diabetics.

References

Jennings, J. Diet, hormones and diabetes. *Prevention* p. 83, December 1971.

Hambidge, M. Chromium nutrition in man. *Amer. J. Clin. Nutr.* 27:505 May 1974.

Mertz, W. Chromium occurrence and function in biological systems. *Phys. Rev.* 49:163, April 1969.

Mertz et al. *Fed. Proc.* 33:659, 1974.

Pecarek, R. S. et al. *Anal. Biochemistry* 59:283, 1974.

——— *Fed. Proc.* 33:660, 1974.

——— Relationship between serum chromium concentrations and glucose utilization in normal and infected subjects. *Diabetes* 24:350, 1975.

Schroeder, H. A. et al. Chromium deficiency as a factor in atherosclerosis. *J. Chron. Dis.* 23:123, 1970.

CHAPTER 27

Tin

Tin was discovered to be an essential life element during the 1960s; however, the nature of its specific functions is debatable. Because of its widespread use in industry, tin has a high potential for atmospheric pollution. Higher levels are therefore found in the lungs than in any other tissues. More lung tin is found in people in highly industrialized areas of the country than in other areas.

Apparently only a mildly poisonous effect results from the inhalation or ingestion of tin salts. Stannous chloride is an example of a tin salt which is found frequently as a chemical preservative. Stannous fluoride is present in some toothpastes. The average daily consumption by man, as indicated by food analysis on a collection of samples, is approximately 2 mg. Attempts to determine normal tissue and body tin content have been hindered by two problems: the destruction of the structure of the chemical complexes of tin during the process of ashing the sample, and lack of adequate research into the nature of tin complexes or molecules in biological samples.

Diets containing high levels of tin can frequently cause anemia unless sufficient amounts of iron are given. Experiments have shown that in rats, 0.3 percent tin in the diet caused growth depression and lowered the amount of hemoglobin synthesized. In this study, some histological changes occurred in the liver. These effects were diminished by administration of copper and iron. Therefore, one might conclude that tin does not work in the body system in isolation but is affected by other trace metals, particularly iron and copper.

Since tinplate is widely used in the canning of foods, continued research efforts should be made to determine whether tin is entirely innocuous. One report has stated that asparagus spears had a different taste when canned in glass jars. The preferable taste was restored when traces of tin were added to asparagus in glass jars.

References

Dekker, M. *Newer trace elements in nutrition.* New York: Mertz and Cornatzer, 1947.

Hiles, R. Absorption, distribution and excretion of inorganic tin in rats. *Toxicity and Applied Pharmacology* 27:366-379, 1974.

Trager, J. *The bellybook.* New York: Grossman, 1972.

CHAPTER 28

Cobalt

Cobalt is essential for life as a vital part of the vitamin B-12 molecule. No other function of cobalt in animal or man is known. Dr. Henry A. Schroeder believes that humans do not need to worry about cobalt deficiency because humans require very little of this trace metal and we receive adequate supplies from animal sources. Thus, we need only worry about B-12 deficiency in strict vegetarians and older people. No evidence of cobalt insufficiency has been observed in humans, even in cases where there was not enough cobalt in the soil to keep plant-eating sheep and cattle healthy.

Beginning in 1935, mysterious wasting diseases afflicted cattle and sheep in areas of Australia and New Zealand. After a long and exhaustive investigation, a chain of nutritional insufficiencies was traced. In 1948, vitamin B-12 was discovered to contain cobalt. The soil in the areas of affliction was found to be deficient in cobalt. Local plants, therefore, were deficient in that mineral and the plants failed to supply the animals with amounts of cobalt needed for sufficient B-12 production.

Cobalt Excess

In 1966, another strange new disease, which culminated in heart failure, struck heavy beer drinkers in Quebec City, Canada; Leuven, Belgium; Omaha, Nebraska; and Minneapolis, Minnesota. Various physicians and researchers voiced opinions as to the cause. Some attributed this disease of the heart muscle to an excess of cobalt. Others thought other dietary factors were involved and that cobalt was not solely responsible, and Dr. C. A. Alexander noted that many of the victims had inadequate diets, especially low in protein. These tragic victims were consuming between six and thirty bottles of beer per day, and the *Annals of Internal Medicine* reported that 1.2 ppm of cobalt were found in the Canadian beer. The film left on the glassware by synthetic detergents kills the foamy "head" of beer. Therefore, cobalt was added to beer to preserve the foamy head and keep the product aesthetically pleasing.

As "beer drinkers' cardiomyopathy" illustrates, too much cobalt can be toxic. Administering too much cobalt has caused polycythemia (too many red blood cells) in rats, mice, guinea pigs, ducks, chickens, pigs, dogs and humans.

It is interesting that G. S. Wiburg et al. have found that a high-quality protein diet gave considerable protection against the toxicity of cobalt. Nutrition must continue to be a complete picture, not just a couple of spotlighted items.

References

Alexander, C. A. Cobalt-beer cardiomyopathy. *Amer. J. Med.* October, 1972.

Cobalt and the heart. *Annals of Int. Med.* 70:2, February 1969.

Wiburg, G. S. et al. Factors affecting the cardiotoxic potential of cobalt. *Clinical Toxicology* 2(3):257-271, September 1969.

CHAPTER 29

Fluoride

Elemental fluorine is a highly reactive, greenish-yellow gas and therefore never occurs alone in nature; the fluoride ion, however, is common and occurs in minerals bonded to metals to make binary fluoride salts. The wide distribution of these salts in the ocean and soil is responsible for the presence of fluoride in all body tissues. Fluoride has never been proven essential to life, but it is important in human nutrition to help maintain normal bone and tooth structure and resistance of teeth to decay. Fluoride has been administered alone to curb osteoporosis (a decrease in bone density) and to stop the loss of hearing associated with otosclerosis. Its most extensive and widely publicized use has been as an additive to public drinking water.

The Fluoridation Debate

Fluoridation may be traced back to Colorado Springs and the year 1916. There, a dentist named Frederick S. McKay noticed mottled teeth, but few cavities, in his patients. The city's water supply was analyzed and found to contain 2 ppm of fluoride as soluble salts. (Optimal for good tooth structure is 1 ppm.) Subsequent surveys throughout the world revealed a definite inverse relationship between incidence of dental caries and fluoride concentration in drinking waters. Excessive fluoride intake, however, was found to cause mottled teeth. This condition is characterized by chalky white splotches over the surface of the teeth combined with intermittent yellow-brown staining. In severe cases, there is pitting of the enamel which causes the teeth to appear corroded.

The incidence of dental caries and the incidence of mottling as functions of fluorine concentration were carefully plotted on a logarithmic scale. The two lines crossed at 1 ppm, which became the standard value for "eufluorosis." This condition occurs when there is optimum protection against dental caries with a minimum of mottling. Now hundreds of municipalities have fluoridated their water supplies to maintain fluoride levels of 0.8 to 1.2 ppm. For areas of higher mean temperature (more sweating and therefore more drinking) less fluoride is needed. Fluoridation has produced average reductions of 40 to 70 percent in the incidence of dental caries in children born after the treatment started.

Still, hundreds of communities refrain from adding fluoride to their water. Opponents of fluoridation maintain that we already receive enough fluoride from other sources. Tea, for example, is rich in fluorine, and many industries emit fluorine fumes in processing minerals. Opponents cite cases where cows have grazed on fluoride-rich pasture and have become exceedingly crippled. They also cite cases where tooth mottling occurs. Tooth decay, they maintain, is a disease of civilization caused by our excessive intake of sweets and carbohydrates, and fluoridation is only a ploy to keep soft-drink and candy industries in business. Those who sweat excessively and drink only soft drinks are apt to be fluoride-treatment failures.

On the other hand, statistics show that the benefits of fluoridation far outweigh their costs; fluorosis (fluoride poisoning), mottling and other ill effects have been minimal as long as fluoride levels are monitored, supervised and maintained in the neighborhood of 1 ppm. Anthropologists have demonstrated that tooth decay has occurred in all agricultural people throughout history, whether they had access to sweets and junk foods or not. And finally, the foremost trace elements experts universally and independently concur that fluoridation of water supplies is generally beneficial. These scientists are Navia of Alabama, Schroeder of Vermont, Mertz of Maryland and Underwood of Australia.

Fluoride in toothpaste is most effective before it is diluted by saliva, when it comes directly in contact with teeth and can inhibit bacterial growth. Direct contact with the teeth is also the means by which fluoridated waters reduce caries. Good food sources of fluoride include fish, cheese, and meat as well as tea.

References

Shupe, J. L., Olson, A. E., Sharma, R. P. Fluoride toxicity in domestic and wild animals. *Clinical Toxicology* 5:195, 1972.

Sodium fluoride halts otosclerosis hearing loss. *JAMA* 224:1482, 11 June 1973.

Underwood, E. J. *Trace elements in human and animal nutrition.* New York: Academic Press, 1971.

CHAPTER 30

Nickel: An Essential Trace Metal but Where?

In the 1920s the trace element nickel was discovered in animal tissues. At one time, nickel was thought to be the only element in the periodic table not essential to animals; this belief resulted from the difficulty in preparing nickel-deficient diets, since nickel is ubiquitous. (It occurs in the air, in plants and in animals, including the newborn.) Until recently, researchers were also handicapped by the lack of appropriate environments for the raising and maintaining of laboratory animals. However, nickel has been found to have a physiological role both in animal and human metabolism.

More is known about the effects of nickel in certain animals than in man. Nickel in tissues outside the intestine intensifies the hypoglycemic effect of insulin in both the rabbit and the dog. Large doses alter lipid (fatty substance) metabolism, and injection of nickel amino acid complexes into rabbits increases plasma lipids. In humans, it has an antidotal effect on the hypertensive action of adrenalin (the hormone found in the adrenal medulla area of the brain) which acts as a vasoconstrictor and cardiac stimulant. Its possible physiological function, therefore, may involve hormone, lipid and also membrane metabolism.

In human blood serum a concentration of nickel is maintained within a characteristic range. High levels may occur in patients who suffer from a blockage of blood flow to the heart (myocardial infarction), in patients with strokes and severe burns and in women with toxemia of pregnancy or uterine cancer. Low levels occur in patients with cirrhosis of the liver or chronic kidney failure. Significant concentrations of nickel are found in DNA and RNA and may contribute to the stabilization of nucleic acids.

Contradictions

Evidence concerning the potentially harmful or beneficial effects of nickel seems contradictory. Although nickel is essential in the diet of chickens, it can be toxic to humans when absorbed in large quantities. Nielsen and Sauberlich reported in 1970 that young chicks fed a regulated diet consisting of 40 ppb of nickel (high dose) developed symptoms of pigmentation changes in the shank skin, swelling in the legs, dermatitis, fat- and oxygen-depleted livers (and thus suboptimal function of that organ) and a small accumulation of nickel in the liver, bone and aorta.

The ill effects of nickel and nickel-containing compounds in humans probably range from dermatitis to lung cancer. Exposure to nickel is widespread, since it is found in such common articles as nickel coins, eyeglass frames, costume jewelry, kitchen appliances, pins, scissors and hair clips. Nickel can be most dangerous when present in combination with carbon monoxide. The resulting substance, nickel carbonyl, which is encountered in many industries, can be lethal. Recently, thirty-one men working in an oil refinery were exposed to nickel carbonyl and required hospitalization; three died as a result. Symptoms of this poisoning are frontal headache, vertigo, nausea and vomiting. Delayed reactions may also include constrictive chest pain and cough.

A final warning to cigarette smokers: nickel and its carbonyls are suspected of causing cancer, and nickel carbonyl is found in tobacco and is present in cigarette smoke. It has been shown that the amount of nickel capable of inducing lung cancer in rats is equivalent to that of fifteen cigarettes a day smoked for one year.

Nickel may be used in an organic complex, as cobalt is in vitamin B-12, or as chromium is in the glucose tolerance factor. This conjecture needs further study.

References

Nielsen, F. H. and Ollerich, D. A. Nickel: a new essential trace element. *Federation Proceedings* 33:6, June 1974.

Nielsen, F. H. and Sauberlich, H. E. Evidence of a possible requirement for nickel by the chick. *Proc. Soc. Exp. Biol. and Med.* 134:3, July 1970.

Studies show nickel could play major metabolic role. *JAMA* 214:4, 26 October 1972.

Sunderman, F. Jr.; Nomoto, S.; Pradhan, A. M.; Levine, H.; Bernstein, S. H. and Hirsch, R. Increased concentrations of serum nickel after acute myocardial infarction. *New Eng. J. of Med.* 283:896-899, 22 October 1970.

Sunderman, F. Jr.; Nomoto, S.; Morang, R.; Nechay, M. W.; Burke, C. N. and Nielsen, S. W. Nickel deprivation in chicks. *J. Nutr.* 102:259-268, February 1972.

Trace metals—medicine's newest alchemy: II, an essential role for nickel? *Medical World News,* 21 April 1972.

von Mertz, D. P., Koschnick, R. and Wilk, G. The renal excretion of nickel by humans. Studies on the metabolism of trace elements, IV. *Z. Klin. Chem. u. Klin. Biochem.* Berlin: Walter de Gruyter, 1970.

CHAPTER 31

Aluminum

Aluminum. What is it and how is it used? If a layman were asked what aluminum is used for, he might say that it is used as foil to wrap foods and to make pots and pans. A scientist might reply that it is used in antacids, deodorants and baking powder. However, when asked what aluminum's function is in the human body, most people probably would not know. Scientists don't know either! There is still a great deal to learn about it.

Although aluminum is plentiful in the earth, relatively low concentrations are found in the tissues of plants and animals. Dr. Henry Schroeder, a foremost authority on the relationships between trace elements and man, believes that there may be more aluminum in modern man than was present in primitive man; one of the principal causes may be food additives. For example, sodium aluminum phosphate is used as an emulsifier in some processed cheeses. Table salt often contains sodium silico aluminate or aluminum calcium silicate to prevent the salt from caking. One of the bleaching agents used to whiten flour is potassium alum, an aluminum-containing compound.

The body stores its highest concentrations of aluminum in the lungs, liver, thyroid and brain. Usually, most of the aluminum taken into the body is later excreted. Although concern has been expressed about the ingestion of aluminum from cookware and aluminum-containing baking powder, some authorities such as E. J. Underwood and H. A. Schroeder contend that no harmful effects or dangers result from using these things in the preparation of food.

Dr. Schroeder discovered that mice and rats fed 10 ppm aluminum in their drinking water during their lifetime did not develop ill effects either in their growth or lifespan. Ehrismann reported in 1939 that rabbits and guinea pigs exposed to aluminum dust six hours daily for several weeks showed no abnormalities except for irritation of the lining of the nose and throat with the larger doses.

However, the stomach antacid, aluminum hydroxide gel, which has many trade names, can greatly reduce blood phosphate, according to L. R. I. Baker of London. With low serum phosphate the bones dissolve, the muscles ache and are extremely weak. In a patient on regular dialysis therapy for his poor kidney function, bone pain and the muscle weakness disappeared six weeks after the aluminum hydroxide therapy was stopped. The porosity of the bones was healed in three months, as judged by X-ray examination. Older patients, who are particularly subject to osteoporosis, should therefore limit their use of aluminum hydroxide gel.

To date, there is no conclusive evidence that aluminum is essential for the life of microorganisms, plants, animals or man. On the contrary, aluminum may be harmful.

Aluminum's Ill Effects

Many aluminum salts have antisweat effects when used with other chemicals. Because of this, many deodorants contain aluminum salts which can produce a contact dermatitis and irritation. The skin rash disappears when the deodorant is discontinued. This rash is minor compared with the possible brain damage which can result from too much inhaled or ingested aluminum.

Kopeloff et al. reported in 1942 that in animals the application of trace amounts of aluminum to the surface of the brain will initiate the electrical activity of seizures or fits. According to Klatzo et al., the injection of aluminum salts into the fluid surrounding the brain will initiate the degeneration characteristic of some types of senile dementia. Crapper et al. at the University of Toronto have found that aluminum-injected cats are slower learners in a simple conditioned avoidance task. The level of aluminum in the cats' brains is exactly equivalent to the high level of aluminum (12 mcg per gm) found in the brains of patients suffering from Alzheimer's disease, which is one type of senile dementia. The authors point out that this comparably high level in the two instances suggests that aluminum may be a poison in human senility. Aluminum therefore may be implicated as a factor in at least one brain disease.

As investigation of the rarer trace elements opens new vistas, uncharted regions appear that need to be explored. Aluminum is a prime example. More research needs to be done on the presence of high levels of aluminum in the brains of senile individuals and epileptics. In the meantime, aluminum pans should not be cleaned by cooking acid fruits, such as rhubarb, in them. The cleaning water goes into the rhubarb and hence into the unsuspecting consumer.

References

Adams, R. and Murray, F. *Minerals: Kill or cure?* New York: Larchmont Books, 1974.

Baker, L. R. I. et al. *Br. Med. J.* 3:150-151, 20 July 1974.

Crapper, D. R., Krishman, S. S. and Dalton, A. J. Brain aluminum distribution and experimental neuro-fibrillary degeneration. *Science* 180, May 1973.

Furia, T. E. *Handbook of Food Additives.* Cleveland; The Chemical Rubber Co., 1968.

Klatzo, I., Wisniewski, E. and Streicher, J. *J. Neuropathol. Exp. Neurol.* 23: 187, 1965.

Kopeloff, L., Barrera, S. and Kopeloff, N. *Amer. J. Psychiat.* 98:881, 1942.

McLaughlin, A. I. G.; Kazantzis, G.; King, E.; Teare, D.; Porter, R. J. and Owen, R. *Brit. J. Ind. Med.* 19:253, 1962.

Schroeder, H. A., *The trace elements and man.* Old Greenwich, Connecticut: Devin-Adair, 1973.

Sollman, T., *A manual of pharmacology*. 8th ed. Philadelphia: W. B. Saunders, 1957.

Underwood, E. J., *Trace elements in human and animal nutrition*. London: Academic Press, 1971.

PART FOUR

Toxic Effects of Heavy Metals

INTRODUCTION

The heavy metals, mercury and lead, have been known to produce psychotic behavior which has sometimes been diagnosed as schizophrenia. Thus, in the 1930s, when the wool-felting industry used mercury salts for sizing, some of the workers in the hat industry became known in medical literature as the "mad hatters." When mercury was discovered to be the poison, this disease of the hatters was controlled. Similarly, lead poisoning can produce a variety of nervous and mental symptoms as a result of which a patient may be labeled hyperactive or possibly even schizophrenic. Cadmium has not been studied for its effect on behavior. We do know, however, that cadmium increases the sense of pain, particularly in the bones that are malformed and painful in "Itai Itai" or "Ouch Ouch disease" which occurred in Japan after people had eaten fish raised in a cadmium-poisoned river.

Cadmium, in contrast with lead and mercury, does not pass the body's membranal barriers. Infants, in the uterus, are not affected by cadmium poisoning in the mother. Also the mother's milk is free of cadmium. Perhaps the blood-brain membranal barrier protects the brain from cadmium poisoning.

CHAPTER 32

Lead, Mercury and Cadmium

Lead Poisoning

Investigators are now busy assessing the role of lead and methyl mercury in hyperactivity and mental retardation in children and poisoned animals. To date, most of the available data are on lead poisoning. The pioneer article appeared in *Lancet* in 1972. Dr. Oliver David and his colleagues at the Downstate Medical Center in Brooklyn set up a study which employed a challenging dose of penicillamine in three groups of children. Penicillamine, a chelating agent, promotes the excretion of lead via the urinary pathway. The first group of children in the study were known to have been lead poisoned, the second were hyperactive children and the third were "normal" children. The individuals of each group were challenged with a 500 mg. dose of penicillamine at bedtime and the morning urine was collected from each child. The lead level in the urine was determined under blind test conditions. The excretion of lead was highest (325 micrograms per liter—mcg/l) in those children diagnosed as lead poisoned but in remission. The next highest urinary lead excretion was in the hyperactive children (146 mcg/l) and their lead excretion was significantly different from that of the "normal" children (77 mcg/l). All children were from poorer sections of Brooklyn and had been exposed daily to the usual hazards of lead intoxication from auto exhaust and old paint dust.

Drs. Michaelson and Sauerhoff of Cincinnati fed 4 percent lead carbonate to rats and found that the animals became hyperactive. Drs. Silbergelb and Goldberg of Johns Hopkins in Baltimore fed mice lead and again found hyperactivity. This abnormal activity was reduced by deanol or amphetamine therapy and made worse by phenobarbitol, a correlation with the known drug response in hyperactive children. Others have studied the effect of lead in rhesus monkeys and very young baboons. However, the degree of hyperactivity in these larger species was not measured.

Finally, Drs. Niklowitz and Yeager of Cincinnati have exposed rats to tetraethyl lead and analyzed the brains for levels of the more common trace elements zinc, copper and iron. All three of these essential trace elements were significantly decreased by lead exposure. Results of the study strongly indicate that the specific toxic property of lead which causes abnormal brain function is its ability to interfere competitively with the trace metal components of zinc, copper and iron dependent enzymes which regulate mental processes.

Many sources of lead in the environment are potentially hazardous. A major source of environmental lead is pollution from auto exhaust. Tetraethyl lead is added to most high-test gasolines to improve acceleration and as an antiknock. The concentration of lead in the atmosphere of large cities and in the air near interstate highways is so high as to cause toxic reactions in some particularly toxicity-prone individuals. Toll booth collectors have been known to exhibit toxic blood levels of lead. Caprio and his colleagues at the New Jersey College of Medicine in Newark studied inner-city children who lived near arterial highways. They found blood lead levels to be higher in children who lived closest to these roads. Many of the children had lead levels above 60 mcg percent—a level which indicates lead poisoning.

Darrow and his colleagues at Brattleboro, Vermont have found that sweepings from parking lots are sufficiently high in heavy metals as to retard the growth of young animals when these sweepings are added to the diet. The most likely poison from parking lots is lead from auto exhaust. Lead also often appears in the vegetation beside well-travelled highways. Cows who subsist on this vegetation alone can have lead-induced abortions. Vegetables grown beside busy highways should not be eaten unless their lead content can be proven safe for consumption.

The latest in a long series of smelter pollutions has occurred in Kellogg, Idaho where the Bunker Hill zinc smelter may have polluted the downwind environment with lead dust. Some of the children of Kellogg have developed lead poisoning for no apparent cause. Houses closest to the smelter had more children with lead poisoning. While the smelter may not be entirely to blame, the cumulative effect of smelter lead and auto exhaust lead can add up to clinical lead poisoning. When discovered, such communities should be labeled disaster areas with funds available for cleaning or relocation of homes and other buildings.

Lead may also enter our ambient air through cigarettes, due to the lead arsenate applied to the tobacco as an insecticide, through the burning of coal, and through the fumes and ash produced by the burning of lead battery casings. The decay products of gaseous radon, which enter the atmosphere through natural volcanic activity, contribute to the lead content of ambient air. At present, however, the chief source is exhaust from autos burning leaded gasoline.

In urban areas, the concentration of lead in polluted air varies inversely with altitude. This is only logical since lead is such a heavy element. Consequently, we find that lead poisoning occurs frequently in small urban dogs. Epilepsy is usually the first symptom. Unfortunately, it is also frequent among young urban people who toddle about close to the ground. In these, hyperactivity may be the first presenting symptom.

Another dangerous environmental source of lead is from the drinking water in soft water regions which courses through lead plumbing systems. Soft water is more acidic than hard water. Because of its acidity, soft water will erode lead from lead piping and become contaminated with this heavy metal.

A group of investigators in Glasgow, Scotland, directed

by Dr. A. D. Beattie of Stobhill Hospital, have established a significant correlation between lead ingested from contaminated soft drinking water and mental retardation in children. Dr. Beattie and his team studied 154 Glasgow children. Seventy-seven of the children were attending clinics in Glasgow because of retardation in mental development while the remaining seventy-seven were nonretarded healthy youngsters forming a control group matched for age, sex and geographic location in the city.

The investigators collected water samples from the taps of the homes where the children lived and also collected blood samples from their subjects. Analysis of the samples revealed significantly greater amounts of lead in water from the homes of the retarded children as compared with that from the homes of the normal children. Blood levels of lead were also higher in the retarded group than in the control group, strongly implicating tap water lead as the cause of brain damage.

Dr. Beattie and his colleagues further postulate that tap water lead poses a serious threat to children even before birth. Lead ingested by mothers drinking contaminated tap water is capable of crossing the placenta to the fetus. Since the blood-brain barrier in the fetus is less developed and therefore more permeable to toxic substances than it is in the full-term infant, the prenatal hazards of lead poisoning would indeed be probable.

On the basis of their findings, Dr. Beattie and his team emphasize the need to remove lead from plumbing systems (e.g. water tanks and pipes). Although this would be the most satisfactory solution, several years will be required to accomplish this goal. In the meantime, water reservoirs supplying Glasgow will be treated with calcium salts. By decreasing the acidity of the soft water, calcium salts will protect the water supplies from lead contamination.

Furthermore, sufficient dietary calcium has been found effective in preventing the accumulation of lead in body tissues. Two researchers, K. M. Six and R. A. Goyer, discovered that reducing dietary calcium in rats greatly enhanced the body burden of lead as evidenced by increased levels of lead in blood, bone and soft tissues. Professor C. Snowden of the University of Wisconsin also found that in calcium-deficient rats given water containing lead, lead replaced the lacking calcium in bones and teeth. Experimental studies conducted by L. G. Lederer and F. C. Bing, again using rats, indicated that adequate dietary calcium prevents accumulation of lead in body tissues by reducing absorption of ingested lead from the intestinal tract, a finding supported by the research of Professor F. Hsu and his colleagues at Cornell University using weanling pigs. Since calcium protects both water and body tissues from lead contamination, the addition of this trace element to drinking water supplies in high risk areas such as Glasgow will be highly beneficial.

Lead-based paints are another source of lead poisoning. A New York psychiatrist, Dr. William Niederland, speculates that a mysterious mental illness which struck the Spanish painter Goya at the age of 46, was lead poisoning caused by the artist's use of lead-based paints. For years, art historians have considered this illness to be the cause of an abrupt change in the subject matter of Goya's work—from pleasant court portraiture to grotesque social commentary. Dr. Niederland points out that Goya used large quantities of white paint made from lead carbonate in his work and, unlike other painters, often completed an entire painting in a single afternoon. Lead carbonate will seep through the intact skin and also give off noxious vapors. As a result of consistent and prolonged periods of exposure to a toxic lead compound, Goya could have absorbed into his bloodstream amounts of lead sufficient to produce brain damage. According to Dr. Niederland, the symptoms of Goya's illness—vertigo, mental confusion, hallucinations and impaired balance, hearing and speech—are characteristic of fulminating lead encephalopathy.

Three- or four-year-olds who cut their milk teeth on peeling lead-based paint or plaster in old dilapidated housing frequently develop lead poisoning. School children who chew on the lead-containing paint coatings of pencils can develop lead poisoning. Adults who attempt to remove old lead-based paint by the usual dusty mechanical methods can also get lead poisoning—only wet methods should be used.

The home craftsman (or woman) should be especially careful of certain lead-containing pottery glazes. If fired at too low a temperature, the lead in the glaze is not fixed and can leach out into foods.

Young children are highly susceptible to lead poisoning from a wide variety of sources. Pica—the consumption of such items as dirt, paper and paint, all of which contain lead—is often the cause of lead intoxication in youngsters. Even babies, who are not yet subject to the range of exposure possible with more mobility, are not safe. The lead plugs used to seal evaporated milk cans are an occasional source of lead for infant formulas. Lead seams of fruit juice cans are a more frequent source.

Pet owners who dote on their precious furry friends might well become enraged at the news that poor Fido may be consuming toxic amounts of lead in his canned dog food. Others, less concerned with the welfare of the animal population, might simply shrug and say, "Well, I'm glad I don't eat dog food!" until acquainted with the full implications of this recent discovery. Researchers Hankin and Heichel of the Connecticut Agricultural Experiment Station, who determined that canned pet foods contain as much as 5.6 ppm lead, traced the lead contamination of such products to the processed organ meats which constitute the main ingredient of Fido's feed. With a daily ingestion of 170 gm (6 oz.) pet foods could contribute up to 1.19 mg of lead to the animal or human diet—about four times the dose of lead (0.3 mg per day) potentially toxic for children. Still convinced that only Fido faces the danger of lead poisoning, one must recall that humans, too, consume processed and fresh organ meats. Liver, for example, is a principal constituent of liverwurst, sausage and popular sandwich spreads. Upon examining seven samples of commercial liverwurst, Hankin and Heichel found lead levels ranging between 1.8 and 7.6 ppm. On the basis of a daily consumption of 113 gm (4 oz.) these products could contribute 0.20 to 0.86 mg lead to the human diet—about 0.6 to 2.9 times the dose of lead potentially toxic for children. Market samples of fresh beef and pork liver examined by the two researchers showed lead levels ranging between 1.4 and 1.6 ppm and levels as high as 5.6 ppm in pork, 7.6 ppm in beef and 10.9 ppm in turkey have been reported. Such meats, then, would contribute even greater quantities of lead to the human diet. On the basis of these findings, fresh liver sausage would be a doubly hazardous food. Farmers may supplement their hogs' feed with copper sulfate in order to accelerate the animals' weight gain. Copper, like lead, is a toxic heavy metal and liver already contains lead, so the poor sausage-lover is threatened on two counts!

Thus, even though most people do not consume pet food, liver and other organ meats are normal components of the human diet and the inadvertent ingestion of lead (and copper) by humans eating liver products is yet another insidious environmental source of heavy metal poisoning.

Because of increasing evidence linking excess blood and tissue lead with hyperactivity and mental retardation, researchers have sought simple, valid methods for determining the presence of toxic amounts of lead in the body. Although it is possible, direct analysis of blood for lead, which demands expensive equipment, skill in analytical technique and great care to avoid the risk of sample contamination from environmental lead, is unsuitable as a general diagnostic procedure.

Recently, Dr. A. A. Lamola and his colleagues at the Bell Laboratories in New Jersey successfully devised a simple, inexpensive diagnostic screening test for lead poisoning. Together with his coworkers, Dr. Lamola found that the metabolite zinc protoporphyrin (ZPP) accumulates in erythrocytes (red blood cells) as a result of lead interference with heme synthesis. ZPP is a fluorescent compound which can be measured directly and accurately by means of a spectrofluorometer, thereby offering a valid indirect means of monitoring blood lead concentration. Bell Laboratories has designed a small inexpensive fluorometer which is currently undergoing field testing. If approved for use, this instrument will allow frequent examination of children in high risk populations, thus increasing the public health benefits of this new test.

The Mercury Threat

Pesticides and some large fish are the most notorious sources of mercury. If fish are poisoned by mercury, the extent of poisoning is directly proportional to the size of the fish, and therefore the large tuna such as yellow fin and big eye will then be much more likely to poison people who eat them daily than albacore or skipjack. The mercury menace in swordfish is enough to keep this large fish off the market. Swordfish used for commercial meat weigh as much as one hundred pounds.

The process known as organic complexing is responsible for the spread of the culprit compound, methyl mercury, throughout the aquatic world. Mercury-containing bacteria are first consumed by algae, and eventually the fish eat the algae and men eat the fish. At each step upward on the food chain, the concentration of methyl mercury increases. The amount of poison concentrated in the fish is thousands of times the amount concentrated in the algae. This is due to a half-life retention of mercury in fish of 200 days (i.e. every 200 days, a total of one-half the previous amount of mercury is dissipated). Fish balance their mercury with a higher level of selenium than man. Mercury selenide is not toxic because it is excreted.

Mercury enters rivers and lakes in a number of ways. Chemical companies use it as an electrode in the production of chlorine and it ends up in places like Lake St. Clair (which is closed to commercial fishing) where a large company has a chloralkali factory at Sarnia, Ontario. Paper pulp mills use mercury compounds as slimicides in their paper-making process. (Slimicides inhibit the growth of slime molds.) In 1970, the U.S. government urged fishermen not to eat or sell fish caught in Lakes Erie, Ontario, and Champlain and the Oswego and Niagara Rivers, because of the mercury threat.

Accounts of mercury poisoning have appeared throughout history, dating back to the time of Hippocrates. In 1700, Ramazzini recorded mercury poisoning in surgeons using mercurial ointment. But it was not until the Minimata Bay disaster in Japan (1953-60) that the mercury content of foods was considered a serious problem. In that disaster, 111 persons died or were severely disabled after eating fish which had been contaminated with a methyl mercury-containing effluent from a local plastics factory.

Among the most striking case histories in recent times is that of the New Mexican laborer who fed seed grain sweepings to his hogs. The grain had been treated with Panogen, an organic mercury-containing antifungal agent; the hogs were eventually butchered and fed to the laborer's family. Within two weeks three out of the family of ten were stricken with a derangement of the brain and spinal cord. One girl lay unconscious for eight months in the hospital before waking totally blind and unable to speak. Her sister could walk and talk with effort, but the younger brother tumbled into a four month coma. The problem was eventually traced back to the organic mercury compound used as a fungicide. This mercury compound had passed into the hogs and the pork poisoned the family!

The use of mercurial fungicides on seed grains has caused numerous poisonings around the world. Frequently the poison warning on the side of the sack is only in English. A hungry Asiatic is not apt to take lessons in English in order to learn the meaning of words on a sack of potential food.

Mercury can accidentally originate from a variety of sources such as electric batteries, mercury vapor lamps, mercury switches and coal burning. Mercury from all coal-burning sources amounts to 3,000 metric tons per year, whereas natural sources of weathering rock and soil contribute 230 metric tons per year. Other sources include accidental breaking of thermometer and barometer bulbs and silvering pennies.

Calomel (mercurous chloride), widely acclaimed during the nineteenth century as the "Samson of the *Materia Medica*" due to its alleged effectiveness in the treatment of every infectious disease from smallpox to malaria, typhoid fever and even rheumatism, acts as a most insidious cause of mercury poisoning. As early as 1825, a poem appeared in a Virginia publication depicting the dire consequences of mercury poisoning which resulted from the use of this chemical and urging physicians to stop using calomel:

> How'er their patients do complain
> Of head, or heart, or nerve or vein,
> Of fever, thirst, or temper fell,
> The Medicine still is Calomel.
> Since Calomel's become their boast,
> How many patients have they lost,
> How many thousands they make ill,
> Of poison with their Calomel.

Since in recent times, calomel's laxative properties have rendered it an active ingredient in several commercial remedies, the threat of mercury poisoning remains. Dr. J. R. Wands and his colleagues have found that continued use of the "insoluble" mercurous chloride as a laxative will result in severe poisoning. In two patients with chronic kidney failure, tremor, watery diarrhea and dementia who finally died, autopsy revealed exceedingly high levels of mercury in both the colon and kidney. Mercury levels above normal were found in all organs tested including the brain.

Damage due to orally administered mercurous compounds became apparent when it was discovered that acrodynia (pink disease), a once-common disease of young children, was due to the use of teething powders containing calomel. In spite of the recognition of these hazards, mercurous chloride can still be purchased over the counter.

It is clear that man, like experimental animals, can absorb mercury from the intestine when it is ingested as mercurous chloride. Mercury accumulates within the brain, preferentially located in certain neuronal populations. Eventually, it reaches concentrations that damage neural elements, resulting in a variety of clinical manifestations. Mercurous compounds taken by mouth must therefore be considered potentially toxic.

Industrial workers are exposed to mercury in the manufacture of thermometers, mercury-arc rectifiers and other scientific equipment, the manufacture of dry cells, and the cleaning and packing of mercury compounds. Dental workers are exposed to the dangers of mercury in mercury-amalgam fillings, which contaminate the hands and atmosphere. Finally, travellers on their way to the Aland Islands might make a travel note to beware of the mercury-containing goosander eggs.

Mercury poisoning can be helped if treated quickly with a chelating agent such as penicillamine. Approximately 10 percent of ingested mercury goes to the brain. In the cases of methyl and phenyl mercury, the brain may be quickly depleted of its zinc. Methyl mercury can cause neurotoxic effects and produce birth and genetic defects; it can produce excessive salivation, loss of teeth, gross tremor, and serious mental disturbance (e.g. "the mad hatters"). As the endpoint of its deleterious effects, overt neurological impairment or death may occur. Organic mercury compounds may irritate the skin, cause redness, irritation and blistering. Skerfring, Hanson and Lindsten (in 1970) found chromosome damage in humans exposed to mercury through consumption of mercury-poisoned fish.

The Cadmium Hazard

A third heavy metal scourge is cadmium. Sources of cadmium include refined foods which may have low zinc-to-cadmium ratios, water and mains and pipes (which may have cadmium content due to the impurities in zinc used many years ago for the galvanizing process, and through which soft water flows), coal burning and tobacco smoke. As we have seen, the outbreak of "Ouch Ouch disease" in Japan was due to cadmium, which appeared as a byproduct in the zinc-refining process.

While an excess of zinc in the body might prevent the accumulation of cadmium, a slight zinc deficiency would enhance cadmium poisoning. Cadmium can replace zinc in the body and cause high blood pressure and cardiovascular disease. Cadmium can interfere with copper metabolism as well.

Cadmium poisoning is a most subtle metal poisoning—probably only exceeded in subtlety by poisoning caused by the trace metals copper and iron. Cadmium deposits in the kidney and arteries raise blood pressure and cause early atherosclerosis. The early zinc used for galvanizing contained cadmium as an impurity. In many old buildings the big galvanized cold water tank was placed in the basement as the building was under construction. After thirty years the tanks start to leak and must be removed. The only possible method of removal is to cut the tank into smaller sections with an oxyacetylene burning torch. Basements are not noted for ventilation, and fresh air masks are seldom available. The tank cutter gets fume fever because of the zinc and cadmium. Since workers know of the discomfort, it usually falls to the lot of the biggest and bravest man to face the danger. In a state hospital system the chief engineer was the one who cut up the tanks in the old buildings and he, in due course, died of hypertension and atherosclerosis of the spinal artery. In cutting down the abandoned elevated line in New York, workers who did not wear their fresh air masks got lead poisoning from old paint.

Those who live downwind from zinc smelters may be exposed to great excesses of cadmium both from air and contaminated soil. Measures are now being taken to prevent atmospheric pollution in the smelting of zinc ore.

The cigarette smoker gets cadmium from each cigarette often in sufficient quantity to produce emphysema—a disease in which the lungs have lost their natural elasticity. Patients with emphysema should stop smoking and take extra dietary supplements of zinc and vitamin B-6.

Trace metals have always occurred in man's natural environment. Consequently, they have played a role in our evolution and many of them are essential in our diet. However, when man began to use metals in manufacturing, the exposure to heavy metals greatly increased. In the four thousand, five hundred years since the introduction of metals in industry, there has not been time for our biological systems to adjust to more than the trace amounts formerly found.

The elements which are toxic are those which accumulate in mammalian tissue as a body burden with age. Other industrially used metal contaminants we have not discussed are: beryllium, silver, antimony, tellurium, barium and gold.

To summarize, heavy metal intoxication of the brain can cause hyperactivity in animals and presumably in some children. This hyperactivity in rats may be accompanied by a displacement of a sedative metal such as zinc from the brain. We know that zinc will antagonize mercury toxicity. Perhaps adequate zinc therapy along with chelators for lead will decrease the behavioral hyperactivity in children caused by lead toxicity. Since hyperactivity is only a symptom and not a diagnosis, we will probably find in the future many other causes of hyperactivity in children, each with its own logical treatment. In the meantime, analysis for suspected lead poisoning is indicated in the hyperactive child.

TABLE 32.1

Hazardous environmental heavy metals

Metal	*Sources*	*Illness*
Lead	**Auto exhaust**	**Anemia**
	Lead-based paints	**Colic**
	Smelter pollution	**Fatigue**
	Lead water pipes	**Convulsions**
	Lead batteries	**Hyperactivity**
		Psychosis
Mercury	**Coal burning**	**Psychosis**
	Batteries	**Blindness**
	Some fungicides	**Paralysis**
	Fish	**Convulsions**
		Kidney damage
Cadmium	**Zinc smelters**	**Hypertension**
	Cadmium plating	**Kidney damage**
	Cigarette smoking	**Atherosclerosis**
Copper	**Acid well water**	**Hyperactivity**
	Soft drink dispensers	**Psychosis**
	Algicide use in reservoirs	**Depression**
	Hemodialysis	**Disperceptions**
		Atherosclerosis
		Hypertension

References

Beattie, A. D. et al. Role of chronic low-level lead exposure in the etiology of mental retardation. *Lancet* p. 589, 15 March 1975.

Caprio, R. J., Margulis, H. L. and Joselow, M. M. Lead absorption in children in relationship to urban traffic densities. *Arch. Environ. Health* 28:195, 1974.

David, L. E. et al. *Arch. Neurol.* 30:428, 1974.

David, O. et al. *Lancet* 2:900, 1972.

Environmental health perspectives. *Experimental Issue 7*, May 1974.

Fellows, L. Color pages in magazines cited as a source of lead poisoning. *The*

New York Times, 25 November 1973.

Goldwater, L. J. Mercury in the environment. *Scientific American*, May 1971.

Hankin, L., Heichel, G. H. and Botsford, R. A. Lead in pet food and processed organ meats: a human problem? *JAMA* 231:484-485, 1975.

Hsu, F. et al. Interaction of dietary calcium with toxic levels of lead and zinc in pigs. *J. Nutr.* 105:112-118, 1975.

Lamola, A. A. et al. Zinc protoporphyrin (ZPP): a simple, sensitive fluorometric screening test for lead poisoning. *Clin. Chem.* 21:93-97, 1975.

Lederer, L. G. and Bing, F. C. Effect of calcium and phosphorous on retention of lead by growing organs. *JAMA* 114:1 457-2461, 1940.

Michaelson, A. and Sauerhoff, M. Hyperactivity and brain catecholamines in lead-exposed developing rats. *Science* 182:725-727, 1973.

Newman, B. Handicraft hazards: pottery made at home can be very harmful. *Wall Street Journal*, 11 November 1971.

Niklowitz, W. J. and Yeager, D. W. Interference of Pb with essential brain tissue Cu, Fe and Zn as main determinant in experimental tetraethyllead encephalopathy. *Life Sciences* 13:897-905, 1973.

Rensberger, B. Goya grotesquery laid to lead's use. *The New York Times*, 28 February 1974.

Risse, G. B. Calomel and the American medical sects during the 19th century. *Mayo Con. Proc.* 48:59, 1973.

Schroeder, H. A. Trace elements in the human environment. *The Ecologist*, May 1971.

Silbergelb, E. K. and Goldberg, A. M. A lead-induced behavioral disorder. *Life Sciences* 13:1275, 1973.

Six, K. M. and Goyer, R. A. Experimental enhancement of lead toxicity by low dietary calcium. *J. Lab. Clin. Med.* 76:933-942, 1970.

Skerfring, S., Hanson, K. and Lindsten, J. *Arch. Environ. Health* 21:133, 1970.

Trace metals: unknown, unseen pollution threat. *Chemical and Engineering News*, 19 July 1971.

Wands, J. R. et al. Massachusetts General Hospital, Boston, 57:92-101, 1974.

CHAPTER 33

Copper: The Fourth Heavy-Metal Intoxicant

Our Body Burden of Copper

As we have seen, the heavy metals lead, mercury and cadmium are poisons which slowly accumulate with age as a body burden, much as barnacles accumulate on a ship at sea. This body burden can shorten life by the production of hardening of the arteries, high blood pressure, kidney disease, psychosis, early senility and numerous other diseases of aging. We now have sufficient evidence to incriminate a fourth metal, copper, as a culpable heavy metal.

Copper Is Too Much with Us

Copper is essential in small amounts to form hemoglobin. This discovery was made by Dr. E. B. Hart of the University of Wisconsin in 1928, but work on the intimate metabolism of copper is proceeding slowly. Copper can be found in all iron salts and in many foods, so that adult man can be considered safe from copper deficiency. Dr. Gubler, in an excellent review published in 1956, states, "It is doubtful that an unquestioned case of copper deficiency has been reported in man. It is also extremely unlikely that copper deficiency could occur in man even on suboptimal diets." We have determined serum copper in more than seventeen hundred patients and have not found a single case of copper deficiency. In our present environment, we are satiated with copper, so that only premature infants and patients on parenteral (intravenous) feeding have shown copper deficiency. Anyone who eats and drinks gets copper!

The body of an adult contains 125 mg of copper; the liver, via the bile, is the main route of excretion of excess copper. The liver has the highest copper content, the brain is second, and other organs and tissues contain much less. Fetal liver at term contains approximately seven times as much copper as adult liver. Five to fifteen years are needed to bring the level of copper down to the adult level. Since copper is a stimulant to the brain, this excess copper may be a factor in the hyperactivity in children which ameliorates with age and slow elimination of the copper burden. This excess of copper in the young is also evident in sheep and cows. Lambs' and calves' livers are much higher in copper than are the livers from the fully-grown animals.

Postpartum Psychosis

We quote as follows from R. Gooch (1820):

> It is well known that some women, who are perfectly sane at all other times, become deranged after delivery, and that this form of the disease is called puerperal insanity. My situation gives me more than the common opportunities of seeing it and, though I am unable to make any important additions to our knowledge of the subject, I have witnessed some things which seem to me to deserve attention: these I will venture to describe, together with what I have observed about the causes, progress, and treatment of this distressing malady.
>
> The most common time for the disease to begin is a few days, or a few weeks, after delivery; sometimes it happens after several months, during nursing, or soon after weaning.
>
> The approach of the disease is announced by symptoms which excite little apprehension because they so often occur

> without any such termination; the pulse is quick without any manifest cause, the nights are restless, and the temper is sharp; soon, however, there is an indescribable hurry, and peculiarity of manner, which a watchful and experienced observer, and those accustomed to the patient will notice; her conduct and language become wild and incoherent; and at length she becomes decidedly maniacal; it is fortunate if she does not attempt her life before the nature of the malady is discovered.

Copper, and particularly ceruloplasmin (a copper-containing protein) is elevated by estrogens; therefore, the levels of copper and ceruloplasmin rise progressively during pregnancy. Serum copper is approximately 115 mcg percent at conception, and reaches a mean of 260 mcg percent at term. After delivery, a period of two to three months is required before the original serum copper level is reached. This high postpartum copper level may be a factor in causing postpartum depression and psychosis; more data are needed in this area. One must also discover the differences in copper metabolism when the pregnant schizophrenic patient carries a male or female child. We know that the incidence of postpartum psychosis is much greater after the birth of a male child. If the estrogen level alone were the cause, one would expect the reverse.

According to Ylastalo and Reinila, the exaggerated rise in serum copper may be a factor in toxemia of pregnancy (preeclampsia level, 287 v. 258 for normals) and in hepatosis (inflammation and enlargement of the liver) or pregnancy (serum copper, 342 mcg percent). Pfeiffer and Iliev have found that the oral contraceptive, with its potent estrogen, raises copper in schizophrenics to a level higher than that of the ninth month of pregnancy. This rise produces activation of their psychoses which may last for several weeks after stopping the pill. The remission of the psychosis corresponds to the slow decline of accumulated copper in the blood and tissues.

Dietary Copper

Copper is an essential element for supporting life, but, in excess, copper can be toxic. Environmental factors can cause copper and iron overloading. The foods we eat and the water we drink affect our delicate balance, depending on the environment and the material of the water piping. The average adult ingests 3 to 5 mg per day. Since the actual adult need is closer to 2 mg per day, an accumulation may occur.

From a biochemical point of view, surplus dietary copper can cause severe physical and mental illness. Although additional copper sulfate may promote growth in various animals, it would be prudent to consider the effect that this dietary supplement might have on those people eating the meat products. Even those who refrain from eating meat may be subject to copper intoxication; soybeans contain a significant amount of copper. Research is now under way on growing soybeans with extra zinc and manganese so that individuals relying on this product for their intake of protein will not be nutritionally deficient or too high in any one trace element.

Deficiency of Zinc Accentuates Copper Excess

Food-processing techniques deprive foods of many nutrients. Wheat, for example, has twenty-three nutrients crushed, ground and squeezed out of it during processing. This processing is designed to reduce trace metal content since such removal prolongs the shelf life. During the freezing process, fresh green vegetables are "blanched with sequestrants" to produce a bright green color when cooked. However, the zinc and manganese content is reduced to 20 percent of the normal range! A European diet provides more zinc and manganese than the American diet. Europeans consume homemade soups and fresh vegetables and drink wines, while Americans seem to favor frozen foods, ice cream, soft drinks and artificial fruit juices. Because the food we eat and the water we drink influence our physical and mental health, we should investigate the possibility that many of the devices used to promote growth in plants and animals and to process our foods may be detrimental to our own minds and bodies.

Copper in the Water We Use

Critical attention is now focused on certain elements in man's drinking water that may, in toxic quantities, cause severe physiological and mental illnesses or death. Pfeiffer and Iliev have shown that in some suburban homes, individual water systems where the well water is usually acid can produce copper intoxication. As an example of the copper in drinking water, look at these data from a suburban home in Peapack, New Jersey. The well water has 0.03 ppm of copper, the upper bath has 0.32 ppm and an outside faucet has 1.62 ppm. In the house, only the upper bathroom tap has drinkable water by United States Public Health Service (USPHS) standards (maximum 1 ppm).

TABLE 33.1

Typical copper content of home waters*

Residence water in Peapack, N. J., 22 June 1974

	Copper content
Well	**0.03 ppm**
Upstairs bath	**0.32 ppm**
Kitchen—Calgon charcoal filter	**1.24 ppm**
Outside faucet	**1.62 ppm**

* The dripping faucets of this home were noted for producing blue deposits on the porcelain. A brass filter containing charcoal was installed in the kitchen. This did not correct the basic fault, namely acid well water which leaches copper from the plumbing and even from the brass of the filter. Some outside, unused faucets can have copper levels of 50 ppm.

A recent report from Australia confirms the gravity of this finding. A new well was bored on an Australian farm and new copper plumbing was installed, complete with a copper hot-water tank. The mother was four months pregnant when the family moved to the farm. At birth, the male infant was not breast fed but rather bottle fed, with water from the tap being used to make the infant's formula. The child died at fourteen months of age with all the symptoms and findings of chronic copper intoxication.

Upon examination the well water had an acid pH of 3.8 to 4.8 (normal 7.0) and a copper content as high as 970 mcg percent. (The upper limit for drinking water set by the USPHS is 100 mcg percent.) The family was tested and all showed normal copper except the mother who, when given penicillamine (a chelating agent) excreted large amounts of copper. This suggests that copper excess could have started in utero. This death is the first to be reported from copper in the drinking water, but many previous deaths have been reported from copper poisoning.

Serum zinc deficiency and serum copper excess have become evident only since the change from galvanized water pipes to copper plumbing. Before copper plumbing, man obtained his needed supply of zinc by drinking water which had coursed through zinc-lined (galvanized) pipes. As a result of the installation of copper plumbing in conjunction with the slight acidity of most drinkable water, we are getting an excess of copper which may be antagonizing the zinc we obtain from food. This is most likely when water is pumped from shale or loam. In some areas of New Jersey, well water will produce pin holes in copper piping in ten years' time. The copper goes into the drinking water! (See Table 33.2.)

In subacute poisoning of rats with copper, Lal et al. have found great increases in liver copper and some deaths. The activity of a zinc-containing enzyme, lactic acid dehydrogenase, was decreased, as was that of the enzyme which destroys amines in the brain when they are no longer needed. Brain copper increased 36 percent in a six-week period, and the turnover of serotonin was apparently reduced. The adrenal glands markedly increased in weight—an index of stress.

Excess copper in the body may play a role in certain diseases. Mildred Seelig, in 1973, researched the role of the copper-molybdenum interaction in certain iron-deficiency anemias and has postulated that a high copper-molybdenum ratio in the American diet may contribute to iron-deficiency anemias and

TABLE 33.2

Copper content of some drinking waters in the eastern United States[a]

Location	*Water source*	*Dwelling*	*Copper content (ppm)*[b]
New York City	**River**	**Apartment**	**0.07**
Long Island	**Well**	**Cottage**	**0.03**
Cleveland	**Lake**	**Motel**	**0.06**
Boston	**Well**	**House**	**0.12**[c]
Greenwich, Conn.	**Well**	**House**	**0.35**[c]
Greenwich	**Well**	**House**	**0.37**[c]
Wilton, Conn.	**Well**	**House**	**1.60**[c]
Wilton	**Well**	**House**	**1.34**[c]
Wilton	**Well**	**House**	**0.68**[c]
Wilton	**Well**	**House**	**0.36**[c]
Wilton	**Well**	**House**	**0.40**[c]
Wilton	**Well**	**House**	**0.18**[c]
New Canaan, Conn.	**Well**	**House**	**0.85**[c]
Redding, Conn.	**Well**	**House**	**4.20**[c]
Belle Mead, N.J.	**Well**	**Clinic**	**0.12**
Bernardsville, N.J.	**Well**	**House**	**0.54**[c]
Princeton, N.J.	**Well**	**House**	**0.05**
Princeton	**Well**	**House**	**0.11**
Princeton	**Well**	**House**	**0.04**
Princeton	**Well**	**House**	**0.06**[c]
Milwood, N.J.	**Well**	**House**	**0.09**
Trenton, N.J.	**Well**	**House**	**5.60**[c]
Stamford, Conn.	**Well**	**House**	**5.20**[c]
Boston	**Well**	**House**	**0.64**[c]
Atlantic City, N.J.	**River**	**House**	**0.01**[c]
Dayton, Ohio	**Well**	**House**	**0.56**[c]
Washington, D.C.	**River**	**Hotel**	**0.01**

[a] All waters were collected in plastic containers and were acidified with copper-free HCL prior to testing. The sample was the first collection of water in the morning.

[b] The USPHS has ruled that water containing more than 1.0 ppm of copper is unfit to drink. In earlier generations with lead plumbing, grandfather, who drank the first cup out of the faucet in the morning, often got lead poisoning. It is now possible in some suburban homes for grandfather or others to get copper poisoning.

[c] Indicates a family in which at least one member has psychiatric problems.

possibly cause iron-storage diseases. There is evidence that elevated serum copper levels decrease iron during pregnancy and also result in a conditioned molybdenum deficiency. According to Butt et al., the trace-metal pattern of iron-storage diseases suggests a relationship of iron, molybdenum, lead and possibly copper to the cause of these diseases. Several anemias that do not respond to iron therapy have been found to be associated with high copper levels.

Copper and Cadmium in Plated Containers

All soluble salts of copper and cadmium are strong emetics (produce vomiting) when taken in sufficient dosage. Zinc and nickel sulfates are milder emetics, in that a larger dose is needed to produce vomiting. This means that epidemics of nausea and vomiting can occur when acid syrups such as cola or lemon drinks are stored in automatic dispensing machines. Since the effect is dose-/body-weight related, the young child who attends the Saturday afternoon matinee may have serious nausea and vomiting if he happens to get the first drink of the day from the soft-drink dispenser. Acid syrup, standing in contact with the tubes and valves overnight, may accumulate a dose of cadmium and copper which is toxic in a 50-pound child. The adult male might only get nausea, while the child may have repeated vomiting. In such cases, both child and adult add to their body burden of copper and cadmium.

We first witnessed this phenomenon in the U.S. Navy, where our duty included the review of all courts-martial proceedings. We had such gems as, "U.S. Navy v. John Doe, Seaman First Class, who did urinate on the deck of the Cruiser Tuscaloosa *while the nation was at war.*" But, more seriously, we had submarines which were forced to abort their Pacific cruises because of epidemic nausea and vomiting. Those who could work manned their posts while the sub went back to Pearl Harbor without firing a single torpedo—hence the court-martial inquiry.

After eliminating the possibility that the cause was arsenic and antimony poisoning from contaminated plates of the storage batteries, we finally found the root of the problem in an ice cream soda fountain that had recently been installed aboard these submarines. In wartime, because nickel was scarce, the syrup containers were *cadmium* plated. The soda fountain was open only once a week, so any acid syrups accumulated great amounts of cadmium from the six days' exposure to the surface. Men who preferred chocolate did not get sick, but the favorite flavor was raspberry (very acid) and all who preferred raspberry sundaes got deathly sick, with nausea and vomiting, from the cadmium content. All epidemics stopped when plastic containers were substituted for the cadmium-plated containers.

The insidious nature of heavy-metal poisoning should alert the consumer, the physician and the epidemiologist to all risk factors of modern life if poisoning is to be restrained to a reasonable level.

Excess Copper as a Possible Cause of Autism

The changes in copper and iron storage which occur during pregnancy, suckling and infancy were reviewed by Linder and Munro in 1973. We know that during the suckling period breast milk is deficient in copper and iron; the amount of excess copper and iron stored in the infant's liver should therefore decrease in the first six months of life. At this time, the liver produces the normal copper protein, ceruloplasmin, which stores copper in the blood serum and prevents excess absorption. Similarly, ferritin, the iron-containing protein, is made. Any abnormality which results in inadequate ceruloplasmin or ferritin could allow excess copper or iron to be absorbed, which would affect the brain. Both of these metals are stimulants to the brain and might produce hyperactivity or autism, with development into adulthood being slow or failing to take place normally. Nothing in the fetal development process protects against excess copper and iron. An alternative hypothesis is that heavy metals such as lead and mercury could interfere with the synthesis of ceruloplasmin or ferritin. This theory is worthy of testing, and can be tested by the usual laboratory methods in autistic children.

Tap Water, Blood and Dementia

The use of tap water as a dialysis substance has probably resulted in many unexpected deaths. "Dementia dialytica" was first described in 1964 by Peterson and Swanson. Patients had psychiatric changes which ranged from stuttering to aphasia (loss or impairment of the ability to use words as symbols of ideas) to unreality and cardiac standstill—with many symptoms in between (see Table 33.3)! Lindner et al. have found that patients subjected to dialysis can develop fulminating arteriosclerosis which could have been caused by cadmium, copper or a great deficiency of zinc. The anemias of pregnancy, rheumatoid arthritis and infection show high levels of ceruloplasmin. Wilson's disease has been associated with the high copper/molybdenum ratio, especially in the liver.

TABLE 33.3

"Dementia dialytica": clinical mystery or diagnostic dichotomy?

Psychiatric, neurological, and medical symptoms of hemodialysis patients using tap water

Psychiatric diagnosis since 1964 (Peterson and Swanson) termed "Dementia dialytica"	*Medical diagnosis since 1969 (Matter, et al.) Tap-water dialysis increases serum copper*
Neurological symptoms	*Medical symptoms*
Speech disorder, slow articulation	**Hemolytic anemia, hematuria (Ivanovich, et al. 1969)**
Stuttering, aphasia, headaches	**Lowered hematocrit with right (liver) or left (spleen) upper quadrant pain (Manzler and Schreiner, 1970)**
EEG: Slow waves with delta waves and spikes. (Alfrey, et al. 1972)	**Green plasma**
Myoclonus, convulsions	**Nausea, vomiting**
Hypertension, restlessness	**Yellow, watery diarrhea**
Increased heart rate and irregularities	**Weakness, syncope**
Cardiac standstill	
Psychiatric symptoms	*Psychiatric symptoms*
Inability to concentrate	**Unreality**
Impaired memory	**Depression**

Personality changes
Psychotic behavior
"Disequilibrium syndrome"
(unknown changes in vasoactive amines)
Journal of the American Medical Association **224:1578 (1973);**
Ibid **226:190 (1973)**

Psychosis

Pathological symptoms

Increased tin in brain at autopsy

Psychiatric Theories (Halper, 1971)

Dependency increases aggressive feelings (dependency on public finances)
Defenses all brittle
Stress: anxiety, depression, paranoia and suicidal tendencies
Denial of aspects of reality
Decreased sex activity

Medical theories

Heavy metal intoxication
Copper intoxication
(Mahler, et al.**, 1971)**

Copper in the tap water may turn the blood plasma green since copper accumulates preferentially in plasma. Symptoms have been described since 1964, but only in 1969 was the syndrome correlated with excess copper or other heavy metals such as tin. In some instances, according to Barbour et al., copper tubing or copperized plastic was involved. Excess copper would appear to be the most likely cause since some schizophrenics improve when their excess copper is removed. Cross-references between the two columns are so rare as to suggest a dichotomy of diagnosis and thinking.

When the quantity of copper-containing protein, ceruloplasmin, is adequate in the blood, it inhibits the intestinal absorption of copper. But if, as is the case in Wilson's disease, the serum contains an insufficient amount of ceruloplasmin, copper is absorbed in excess and diffuses into the tissues, and may accumulate in high levels in the brain and liver, producing severe mental illness and death. Fortunately, Wilson's disease is rare; in more than seventeen hundred psychiatric patients studied for copper levels, we have not found a single case of Wilson's disease.

Copper and Heart Attacks

Cases of myocardial infarction in people under forty is increasing in the United States, which is already the world leader in this disease. The recent studies of Dr. Oscar Roth, of the Yale University School of Medicine reveal that the rate is twenty-seven times higher in men than in women, but that women on oral contraceptive medication may have a much greater risk. He has observed five tragic cases of myocardial infarction in women on the pill. Serum copper is high with use of the birth control pill, and the copper level of the heart is higher than normal in those dying from heart attacks. Copper is also high in patients with high blood pressure and in those who smoke. We therefore postulate that the smoking woman, on oral contraceptives, who lives in suburbia where well water is used and is at the same time under stress (which dissipates zinc) and who has borderline zinc deficiency may have the greatest susceptibility to early heart attacks or strokes.

Copper and One Type of Schizophrenia

Thus far, excessive copper levels have been associated with our bodies' disorders, but in recent studies of the various schizophrenias, Pfeiffer et al. have postulated that excessive copper and iron and/or zinc and manganese deficiency are primary factors in one type of schizophrenia, namely histapenia. Histaminase is a copper-containing enzyme, and both histaminase and ceruloplasm can destroy histamine. Therefore, patients with high serum copper and ceruloplasm have low levels of blood histamine. Histapenic schizophrenia responds to treatment which rids the body of copper and builds up blood and tissue histamine.

Our studies indicate that a possible factor in some of the schizophrenias is a combined deficiency of zinc and manganese with a relative increase in iron and copper, or both—the copper possibly originating from copper plumbing. The urinary copper excretion in schizophrenics is consistently less than in "normal" patients; zinc plus manganese in dietary doses is effective in increasing copper elimination and reducing copper to normal levels. Further research is needed to determine the exact roles of these elements in vascular and brain chemistry. If, in fact, zinc deficiency and copper excess are crucial factors in causation of one of the schizophrenias, then more evidence is needed on the exact causes of these imbalances, so that treatment can be facilitated and prevention provided.

The clinical syndromes (other than Wilson's disease) wherein elevated serum or tissue copper may be an important factor are paranoid and hallucinatory schizophrenia, hypertension, stuttering, autism, childhood hyperactivity, preeclampsia, premenstrual tensions, psychiatric depression, insomnia, senility, and possibly functional hypoglycemia. Postpartum psychosis and the newborn infant's burden of copper have been described.

How to Lower Our Copper Burden

We have said that copper is essential for life, that excess copper accumulated in the body can be dangerous to good health, and that the general knowledge that the metals lead and mercury can cause insanity has now been extended to copper. We must now ask, how does one rid the body of its burden of excess copper?

It has long been held that a well-balanced diet is all that is needed. It is true that a perfectly balanced diet is so replete in all essential minerals that the zinc, manganese and molybdenum content would antagonize copper and prevent any accumulation. However, soil, fertilizers, foods and people are seldom tested for anything other than heavy metals and iron. On the basis of hemoglobin determinations, the teen-ager and the young adult have been labeled iron deficient. We know, however, that pyridoxine (B-6) and zinc are also involved in hemoglobin synthesis. Our deficient soils lower the levels of trace elements in our plants. Food processors continue to remove 90 percent of the zinc, manganese, molybdenum and pyridoxine from wheat grain, while enriching white flour with more iron. More iron without zinc and manganese will result in a higher incidence of gray-skinned siderotic (high-iron) patients. The present white flour should be called "tinkered ersatz" rather than "enriched." Additional tinkering should be in the direction of restoring zinc, manganese and magnesium content to the original level found in the wheat grain.

TABLE 33.4

Selected foodstuffs with appreciable amounts of copper

mg/100gm

Meats

beef liver	2.80
beef heart	.29
calf liver	7.90
duck liver	4.87
lamb liver	5.60
pork liver	1.14
veal chops	.25
pork chops	.31
lamb chops	.24
mutton, leg	.24
chicken breast	.18
chicken wing	.22
bacon	.52

Seafood

crab, canned	1.52
lobster	1.69
oysters	17.14
shrimp, fresh	.60
tuna, fresh	.50

Dairy Products

cream	.11
eggs, fresh	.10
milk, condensed	.22

Nuts and Seeds

brazil nuts	1.53
filberts	1.23
peanuts	.62
pecans	1.14
walnuts	1.39
sesame seeds	1.59
sunflower seeds	1.77
pistachio nuts	1.12

Spices

curry powder	1.07
pepper, black	.58
salt	.44

Dried Fruits

apricots	.35
dates	.22
figs	.28
prunes	.28
raisins	.25

Vegetables

avocados	.39
kidney beans	.84
lima beans	.73
navy beans	.85
mushrooms	1.00
peas	.22
soybeans	1.17
yams	.22

Cereals

bran flakes	.61
Cheerios	.44
Puffed Rice	.39
Rice Krispies	.30
wheat flakes	.44

Breads

brown	.28
rye	.23
wheat	.24
white	.23

Grains

wheat bran	1.45
wheat germ	2.39
corn, white	.24
corn germ	1.01
rice	.28

Sweets

sugar wafers	.84
chocolate (bitter)	2.67
chocolate (sweet)	1.04
jam, all kinds	.31
molasses	1.42
licorice	.39

Condiments

mustard	.40
olives	.34
sweet relish	.50
catsup	.59

Beverages

cocoa powder	3.57
ground coffee	1.26
tea, bag	4.80
tea, instant dry	1.10
Instant Breakfast (Carnation) dry	.50
Instant Breakfast (PET) dry	6.25

Miscellaneous

yeast, dried	4.98
gelatin	1.78

Reference: Pennington, J. T. and Calloway, D. H. Copper content of foods. *Research* 63:143-153, 1973.

Of the trace elements tested, oral zinc plus manganese in a ratio of twenty to one will increase copper excretion via the urinary route. Molybdenum antagonizes copper absorption in sheep to the extent that naturally black sheep may grow depigmented wool when raised on feed with excess molybdenum. Data are not yet available for these three essential elements in Wilson's disease or even milder states of copper intoxication. Because this knowledge is lacking as regards man, patients are treated with more expensive and toxic chelating agents such as penicillamine, acetylcysteine and EDTA (ethylene diaminetetracetic acid).

These chelates are not specific for any one metal, but remove, via the urinary pathway, copper, zinc, lead, mercury and cadmium. This therapy is less than perfect since penicillamine also removes zinc from the body. Certainly, when penicillamine is used, the patient will lose his sense of taste if zinc and pyridoxine (B-6) are not given in adequate supply. The B-6 should be given at noon, while the penicillamine is given morning and night. Penicillamine will cause a two-hundredfold increase in urinary copper excretion. Patients sensitive to penicillin salts are usually also sensitive to penicillamine.

Avoiding Iron and Copper

Advertising campaigns promote iron-containing vitamins as a means of combating "iron-poor blood." As a result of this sales pitch, many vitamin-plus-mineral preparations predominantly contain iron and copper. We should attempt to rid the body of excess copper rather than look for new sources! In spite of this consideration, the large manufacturers of vitamin-and-mineral preparations see fit to follow the ancient Wisconsin patent which gives the dose of copper needed daily as 4 mg. Theragran-M and Geriplex have 2 mg of copper per capsule, while fifty other preparations in the *Physicians' Desk Reference* also contain copper. Many patients have zinc-poor tissues, and their fatigue may disappear when zinc plus vitamin B-6 is given as a dietary supplement.

References

Butt, E. M. et al. Trace metal patterns in disease states. *Amer. J. Clin. Pathol.* 30:474-497, 1958.

Gooch, R. Observations on puerperal insanity. *Med. Trans.* 6:263-324, 1820; *JAMA* 208:1697, 1969.

Lal, S.; Papeschi, R.; Duncan, R. J. S. and Sourkes, T. L. Effect of copper loading on various tissue enzymes and brain monoamines in the rat. *Toxicology and Applied Pharmacology* 28:395-405, 1974.

Linder, M. C. and Munro, H. N. *Enzyme* 15:111-113, 1973.

Peterson, H. and Swanson, A. G. *Arch. Intern. Med.* 113:877-880, 1974.

Pfeiffer, C. and Iliev, V. A study of zinc deficiency and copper excess in the schizophrenias. *Intern. Rev. of Neurobiol.* 141-165, 1972.

Roth, O. Myocardial infarct rate among young rises in U.S. *Int. Med. News,* 15 September 1974.

Schroeder, H. A. Essays in toxicology. 4:107-199, 1972.

Seelig, M. Proposed role of copper molybdenum interaction in iron-deficiency storage diseases. *Amer. J. Clin. Nutr.* 657-672, 1973.

Walker-Smith, J. and Bloomfield, J. Wilson's disease or chronic copper poisoning? *Arch. Diseases in Childhood* 48:476-478, 1973.

CHAPTER 34

Bismuth: The Fifth (Column) Heavy Metal

In addition to mercury, lead, cadmium, and copper, another metal has been discovered to be a cause of mental symptoms. Bismuth is a heavy metal which has no known natural function in man, animals or plants. Primarily in Australia, bismuth subgallate is prescribed to be taken orally, in a powdered form. Bismuth has been used in the past for treating syphilis, and mental symptoms such as are now described were not seen with overdosage.

Patients who have undergone a colostomy (an operation in which an artificial opening is formed in the abdominal wall) are frequently given bismuth salts in order to reduce fecal odor and regulate elimination. Dr. James F. Robertson of Australia has reported cases of bismuth intoxication which could erroneously be diagnosed as mental illness. The use of bismuth subgallate produced a staggering gait, difficulty in memory recall, tremor, disturbances of vision and hearing, and difficulty in estimating time and distance. In some cases, auditory and visual hallucinations occurred. The symptoms disappeared when the salt of bismuth was discontinued.

Other preparations which contain bismuth are certain rectal suppositories for the relief of pain and discomfort, and some antidiarrhea medicines containing bismuth, pectin and paregoric. In light of the potential mental effects, we advise avoidance of repeated oral use of products which contain bismuth in any form.

Bismuth and Zinc

The time course of return of memory and relief of other symptoms would suggest that bismuth may interfere with the absorption of zinc from the small intestine. If bismuth were lodged in the brain, the patient would need extensive chelation therapy to reverse the intoxication. In Dr. Robertson's experience, the symptoms decreased when the dose of bismuth was reduced. The gallic acid molecule is similar to the phytic acid molecule, so that the repeated use of bismuth subgallate could result in zinc deficiency. If bismuth subgallate produces zinc deficiency, this can be proven by blood serum analysis for zinc. Zinc deficiency would produce the reversible intoxication which is described in the following case history from Australia.

Patient Writes

Dear Mr. A.,

Further to our phone conversation of today I outline the main things that I experienced when I nearly died in Prince Henry's hospital and the symptoms that built up on (and in) me during the four years that passed after my colostomy operation under Mr. Hughes till I was carried in a complete coma into Prince Henry's.

Mr. Hughes told me my operation was eminently successful and that in five weeks I should be normal and back at work. I felt lousy at that time and was quite unable to work. No other adjective describes my feeling.

I first noticed a peculiar sensation in the tips of the fingers and toes and a kind of perpetual neuritis. I put it down to the drugs in hospital. I had then been on bismuth subgallate for about a month when these symptoms started.

After six months still feeling rotten I went back to work

at T.P.N.G. thinking that would be therapeutic. To my dismay I found that the control of my heat in my body was in disarray. I was overhot and sweated profusely or overcold and clammy. It was most distressing after 40 years normal life in the tropics.

I stuck at things for 12 months in T.P.N.G. and then resigned and returned hoping that the cold climate and less onerous life would cure me.

I took up work about the home repair and alteration, little mental work and lived simply and healthy. But there was no real improvement. My mental powers deteriorated, memory, reading and writing ability and sight. I twitched all over especially at night. My breathing started to be affected shortness of breath at times and peculiar momentary breath in the inhaling process when my lungs were about half full.

I found my manual work increasingly difficult over three years. I finally had to stop as I could not hold a tool steady. I could not do my buttons or hold a tea cup steady and level except with major concentration. I lost my balance and was continually falling over. This so degenerated that I would fall over twitching and sight all went out of order. My feet swelled so I had to get large shoes.

I lost my ability to laugh or smile. I could not work the muscles of my face. I also became rather moon faced. I could not keep the car off the gravel edge of the road and within the white lines so I gave up driving. I completely lost my sense of direction and geography of Melbourne.

I became a great sufferer from insomnia. I twitched so much and also could not lie still in bed but had to turn from side to side every minute or so. I was put on various drugs but none really helped. I forgot their names, but each drug's effect wore off fairly soon and I had to be given another. In the day time however I could not keep awake. I used to fall into a so-called sleep (though it was not that) even when talking to friends. My wife tried everything to keep me awake in the day time so I might sleep at night. But it did nothing to help me sleep normally. Waking from this "sleep" in the day time was a horrid experience. One seemed to be climbing up and out of a deep unconsciousness. I felt that one day I just would not climb out! I'd be dead. I dreaded each day time as I could not do anything up about the house or rest in bed at night. Too I dreaded the nights also. I was very disorientated and mentally could not remember things and did strange things at times and my wife had to watch me very carefully.

I had a relapse and into Repat., where they cut my intestine back about 4″ and this helped with handling my equipment and comfort. However my general condition which was now diagnosed as a nervous one and possibly of psychological origin did not improve. Finally after 5½ years I fell over in the garden in a coma and was carried into Prince Henry's Hospital. (By the way I had become incontinent.) I was in P.H. about six weeks, violent and strapped to my bed, with a surround to keep me in bed. I can remember patches of the awful nightmares which took hold of me. The doctors told my wife that all the tests made showed that my brain was dying rapidly though my body was relatively strong. After three or four weeks of this I grew quieter and one afternoon I opened my eyes suddenly and saw my wife at my bedside and spoke rationally with and to her. She hurried away and told the doctor and he came and did various simple brain tests and then took my wife away and told her they would have to reassess my case as I appeared to have suddenly become rational. Now the only thing in my treatment that had changed in Prince Henry's was that I had not had any bismuth subgallate. All the other drugs were carried on when they could get them into me. I think I was taking three powerful drugs all the time. I forgot their names.

P.H. decided to keep me on longer as I was rational (fairly) instead of sending me to a nursing home to slowly die. After a fortnight further I went out to Wattle Glen Private Hospital and had 12 weeks there with marvellous nursing. They got me on my feet and restored my balance partly. I was beginning to smile again though somewhat weakly.

I returned home not normal but well enough not to be intolerable burden. Over two years all my symptoms have disappeared slowly. I can work again, breath normally, don't twitch, think again, enjoy books, T.V., my technical skills returned normally and mentally (I have very comprehensive technical training).

My sense of direction and geography returned and my driving skill. I wear my old size shoes again. My sight has returned to normal and I wear my old glasses. This return to health was very slow and gradual but I never looked back. Balance is now quite okay. When I got to the dentist he found my teeth *heavily stained yellow* (with bismuth subgallate?)

and under very bad decay. Previously I had excellent teeth. I am constantly in this man's hands for repairs.

I had a peculiar ache in my arms as though my biceps were affected. My lungs (?) or there abouts also ached in different areas. These aches have all gone after two years at home.

I became very weak, could not walk more than a few hundred yards. I could not carry my grandchild a new baby. I could not last out standing for a hymn in church without a tremendous effort.

Well I think that is enough. I dislike writing about it because it is all about "me" and ego certainly is the very devil. But I only write this thinking it may help somebody. My family doctor told his wife who told my wife he had reported this matter of bismuth subgallate to the proper authorities and I hope he has. I feel it is a slow and insidious poison to those persons who are allergic to it. I also feel that some folk on it after a colostomy though not reacting as we did never the less may be suffering poor health and blaming their colostomy for this. I only use charcoal tablets now and don't take any other drugs except odd vitamins. I found Vitamin C helps the improvement of my salivary system and dry mouth which seems to be one of the few disabilities I still have.

P.S. I call to mind some drugs, Stelazine, Seconal, Vallium and one they take for epilepsy—I forgot that one—Tryptanol I believe was another. But I don't think these caused my troubles as my down hill drive started after my colostomy operation the drugs came much later and I had no withdrawal symptoms as these were all gradually taken away.

I hope you can decipher this and get out of it all the tones of what I say. My writing is never good and I am too lazy to peck away at my typewriter.

With kind regards, A.B.

P.P.S. I should add that I am firmly convinced I am alive today only by the intervention of the Lord in and through my circumstances.

References

Robertson, J. F. Mental illness or metal illness? Bismuth subgallate. *Med. J. of Australia* 1:887-888, 1974.

PART FIVE

Clinical Problems

INTRODUCTION

In this section we attempt to zero in on some disorders of mankind which can benefit from adequate nutritional therapy. After introductory essays, we discuss the hypoglycemias and the schizophrenias. Both disorders are intertwined "waste baskets" insofar as accurate diagnosis is concerned. We sort out some of the schizophrenias and classify headaches in a useful manner. After discussing several other disorders we propose areas for further research.

CHAPTER 35

The Human Brain: Three Pounds of Delicate Hardware

Brains, like cabbages, are beautiful—but in a different way. Cabbage heads are dumb and sterile, whereas brains are personal, intelligent and vibrant. A famous inventor once claimed, "My body is just an angulated device to transport my beautiful brain around!" Beneath the convoluted, pulsing, gray matter is the most delicate, complex computer in the universe. Sir John Eccles, Nobel prize winner for his research on the human brain, has said: "The last thing that man will understand in nature is the performance of his brain."

Myths have attached themselves to this piece of anatomy more than to any other organ. The eating of fish was believed to provide "brain food." Too much reading "tired the brain," when, in reality, a brain uses an equal amount of energy whether working or not. Large-sized heads, "egg heads," indicated intelligence, while "pin heads" signified lack of the "gray matter."

Books and films tell thrilling tales of the struggles between superior and inferior brains. Superior brains could read thoughts, cure people, tamper with nature, or inflict harm—"put a hex on you." Master criminals slip away from stupid detectives, and master detectives foil dim-witted criminals. And, of course, Dr. Frankenstein ultimately destroyed himself through the diabolical transplantation of a criminal brain into his monster.

The mystery surrounding the brain reinforces the truth of Sir John's comment and inspires countless physicians and other researchers to further study of this organization of matter and energy.

If one likens the human brain to electronic hardware, it becomes clear that we have within our skulls the most advanced hardware ever produced. The memory of the instrument is capable of storing all the words in the Bible in proper order—with recall of any verse on signal. Its powers of calculation are infinite, and it can collate and rearrange abstract concepts into useful correlations, laws and theories. An exceptionally good typist can do 100 words per minute. Man, through his brain, speaks at an average of 150 words per minute, but the mind can think four times faster. Frequently, the thoughts are the opposite of the spoken words. Many antagonistic thoughts may ebb and flow as pleasantries and falsehoods emerge. (The muscles of the face plate of this computer may betray the lies and the pleasantries, however!)

In a well-run democracy all persons are born equal before the law. Individuals' brains, however, are unequal. Some can carry a tune; some cannot. Some evoke and recognize perfect pitch; others can sing the song only if given the correct pitch. Still others cannot sing at all. Mozart could compose music at the age of eight; others have great difficulty in learning to speak their native languages.

The head with its ears has built-in super radar; the head will turn accurately in the direction of a sound and focus the eyes exactly on its origin.

If the mind cannot recall a name from long ago, a clue will still remain. A person may say, "I know his name began with an F," when in reality the name began with a G (close to F alphabetically). The pondering mind also recalls that the name had two syllables. After pausing for several minutes the mind may come up with "Gessell," a minute later mysteriously correct itself, and finally come up with the true name, "Gerard." (Again, the letters S and R are close alphabetically.) The mind solved the memory problem by a complex, unknown recall process. What mechanisms within the brain enable us to accomplish such memory feats?

The general learning and memory experiments of biologists study the simple worm *planaria* to discover if extracts of proteins transferred from "educated" worms will produce "education" in recipient worms. Other researchers sew an air bladder onto the belly of a goldfish which must then learn to swim again with the added unnatural buoyancy. The goldfish brain is then analyzed after the learning process to see what new proteins occur in the educated brain. While ingenious, these experiments seem crude indeed by comparison when the capabilities of the human brain are considered!

Man's senses, his mental functioning, and particularly his memory are his identity. Each day he must reach into the vast stores of memory located within his brain to cope with life. The human brain not only classifies and stores our memories but recreates the past and plans the future. The circuitry of the nervous system comprising the brain has the power to create within us feelings of harmony and contentment; tragically, through malfunction, it can also create sensory experiences so profound that reality becomes a myth subordinate to the fantasies that prevail. If a man cannot remember his past or if he cannot utilize his past experiences to organize the present, then, in a very real way, he has lost all personality and does not exist.

A Case History

Not long ago, a man and his wife came to the Brain Bio Center seeking nutritional help to retard the aging process. Both were born in the year 1900 and were enjoying their seventy-fourth year of life in good physical health. Their steady gait, good color and cheerful disposition indicated health; yet, sitting across from the doctor, they revealed that a void had developed; something was missing from their lives.

The first question to the wife, as to her age, quickly disclosed her problem of memory failure. She paused, and turned her eyes toward her husband in a silent plea for an answer.

"You tell the doctor," was his reply.

She could not.

Pursuing the question further, the doctor asked the year of her birth. This is always easier to remember since it does not change as does age.

"1925. . . ." the woman hesitatingly answered.

"No, no," corrected the husband. "That's when we were married."

"Do you know the meaning of a golden wedding anniversary?" the doctor asked.

"Oh, that's fifty years of marriage," she promptly replied.

"When will you celebrate your golden wedding anniversary?"

Again, she looked to her husband, but he remained silent. Confused and fumbling for an answer, she could not reply. A few minutes later the husband proudly told of their arrangements to celebrate the golden anniversary in 1975.

Despite her cheerful mood, good physical health and normal sleep patterns, her memory was almost gone.

What could have happened to the delicate hardware in this woman's head? Had the arteries hardened and decreased the blood supply? Could it be plaque or scar formation, or deposition of foreign material such as aluminum in the brain? Perhaps the loss of neurones (nerve cells) with aging? Finally, statistically speaking, could the memory loss be a little bit of each of the above, so that the total effect was that of borderline performance?

Short-term and Long-term Memory

What do we know about memory, and how is memory subdivided by the experts? Most recent scientific reports deal with two types of memory called short-term memory and long-term or consolidated memory. An easy example of the first is the waitress who remembers who ordered the Peking Duck, the fried shrimp, etc. for a table of six. Within two hours the memory traces of these orders have been erased by those of the different main-course orders of numerous other guests. The only consolidated memory of the evening will be the faces and probably the first names of the two college students who joked pleasantly with her during the long and tiring evening.

The consolidation of memory is the formation of permanent memory traces following a given experience. Each sensory experience travels to the brain, is then coded in specific biochemicals in the nervous system and, if not interrupted, is translated into a permanent memory trace with retrieval upon request.

Facilitated Pathways

Transfer of the electrical circuits to proteins in or on the surface of the neurone (nerve cell) has been suggested as the mechanism for long-term memory. However, most brain proteins are resynthesized every twenty-four hours. How, therefore, can we believe that the ability to ride a bike, which stays with us from age ten to seventy, is turned over every twenty-four hours? Such learned abilities must constitute a third type of memory, the facilitated pathways, that are not interrupted by the biochemical turnover process. Such facilitated-pathway memories are not always perfect after long disuse, since we know that the tennis player can have his facilitated pathways get "out of practice." The fine tuning of the serve or the backhand stroke requires constant repetition.

Conditioned Memory

A fourth type of memory is conditioned memory or "gut memory." When the smell of baked turkey or chili sauce a-cooking brings back gustatory memories, the saliva flows and the gut may rumble. Such memories may play tricks, so that the petting and kissing couple may feel embarrassed by borborygmi or gut rumbling—an onomatopoetic word which needs no further definition! Conditioned memories are the basis for the conditioned response used in behavior modification. (One can get grant money to train an autistic child with rewards and pain responses to pull up his pants after a bowel movement. It is almost impossible, however, to get government grants to learn why the child is autistic.)

Conditioned memories betray the best of us. We forget the names of people whom we dislike, but permanently consolidate the names of our allies in any heated argument. Perhaps this is the basis of the Congressional use of "I yield to the gentleman from Maryland." Adversaries' names are seldom on the tip of your tongue. Conditioned memory might also be called "instinct" and, when repeated to the point of harm, "habit." We seldom brag about "good habits" and we are plagued by the reverse.

What Do We Know About Memory?

In a lifetime, more than fifteen trillion specific memories are coded in the brain, and although much of our sensory input is forgotten, selected events remain permanently engraved onto the periphery of our gray matter, waiting to be triggered into use by some unique event. Consolidated memory, then, consists of two mechanisms: the short-term and the long-term memory.

Short-term memory, lasting from only a few seconds to a few minutes, is useful in many of our daily routines, such as remembering what to buy while shopping or a new telephone number. This type of memory is vulnerable to erasure by gross interference with ongoing brain activity. The length of time involved in creating a short-term memory varies with the nature of the experience and the type of interference. The coding process involves reversible phenomena, such as electrical states or conformational changes in the protein, which can be destroyed by electroshock therapy or by a sharp blow to the head. This short-term mechanism is used by the bridge player who can learn the play of fifty-two cards and later forget it, allowing no interference with his next bridge hand.

Although the brain has over ten billion nerve cells, memory feats could not be accomplished if memory traces were stored between neurones in continuous circuits. Perhaps recent memory is stored in electrical circuits. This would help us to forget—a useful and necessary process.

Long-term memory storage is the second stage in memory consolidation. This is the process allowing for future recall. Gradually, our short-term memories are stabilized and consolidated into long-term memory stores, retrievable on demand. Long-term memory is the last to go with the aging process.

How is it that many immigrants, having mastered the English language, still continue to count in their native languages? Or consider the case of the idiot savant who, with an IQ no higher than 60, can perform amazing feats of calculation or memory. Unable to perform basic mathematics, he can calculate the day of the week for any date into the year 3500; or, unable to read or write, he can fluently repeat words spoken to him in a foreign language. These patients are often unaware of the meaning of their calculations or the methods used to arrive at their answers. No one can explain their unusual skill. Perhaps they possess a specific group of brain cells developed to facilitate their specific abilities. The ability to remember such large quantities of information over long periods transcends simple electrical impulsation. At present, scientists are studying biochemical changes within or on the surface of nerve cells as a possible mechanism of memory consolidation.

Memory must then have four facets or types: (1) facilitated pathways (which are carefully coordinated with the balance center in the cerebellum); (2) some short-term memory which may be electrical; (3) long-term or consolidated memory (which is biochemical and the last to fade); and (4) gut or conditioned memory (which involves emotion). If all this memory storage could be worked into the most modern computer, the instrument might be the size of the Empire State building and the energy consumed equal to that of Niagara Falls!

The brain itself, however, is only the size of a softball. It has only one-fiftieth the weight of the body but uses one-fifth of the heart's blood that is pumped throughout the body. Compared with that of any other species, the surface of man's brain is more creased, presumably to provide more space for the surface neurones. With its creases and infoldings spread out, the brain's surface area would cover the top of a card table.

During the initial phases of theoretical brain research, cyberneticists viewed memory as consisting of reverberatory circuits between neurons. In the nerve-network theory, memory is regarded as originating in fixed pathways in certain areas of the brain. According to this theory, a short-term memory would be created by a reverberatory circuit lasting long enough to be encoded into long-term memory or dissolving due to spontaneous decay of nonrehearsal. This reverberatory-circuit mechanism can be disregarded, because experimental evidence has proven that deep anesthesia and electroshock can blot out electrical activity but that long-term memory returns. Only short-term memory may be impaired.

Two hypotheses currently being tested suggest that new memory stores (short- or long-term) are acquired either by means of RNA as the "memory molecule" or through the action of lipoproteins. Initially an individual must "think" about a pending action: for example, a young child, when she first learns to eat with a spoon, must think about what she is doing or she is likely to forget to open her mouth as the spoon arrives. Eventually, the initial movement of opening her mouth will be unconsciously monitored through established neural pathways to enable the movement to continue smoothly. In essence, the brain is a recording machine which "memorizes" all the complex muscular movements as well as sensory actions involved in skilled movements or passive activities.

Experimental evidence suggests that biochemical changes within a neuron that establish RNA and protein molecules specific to each memory are involved in the consolidation process. Experimental drugs such as puromycin and cycloheximide, which are known inhibitors of RNA translation into protein, have been administered to rats at various stages of the memory process. The results show that both drugs act by blocking the conversion of short- into long-term memory, suggesting that the conversion is dependent upon new protein synthesis.

Other studies suggest that the memory process is a function of the number of memory-protein molecules synthesized and their availability over prolonged periods. Scientists at present conclude that memory consolidation involves the establishment of particular molecules within or on the surface of the neuron. These biochemical changes are permanent and recallable when needed, although some pondering may be needed.

But what does all this mean? The process of memory consolidation is both electrically and biochemically dependent. The brain, like all other body organs, is supplied with nutrients from the blood to allow its cells to grow and function properly. Without the proper nutrients, proteins cannot be manufactured or utilized by the nerve cells to maintain desirable mental functions, including memory. Faulty memory and bizarre thought patterns may be evident in someone whose biochemistry is inherently imbalanced or whose diet does not supply the brain with all the needed nutrients (both vitamins and minerals).

Thus, through proper diet and supplementary doses of essential nutrients, an individual can usually insure body fitness and proper mental function, enabling him to cope with the stresses of everyday living. Because alertness and accurate memory are vital to our survival, awareness of what foods are needed to maintain a healthy mind should be a primary consideration in the mind of every individual.

References

Areheart, J. L. Retaining memory in older people. *Science News*, vol. 101, 18 March 1972.

Campbell, I. M. and Gregson, R. A. M. Olfactory short term memory in normal, schizophrenic and brain-damaged cases. *Australian Journal of Psychology*, vol. 24, no. 2, 1972.

Gibbs, M. E.; Jeffrey, P. L.; Austin, L. and Mark, R. F. Separate biochemical actions of inhibitors of short- and long-term memory. *Pharmacology Biochemistry and Behavior*, vol. 1, 1973.

Gregory, R. L. Origin of eyes and brains. *Nature* 213:5074, 28 January 1967.

Kesner, R. P. and Conner, H. S. Independence of short- and long-term memory: a neural system analysis. *Science* vol. 176, 28 April 1972.

Kobilier, D. and Allweis, C. The prevention of long-term memory formation by 2, 6 diaminopurine. *Pharmacology Biochemistry and Behavior* vol. 2, 1974.

Libassi, P. T. Where the past is present—how does memory reside in the brain? *The Sciences*, October 1974.

Luria, L. R. The functional organization of the brain. *Scientific American* vol. 222, March 1970.

Penfield, W. and Mathieson, G. Memory—autopsy findings and comments on the role of hippocampus in experiential recall. *Arch. Neurol.* vol. 31, September 1974.

Uphouse, L. L., MacInnes, J. W. and Schlesinger, K. Role of RNA and protein in memory storage: a review. *Behavior Genetics* vol. 4, no. 1, 1974.

CHAPTER 36

The Air We Breathe

Air pollution. If those words fill your mind with images of nuclear explosions, a poisonous atmosphere and ultimate human extinction, then you are probably and properly a victim of the pollution paranoia. Prophets of doom may well create a quandary that may lead us helter-skelter, like lemmings, over the brink of irrational cliffs.

The pollution of our environment is a very real and serious threat and is a problem that demands the most thorough research, cooperation and the most careful judgments. We must ask ourselves: Is air pollution just another popular crisis that will eventually fade away, or is it the ominous hurricane that will push us along the same declining path as our Roman ancestors, many of whom died of lead poisoning from the water in the final piping of their glorious aqueducts?

Man has developed in an environment of continually increasing amounts of heavy metals and elements since the first flint-induced combustion. When industrialization began polluting the atmosphere with toxic quantities of these familiar elements, man unwittingly allowed these poisons to infiltrate the water he drank and the food he ate. Certain elements can be readily absorbed and eliminated by the body, while others accumulate in the body with age. Which of these elements are harmless, and which of these invading elements are toxic?

An estimated twenty-seven trace elements are found in the air. Five of these are natural and probably harmless pollutants. Seven others are essential to life, yet toxic in large amounts. The remaining sixteen are industrial pollutants. Of these, lead, mercury and cadmium have been clearly identified as the culprits in air pollution diseases.

Airborne Lead

Lead can be a killer. Dr. Henry A. Schroeder has discovered that Americans take in more lead than they excrete. It is present in industrial smoke and auto exhaust and is derived from myriad other sources. Airborne lead from the "no-knock" lead additives in gasoline has claimed the lives of horses and cows who eat the grass on their side of the fences along the highways. What is happening to humans who eat the corn grown along well-travelled roads?

Young Idaho children living near the Bunker Hill Company smelter developed symptoms of lead poisoning in February of 1974. The resulting extensive federal-state investigation revealed in the following September the startling fact that almost every child (99 percent) within a mile radius of the smelter had high blood levels of lead, and that over 20 percent suffered from "frank lead poisoning." Lead poisoning attacks the nervous system and can produce permanent damage: speech impairment, hyperactivity, nervous disorders, hypertension and even death. To date, there are no federal or state standards on lead emissions or preventive measures to be taken by industrial polluters. We do not know as yet the lead content in the Idaho community's garden soil, crops or adults. . . .

Chromium, cadmium, nickel, beryllium, vanadium and selenium are a few of the industrial contaminants that can cause lung and nose irritation and, in some cases, cancer. Workers with continuous exposure to pollutants are especially vulnerable to disease; yet, as the report concerning the Idaho children so tragically indicates, no one can ward off eventual pollution.

Vanadium

Man can inhale these pollutants from sources other than industry. Vanadium in the atmosphere can be produced from the low-sulfur oil imported from Venezuela and Iran and burned in our home furnaces. This element collects in the lungs with age and may be a cause of methemoglobenemia—the poisoning of hemoglobin that produces a bluish tinge to the skin, dizziness, headaches, diarrhea and anemia. (Vanadium is in short supply in the world and so should also be removed as a conservation step.)

Silicosis

The mineral silicon is inhaled as silicon dioxide, which is frequently used in certain manufacturing processes—for example, in the manufacture of glass, ceramics, abrasives and petroleum products. Prolonged inhalation of the dust can cause fibrosis of the lung, silicosis and increased susceptibility to tuberculosis. Those who sandblast buildings or quarry granite rock are particularly at risk. In tunnelling through granite, water should be sprayed constantly to control the fine, inhalable granite dust.

The Flameproof Mineral, Asbestos

Asbestos, a compound which resembles fine, slender, flaxy threads of fiber, is commonly used where a flame-proof, resistant fiber is required. Asbestos is used by construction workers to coat steel trusses and is found in fireproof clothing and curtains, roofing and brake linings. Although the processing of certain materials with asbestos has been discontinued, some three thousand asbestos-processed products are still in use. That innocent bystander, the pedestrian, breathes in asbestos every time a car is braked. Once in the body, these fibers remain for life. The tiny particles accumulate chiefly in the lung, but can also become lodged in the body tissues, the intestine, pancreas, kidney, spleen and liver. No one knows as yet if there is an amount of asbestos which is considered "safe" for the body, but we do know that asbestos can cause mesothelioma—a rapidly spreading cancer of the lung and abdomen.

Cigarette Smoking and Polymer Influenzoid Illness

Some workers in polymer factories (particularly those manufacturing Teflon) are subject to polymer fume fever, which can masquerade as influenza. The symptoms are cough, fever, chills, muscle aches and weakness. Those afflicted are smokers. The 875°C temperature of smoking produces a toxic pyrolysis of the plastic dust on the cigarettes they carry in their shirt pocket or on their hands as they smoke. Washing the hands before smoking and storage of cigarettes in a tight case in clothes lockers prevents this influenzoid illness. Since the plastics which produce this effect are chlorinated and fluorinated, the long-term effect of these repeated influenzoid illnesses could be harmful.

Chromium and the Tobacco Plant

Chromium is selectively absorbed by the tobacco plant, whose leaves are later picked and wrapped in cadmium-containing paper. The smoker, therefore, is increasing his intake of these poisons and his chance of developing disease.

Cigarette smoking is, in itself, a dangerous air pollutant. It is widely believed to be a leading cause of cancer of the lung, stomach and bladder; chronic bronchitis and influenza; ulcers and heart disease. On the average a cigarette shortens a person's life span by about the time it takes to smoke it. So the next time someone asks you if you would mind if he smokes, speak up—say, "YES!"

Carbon Monoxide

A smoker in the car can be as hazardous as the traffic outside.

The major gas pollutant found in cigarette smoke and in traffic is carbon monoxide. This odorless, colorless, tasteless gas is like a thief in the night. It can slip into your bloodstream, preventing the blood from carrying oxygen to the brain, and steal away your health—or your life! Carbon monoxide poisoning is capable of producing bursting headache, mental dullness, dizziness, nausea, irritability, loss of consciousness and death. This type of poisoning can be hard to diagnose and its symptoms are often misdiagnosed. Unfortunately, air filters in air conditioners do not remove carbon monoxide.

Carbon monoxide poisoning is a dangerous surface hazard for most city dwellers. Despite this fact, many pollution-monitoring stations are located well above street level. Carbon monoxide has the same density as air, so upward diffusion is negligible. In New York City, angina (sharp chest pain) has been produced simply by exposing coronary patients to freeway traffic. Could this account for serious symptoms in some of the hundred and sixty thousand heart patients in New York City?

Levels of blood monoxide can be elevated by exposure to the pollutant at street level. City dwellers can aggravate this situation by heavy exercise, smoking, riding in a bus or car, eating lunch at a street-level restaurant or working in auto tunnels. How strenuously the body is working and the duration of inhalation at street level can affect the degree of poisoning as well as the chance of survival in a mechanized world. Could carbon monoxide poisoning perhaps be a cause of the crabbiness and fender-bending among taxicab (and other) drivers?

The dark, cavernous subways below street level may be snatching the light from the city dweller's life. Various forms of polluted air stagnate in the tunnels, creating an atmosphere worse than that at street level. Subway air wafts in from the curbside vents—already heavily laden with auto exhaust and brake-lining dust. Peter Scheiner of the City University of New York believes ozone may be produced by the electrical sparks at track level, and when the ozone reacts with the auto exhausts in the air, photochemical smog is created. In addition, iron and steel dust in the subway air has been found to be above emergency levels. Since we can develop angina, genetic damage, premature aging and any number of pollution-related diseases from these poisons, sources of clean air must be found for our subways.

The Freons and Our Ozone Layer

From the subway tunnels about thirty feet below street level to the stratosphere some thirty miles above the earth, man is travelling and leaving pollution in his wake. Recent studies under the direction of Dr. Michael B. McElroy, Professor of Atmospheric Science, and Dr. Steven C. Wofsy, atmospheric physicist, of Harvard University, have revealed that man has been unknowingly spraying away the ozone layer in his stratosphere. Previously, nuclear explosions were criticized and supersonic transport systems were banned in defense of the earth's ozone layer. Who would have suspected the ubiquitous little aerosol can to be a threat to our huge, upper stratosphere?

The mysterious ozone layer filters out the lethal forms of ultraviolet rays from the sun, protecting the earth below. The gases found in aerosol cans and refrigerators, commercially known as Freons, are stable as they float through the lower atmosphere. But in the stratosphere, they absorb the ultraviolet rays, collapse and release chlorine, a chemical that is highly efficient in destroying ozone. The production of the Freons has grown into a major industry. Two million tons are released into the atmosphere yearly. The frightening aspect of this fact is that almost all such gas produced by world industries to date still remains within our air.

Drs. McElroy and Wofsy believe that even if the production of these gases is banned by 1980, the residue gases will continue to work their way up to the stratosphere. The ozone depletion by the year 2000 could reach 14 to 15 percent. and recovery would be slow.

As the statistics mount, the debate is intensified. Industry spokesmen and scientists argue the validity of the Harvard group's ozone theory. Scientific committees are assembling in urgent meetings to study the possible threat of aerosol can propellants. And millions of people continue to spray out more and more potentially destructive gas, most of them either unaware of the danger or not fully comprehending it.

The Pigeon Doesn't Always Pollute Straight Down

Another, rather unsuspected, source of airborne pollution is the pigeon. This seemingly innocent fowl can foul our environment with its droppings, which can contain as many as one million organisms. The pigeon carries the dangerous cryptococcus bacteria which produce cryptococcus meningitis. Although a rare disease—our body's natural defenses are good against this host—it can kill viciously. People who have an immunologic problem or who take cortisone-like drugs are especially susceptible. All people, however, who live or work near a pigeon-infested area (city halls, churches, etc.) are at risk.

What Can We Do to Fight Air Pollution?

The problems caused by air pollution are not entirely new. Cases of rickets were widespread in the early days of the Industrial Revolution due to the scarcity of sun in the smoky atmosphere. Today, we know that vitamin D would have ameliorated this suffering.

Researchers are discovering that dietary methods can help protect our bodies from environmental abuse. A high-protein diet, especially sulfur-containing amino acids, can reduce the toxicity of pollution. People living on a low economic level and who maintain a poor diet are highly susceptible to air-pollution diseases. Roehm et al. have shown the protective qualities of vitamin E against oxidant air pollution. Vitamin E has no known human toxicity and should be considered by all those exposed to oxidant air pollution. Clinical studies are continuing to determine an optimum dose.

Pollution from toxic metals can and must be eliminated from our environment. Strict adherence by industry to antipollution methods, such as specifically treated smelter and refinery stacks, emission control and the elimination of nickel and lead additives to gasoline could effectively combat the threat of metal-caused air pollution.

Dr. Irving Selikoff, an authority on environmentally related illness, believes that "80 to 85 percent of all cancer comes from the environment." Clearly, effective pollution controls must be enforced.

Fruits and vegetables should be washed thoroughly. The use of aerosol cans should be avoided. It can be worthwhile to try to kick the smoking habit and to help ecological groups fight against air pollution, clean out air conditioner filters and stop feeding pigeons!

Man has met and conquered other problems in his history, but never before has a problem assumed the awesome proportions of pollution. It is not only an individual or even a national crisis. It is a worldwide concern that must be met collectively. Our economic policies, our political philosophies, our individual lifestyles all must change together in support of one principle—the preservation of the species and the good life on earth.

Man can only conquer this problem of environmental pollution with determined efforts, unbiased research, rational actions, and most importantly, consistent cooperation.

References

Lawson, H. G. Specter of lead poisoning. *Wall Street Journal* 27 September 1974.

Levin, A. City diseases that can kill you. *New York Magazine* 7:399, 1974.

Roehm, J. N., Hadley, J. G. and Menzel, D. B. The influence of vitamin E on the lung fatty acids of rats exposed to ozone. *Arch. Environ. Health* 24:237, 1972.

Schroeder, H. A. *Trace elements and man.* Old Greenwich, Connecticut: Devin-Adair, 1973.

Sholman, R. A. Nutritional influences on the toxicity of environmental pollutants. *Arch. Environ. Health* 28:105, 1974.

Wegman, D. H. and Peters, J. M. Cigarette smoking and polymer influenzoid illness. *Ann. Intern. Med.* 81:55-57, 1974.

CHAPTER 37

Milk Problems: Lactose and Lactase

Milk is praised by many nutritionists for its protein, calcium, riboflavin, vitamin and mineral content. Because nonfat, dried milk has a high quality of protein, is nearly a complete food, is cheaper to buy than whole milk and can be conveniently stored and shipped long distances without refrigeration, milk is included in most nutritional aid programs abroad as well as in America.

But why do the West Africans believe that milk from America is evil? Why do the Navajo Indians shun the Commodity Surplus milk? Why is milk avoided by most ethnic groups the world over? Many of the recipients of milk programs and ethnic groups which exclude milk from their diets have been found to be intolerant to lactose, milk's principal carbohydrate. This development has prompted many U.S. agencies, research groups, and the Protein Advisory Group of the United Nations to examine the evidence and to conduct further studies concerning lactase enzyme deficiencies.

Milk contains three major solid components: protein, fats and carbohydrate. Milk's carbohydrate, lactose, is a disaccharide that must be split by the enzyme lactase into monosaccharides (glucose and galactose) in order to be absorbed by the body.

The intestinal secretions contain three enzymes that hydrolyze the disaccharides. The first of these is a maltase that converts maltose into glucose. The second is a lactase that splits lactose, or milk sugar, into glucose and galactose. Finally, an invertase is present that hydrolyzes sucrose, or cane sugar, into glucose and fructose.

Lactase breaks down lactose primarily in the jejunum, the second of the intestine's three main segments. When the body is lacking the enzyme lactose, the unabsorbed lactose passes to the lower digestive tract, where the milk sugar ferments and produces organic acids and gases that irritate the intestine. This results in flatulence (gas), bloating, abdominal cramps and, occasionally, diarrhea.

Lactose Intolerance

Lactose-tolerant people do not have a higher quality of lactase in the intestine; there is simply very little lactase found in the intestine of lactose-intolerant people.

More people are lactose intolerant than tolerant. Intolerance to lactose appears to be the normal trait in adult blacks, lactose tolerance abnormal. There are two basic explanations of adult tolerance to lactose. The first suggests that people with a history of continued milk drinking can tolerate lactose. The milk in the diet may stimulate either lactase activity or the enzyme gene. The second explanation involves a Darwinian adaptation—the possibility of transferring lactose tolerance genetically. The studies of the Yoruba and other African tribes by Dr. Norman Ketchmer et al. tend to confirm the genetic view.

In the United States, the majority of nonwhite citizens have symptoms when they drink the recommended three to four glasses of milk per day. Roughly fifty million people are lactose intolerant: twenty-five million blacks (70 percent of the black population), thirty-four million whites (about 15 percent of the white population), and 80 to 97 percent of the adult Ashkenazai Jews and Oriental ethnic groups in the United States. In addition, adult Eskimos, certain African groups, and South American Indians are especially lactose intolerant. This explains why many pregnant women and people on high-milk ulcer diets become ill after drinking the recommended quart of milk per day. However, small quantities of milk, such as an 8-ounce glass, usually can be tolerated, and the milk proteins will be used by the body even if the milk sugar cannot be used.

Lactose digestion is not a problem during infancy, but in lactose-intolerant people the lactase enzyme disappears during early childhood. A Johns Hopkins University study in 1971 involving 312 black children and 221 white children in Baltimore elementary schools revealed that 58 percent of the black children were intolerant to lactose, as compared with only 18 percent of the white children. These lactose-intolerant children were not allergic to milk, nor had they had milk-digestion problems during infancy.

Alternatives to Milk?

The arguments for and against the nutritional benefits of milk continue to wax and wane. Dr. David M. Paige of Johns Hopkins University suspects that lactose-intolerant people may suffer specific deficits as a result of not drinking milk. For these people, he suggests leafy greens as a calcium source and legumes and cereals with meat and eggs as a protein alternative. However, Dr. Michael C. Latham of Cornell University has concluded from his studies that lactose-intolerant people can drink sufficient quantities of milk to supply useful proteins and vitamins without symptoms. Nutritionists argue that the excessive dose of lactose (equivalent to 2 quarts of milk) generally administered for the lactose-intolerance test is an overload and that lactose-intolerant people can digest smaller amounts of this important food without gastrointestinal symptoms.

Milk is a nutrient-rich food, and for many people the daily drinking of milk supplies these nutritional benefits with no ill effects. Nevertheless, studies concerning lactose-intolerant subjects and research to develop lactose-free milk products should be encouraged.

The lactose-intolerant person can enjoy products containing only a trace, if any, of lactose, such as naturally processed yogurt (some commercial yogurts contain lactose), buttermilk, soy milk, cheese and homogenized bone meal. People who are allergic to the protein in cows' milk may substitute these products and drink goats' milk as well.

Programs that distribute large amounts of milk powder, such as school lunch programs and national and international programs that use milk as a major weapon against protein starvation, must reassess the advantages and problems of the age-old dietary staple, milk.

References

Ketchmer, N. Lactose and lactase. *Scientific Amer.* 227:70, 1972.

Simoons, F. J. New light on ethnic differences in adult lactose intolerance. *Digestive Dis.* 18:7:593, 1973.

The etiology and implications of lactose intolerance. *Nut. Rev.* 31:6:182, 1973.

There's a fly in the milk bottle. *Med. World News* 30, 17 May 1974.

CHAPTER 38

Alcoholism: The Major Drug Addiction

For centuries alcoholism has been hidden under social stigmas, considered a vice or crime and generally ignored in the medical field. Today, great strides are being made in defining and treating this perplexing condition.

In 1956, the American Medical Association (AMA) declared alcoholism a long-term, treatable disease, and accepted the challenge this statement entails. The AMA has stated as follows:

> Alcoholism is the 4th most serious public health menace, following heart disease, cancer, and mental illness.
>
> An estimated 9 million people need treatment for alcoholism, and contrary to popular belief, less than 5 percent are skid-row derelicts.
>
> The alcoholic's life span is shortened by 11 years.
>
> The alcoholic kills or injures both himself and others. Suicide is 58 times more common in alcoholics than in non-alcoholics, and approximately 28,000 auto deaths per year are attributed to excess alcohol.
>
> The national cost of alcoholism is $15 billion dollars per year.

Ethyl alcohol is a drug that can anesthetize the brain cells. Once ingested, it travels first to the areas of the brain cortex and acts as a relaxant—but larger doses can distort learning ability, memory, control, judgment, and regulation of behavior. Alcohol also travels to and affects other areas of the body. Alcohol will dilate the kidney blood vessels, and thus increase urination. The liver may also be jeopardized by excess alcohol, regardless of the vitamin content of the diet.

The controversy concerning whether liver damage is caused by the alcohol itself or by the associated malnutrition was studied by Dr. Charles S. Lieber of New York's Mount Sinai Hospital. His controlled experiments were conducted on baboons because their livers are morphologically similar to the human liver. Dr. Lieber's studies conclusively showed that although some liver damage can be attributed to a low-protein diet, the cellular changes which result in fatty livers, inflammation and cirrhosis (a chronic disease which leaves the liver a mass of scar tissue) resulted from long-term alcohol consumption. (Dr. Lieber may not have had adequate trace metals such as zinc in the baboons' diet.)

The ravages of the hangover—headache, heartburn, nausea, and thirst—are side-effects of alcohol that are well known to all heavy drinkers. Yet the exact definition of the hangover is subject to debate. The celebrated W. C. Fields spent a lifetime nursing the bottle. "Always carry a flagon of whisky in case of snakebite and furthermore always carry a small snake," he advised. Despite bouts with the wrath of his overindulgence, Fields remained faithful to the martini. "A woman drove me to drink," he confessed, "and I never even wrote to thank her." Fields, of course, died of the complications of alcoholism.

The hangover headache can be brought on by relaxation or vasodilation (the opening of blood vessels in the brain). Because nicotine acts as a vasoconstrictor (shrinking blood vessels in the brain), some have suggested smoking to alleviate the throbbing. However, it is important to note that nicotine and alcohol release adrenalin, which subsequently causes a depletion of sugar in the blood—or hypoglycemia. This condition produces shakes, tremors and extreme fatigue.

The most tragic side-effect of alcohol abuse afflicts children born of alcoholic mothers. In the eighteenth century, after

Queen Anne gave gin distilling and drinking a royal nod, a higher incidence of birth defects was noted in children from gin-drinking mothers. The disastrous effects of alcoholism on the population brought sharp criticism which eventually curtailed the use of gin. Critics such as the artist William Hogarth helped. His etchings *Gin Lane* and *Beer Street* are famous. In *Gin Lane* all is bad, while in *Beer Street* all is paradise. Today, at the University of Washington in Seattle sufficient data has been accumulated to establish a link between alcoholism and serious prenatal and postnatal developmental deficiencies: limb, facial and heart defects. These infants were smaller than average at birth, and failed to catch up afterwards. The deformities are due to the alcohol, or the toxic agents sometimes found in alcohol, congeners. The congeners (fusel oils) in some alcoholic beverages are small molecules that are produced in part from the wooden barrels during aging. Found in small quantities in aged alcoholic beverages such as cognac, whisky and bourbon, these congeners, in large quantities, can be lethal.

The fact that alcoholism is often accompanied by nutritional deficiencies and neurologic syndromes leads to dichotomous approaches in treatment. Psychiatry will attempt to stop the drinking through talk therapy, while medicine will seek to treat the illness first and later approach the psychological problems. Psychotherapy alone is not generally successful in the long term, while the medical approach has brought some positive results. The alcoholic must be "dry" before the psychological causes can be treated. "Never mind who stole my little red wagon when I was three," one alcoholic retorted. "I need help now."

Extreme Value of AA in Treatment

Social groups such as Alcoholics Anonymous (AA) are very effective in beefing up the morale of the alcoholic and thus preventing a recurrence. The patient must want to be helped and must realize that to him alcohol and other "downers" are poison. Most AA groups have come to realize that nutrients of all kinds can come in tablet form and should be allowed as part of the continued therapy. Only AA can provide the person-to-person coverage which the backsliding alcoholic may need from time to time. Most cities have AA groups which meet every night so that time never hangs heavy on the alcoholic's shoulders. Participation in AA helps to ease the great burden of selfishness which is part of the personality of the alcoholic.

The family physician can be effective in the early diagnosis of alcoholism. However, because the alcoholic will often deny that a problem exists, this disease is easily overlooked. For this reason, the doctor must familiarize himself with the warning signs of alcohol abuse. Common problems are gastrointestinal complaints such as anorexia (loss of appetite), nausea, difficulty in swallowing, heartburn, complaints of chronic cough, heart palpitations, headache and edema. The alcoholic is usually suffering from dehydration, nutritional deficiencies and hypoglycemia.

The disease is sometimes politely ignored to avoid embarrassment. The stigma attached to alcoholism is being erased, and any feeling of shame should be eliminated. "We are not moralists and judges—but physicians," says Dr. M. E. Chafetz, an authority on alcohol abuse and its prevention. Once the suspicion of alcoholism is confirmed, a personalized treatment program should be designed and started immediately.

What Form of Treatment Is the Most Effective?

Recent research into this question has produced a plethora of drug- and nutrient-based solutions. One radical approach, the use of LSD-25 and similar psychedelic substances, has been tested and debated for over two decades. Cheek and Osmond et al. conducted controlled experiments with LSD-25. Their results did not indicate any long-term positive effects in terms of sobriety.

Metronidozole (Flagyl) as a treatment for alcoholics was discovered in 1964. It was maintained that this drug produced a reduced desire for alcohol without ill effects. However, once the drug has been administered, any alcohol ingestion will produce abdominal cramps, vomiting and nausea, as well as possible health hazards. Therefore, the patient should be thoroughly examined prior to administration of metronidozole. In 1966, the Carrier Clinic in New Jersey conducted a four-year follow-up program on metronidozole treatment for alcoholism in which the drug was found to produce no lasting effects in the alcoholics.

Antabuse, the trade name for disulfiram, is generally accepted and is used by many alcoholism treatment centers and hospitals. Antabuse will not cure the disease, but it acts as a deterrent by producing startling and very severe symptoms after ingestion of even small amounts of alcohol for days after the last dose. Therefore, Antabuse acts as an aid only to the alcoholic who has firmly resolved to recover. The drug should not be prescribed for anyone who lives alone, should only be used during supportive and psychotherapeutic treatment, and the patient must be given a clear and detailed description of the symptoms produced by the reaction.

Sedative and antianxiety drugs may be useful in getting the patient off alcohol. This may merely substitute a dry drug addiction for the original wet addiction. Dry drug addiction can be worse than alcoholism, since many dry drugs such as barbiturates, Librium, Valium and even chloral hydrate have a quicker effect and a deeper narcosis. A formerly alcoholic physician stopped drinking alcoholic beverages but used Seconal instead. On large doses of Seconal he had hallucinations and was barely able to function as a physician. On a trip out of town he smoked in bed after taking his usual whopping dose of Seconal. The red diving bomb caused rapid sleep and he set the bed afire and died later of his serious burns, malnutrition and Seconal withdrawal. Most hotel-bed fires are probably the result of barbiturate addiction.

Valium is only better than a barbiturate in that it has, in most individuals, a twenty-four-hour duration of action compared to the four-to-six-hour duration of Seconal. Librium is intermediate. The dry drugs also are easier to reduce and count out than are the alcoholic drinks when we proceed carefully to reduce the dose each day to get the alcoholic patient off his addiction.

Lithium, the alkaline metal compound, has been successful in preventing both manic and depressive mood swings. The current studies of Dr. Nathan Kline at Rockland State Hospital in New York point to lithium as a method of controlling the compulsive drinking syndrome as well. In order to examine the effects of lithium on alcoholism specifically, alcoholics suffering from severe depression were not included in Dr. Kline's study. Although still in the preliminary stages of research, the use of lithium offers an alternative to the total abstinence and serious physical reactions to drinking involved in other drug programs. The evidence as to how lithium works in the body is not entirely clear. However, data clearly suggest that lithium changes drinking patterns by directly affecting or countering the actions of alcohol on the brain cells, rather than by diminishing underlying depression.

Drug-related attempts at conquering the problem of alcoholism, however, are designed to stop or control the drinking, rather than to discover why the alcoholic craves alcohol. The alcoholic often indulges in drinking to alleviate the stressful symptoms of anxiety and depression brought on by the normal vicissitudes of life. However, this is a maladaptive response which may stem from the disease. The popular misconception that alcoholics harbor an "addictive personality" is slowly being dispelled. The disease is beginning to be approached as a biochemical deficiency rather than a psychological or moral problem.

Alcoholism and Diet

Tests have repeatedly shown that diet can affect alcoholism regardless of genetics or environment. A rat placed on a typical American diet of coffee, refined foods and soda, will eventually avoid the bowl of water in his cage and selectively drink from the bowl of whisky. A diet high in carbohydrates, especially of the refined variety, can produce a drunken rat whether or not he has a mean mother or an alcoholic father! This pattern has been discovered in humans as well. Biochemical deficiencies may also provoke some people to alcohol abuse. Furthermore, the studies in rats indicate that drug- and alcohol-metabolizing enzymes in males and females may be different.

Alcoholism has been successfully tackled when considered in the light of nutritional deficiencies. Niacin (vitamin B-3) appears to contribute to the alcoholic's ability to attain and maintain alcohol abstinence by helping to prevent the craving for alcohol.

Nutrient programs involving a high-protein diet, large (mega) doses of niacin, and vitamin C, vitamin B-6 and occasionally vitamin E have been successful in treating more than five thousand alcoholics, in all stages of the disease.

Three reoccurring problems that can complicate the patient's recovery are concurrent drug use, previously undetected hypoglycemia (because the low blood sugar creates nervousness) and perceptual distortions—distortions of taste, hearing, sight, personal awareness, time and space.

These perceptual disorders and the general personality characteristics of alcoholics are similar to many experienced by schizophrenics: inappropriate affect, anxiety, hostile behavior, somatic complaints, delusions or hallucinations, and depression. The gradual development of serious depressive symptoms produces the high rate of suicide among alcoholics.

The studies of Dr. David Hawkins in New York suggest that the cause of some patients' failure to respond to orthomolecular (nutrient) treatment may be "permanent brain damage on a biochemical basis—because of the body's misuse of adrenalin, a hormone of the adrenal glands which is involved in the body's reaction to stress." A question raised is: does alcoholism complicate some schizophrenias or do the schizophrenias complicate alcoholism?

Alcoholism and Histamine

Our observations suggest that the patient high in histamine tends to be the "hard-core" drinker whose suicidal tendencies are satisfied by the slow, self-destructive process of alcohol abuse. We believe that the brilliant American playwright, Eugene O'Neill, may have been a high histamine person. His illness was hereditary; his immediate family tree, from both his paternal and maternal grandparents to his own two sons, was marked by drug/alcohol addiction, severe depression, and in two cases, suicide. O'Neill harbored a compulsive personality, guilt, and phobias related to thunderstorms and crowds. He was preoccupied with a fear of insanity and endured deep and prolonged periods of depression and a volcanic inner tension. Suicidal tendencies were manifested in his self-killing, hard-core drinking and one suicide attempt.

The person low in histamine is vulnerable to cyclic periods of depression and anxiety. He is frequently the periodic alcoholic who will get intoxicated for the weekend as the stimulation of a job becomes unbearable by Friday night or, perhaps, indulge in a once-a-month binge. On the other hand, patients with pyroluria (the mauve factor) are usually on the verge of nausea and therefore intolerant of alcohol or barbiturates. This condition makes them better able to resist the sedative lure of alcoholic beverages.

When any short-acting depressant, such as alcohol, a barbiturate or other sleeping pill is used to treat the schizophrenic who is a periodic alcoholic, the rebound from the alcoholic binge adds fuel to the already blazing fire of overstimulation. These depressants are potentially habit-forming so that often the patient cannot abruptly stop taking them without becoming seriously ill. Finally, barbiturates are dangerous because they are often used for suicide, or are the causes of accidental death through overdosage. Their effects are additive with those of alcohol, and the combination has killed many. In contrast, the antipsychotic drugs are not habit-forming, nor are they lethal in overdose.

St. Basil writes in his homilies, "Drunkenness is the ruin of reason. It is premature old age. It is temporary death." With the use of nutrients to combat the illness, and counselling to alleviate the psychological problems, modern man can meet and defeat this two-headed monster and restore the millions of suffering alcoholics to a useful life.

References

Cheek, F. E. and Osmond, H. Observations regarding use of LSD-25 in the treatment of alcoholism. *J. Psychopharmacology* 1:56-74, 1966.

Lieber, C. S. and Rubin, E. Alcoholism, alcohol and drugs. *Science* 172:1097-1102, 1971.

Lithium: antidote to alcoholism. (Discussion of Nathan Kline's work.) *Medical World News*, December 1973.

CHAPTER 39

The Hypoglycemias: Low Blood Sugar

The hypoglycemias have now gained widespread attention. You may have heard of the most common one, functional hypoglycemia (FH), which has been pinpointed as the cause of many everyday emotional problems such as fatigue, depression and irritability. Many physicians who specialize in metabolic disorders believe it affects at least ten million people in the United States alone, and some estimates range much higher. FH may affect as many people as diabetes (the opposite condition) and can be as serious. A high incidence of FH is found in people with such disorders as schizophrenia, neurosis, alcoholism, drug addiction, juvenile delinquency, childhood hyperkinesis and obesity. The development of FH is associated with heredity; its onset is precipitated most often by inadequate diet.

Probably the most aggressive and hostile people in the world are the Qolla, who live in the area around Lake Titicaca between Peru and Bolivia. The incidence among these people of fights, theft, rape and murder is staggering. Ralph Bolton, an ethnographer from California, visited the Qolla and found that 55 percent of the men in a sample tested suffered from mild or severe hypoglycemia! (Estimates for the United States range from 2 to 30 percent.) Bolton believes the hypoglycemia to be the cause of the Qolla's hyperaggression.

Perhaps FH is at the root of much of the antisocial and aggressive personal behavior in our own country. No one can say for certain, but hypoglycemia and schizophrenia have been found to occur in juvenile delinquents and in convicted offenders. The discussion which follows will expound the nature and causes, diagnosis and treatment of the hypoglycemias. The reader will then be fundamentally equipped to understand this complex but common disorder which afflicts many Americans as well as the Qolla.

The Nature of the Hypoglycemias

Hypoglycemia means low blood sugar (glucose). It is a condition of low cell fuel, resulting from an abnormal glucose metabolism; each of the body's cells needs glucose to carry on its work. The state of low cell fuel has many physical and psychological consequences, as we shall see. The considerable lowering in mood due to lowering of the blood glucose level when the patient is hungry or following a nutritionally insufficient diet, as compared with the mood experienced when the glucose level is elevated after eating, has been experienced by almost everyone. However, in the hypoglycemias the lowered blood sugar is chronic or continuous.

The hypoglycemic disorders are classified according to whether symptoms occur after eating (reactive or fed hypoglycemia) or when food is withheld (fasting hypoglycemia). (See Table 39.1.) Reactive or fed hypoglycemia represents about 70 percent of the adult symptomatic hypoglycemias. In adults, fasting hypoglycemia is produced by only a few rare conditions. It can result from liver disease, adrenal or pituitary insufficiency, excessive alcohol consumption, some tumors or an excessive dose of insulin or other antidiabetic agents in the diabetic. Fasting hypoglycemia is probably most commonly found in patients with islet-cell tumor of the pancreas.

TABLE 39.1

Classification of hypoglycemias

Fasting hypoglycemias

UNDERPRODUCTION OF GLUCOSE

Liver disease

Adrenal or pituitary insufficiency

Alcohol hypoglycemia

OVERUTILIZATION OF GLUCOSE

Insulinoma (pancreatic islet-cell tumor)

Extrapancreatic tumors

Overdosage of insulin or oral hypoglycemic agents

Fed hypoglycemias

Alimentary hypoglycemia (due to previous gastrectomy or other surgery)

Functional hypoglycemia (FH)

In such an organically caused condition, the severe and prolonged low blood sugar level can lead to permanent brain damage and death. However, the majority of hypoglycemias are functional (FH), one of the classifications of fed hypoglycemia (see Table 39.1) and symptoms occur in response to eating. FH is the hypoglycemia so widely publicized as causing all of our everyday problems and the one to which this chapter is devoted.

The functional hypoglycemias are associated with many other disorders and conditions. Functional hypoglycemia is known to contribute in some people to epilepsy, allergies, asthma, ulcers, arthritis, lack of libido in women, impotency in men, suicidal intent, underachievement in school, and hostile or asocial behavior. Conditions which display a high incidence of FH include alcohol or drug addiction, obesity and mental illness.

Alcoholism can cause alcohol FH (a fasting hypoglycemia) as a result of lack of food intake and substitution of alcohol for essential calories and nutrients. However, there is sufficient evidence that in some alcoholics the FH precedes and causes the excessive drinking. Dr. Robert Meiers has found FH in 95 percent of alcoholics. This type of alcoholic finds that the ingested alcohol provides energy and temporary relief from his hypoglycemic difficulties, and thus he drinks more and more. He makes his FH worse by substituting alcohol for food that would keep his blood sugar level high, and is thus caught in a vicious circle. The hypoglycemic diet and nutrient therapy provide relief for these people.

Another complication associated with FH is obesity. This may result from constant nibbling on sweets and junk carbohydrates; hypoglycemics often have cravings for sweets, and the sweets will alleviate their symptoms and give them a quick pick-up temporarily. So they eat more sweets which, like the alcohol in the alcoholic, worsen the hypoglycemia, make the person hungry again, and thus create another vicious circle.

Incidence of FH

Blood sugar level plays an important part in our mental as well as our physical health. FH can cause abrupt mood swings and even mimic serious mental illness. It is often misdiagnosed as a psychiatric disturbance because of psychopathological symptoms. The symptoms of fatigue, depression, confusion and anxiety that usually occur with hypoglycemia also appear, in many cases, as the first early symptoms of schizophrenia. FH may even produce acute and chronic psychiatric dementia. Carbohydrate metabolism abnormalities (hypoglycemia and diabetes) have been reported in mental illness for more than fifty years. FH has been found to exist in patients with schizophrenia, psychoneurosis, manic-depressive psychosis, presenile and senile psychosis and other chronic psychiatric maladjustments. Dr. Meiers also pointed out that psychiatrists, if they test for it, find FH in from 30 to 70 percent of their psychiatric patients of *all* diagnostic categories.

In the experience of Dr. Jack Ward at the Mercer Hospital, Trenton, New Jersey, about half of the people he counsels for psychiatric problems have abnormal blood sugar metabolism; he has found that about 60 percent of his schizophrenic patients, 80 percent of manic-depressives and 70 percent of neurotics have FH. (Meiers found FH in about 70 percent of schizophrenics tested.)

The occurrence of FH with mental illness is thus sufficiently common to justify such testing. Although not specific to schizophrenia, FH can be an aggravating or precipitating factor in anyone predisposed to schizophrenia. Treating the FH of a schizophrenic can be a valuable addition to the treatment program, in that patients attain a higher level of mental functioning and fewer relapses occur. Furthermore, inadequate nutrition exists in most schizophrenias. The diet used in the treatment for FH is more natural and improves nutrition in general, and is found to be a valuable adjunct in the treatment of all patients with schizophrenia.

Symptoms of FH

Many of the symptoms manifested in FH are common in everyday life, but one should not leap to the conclusion that FH is the cause of all of life's problems. Truly hypoglycemic symptoms are often difficult to distinguish from emotional problems.

However, FH is one of the most important causes of exhaustion, chronic nervous fatigue, depression and irritability, and prevents many from achieving happy, productive lives. It affects different people in varied ways; no two cases are exactly alike. None of the symptoms are specific for FH, and their wide variety and common nature complicate diagnosis. When no physical or mental malfunction can be found, the patient should be checked for this disorder. FH affects more women than men, and the highest incidence is between the ages of thirty and forty. FH is more likely to be found in the person with a family history of obesity, diabetes, mental illness or alcoholism.

Symptoms in FH are episodic and directly related to the time and content of the last meal. In the early stages, the person may experience recurring feelings of light-headedness, usually at mid-morning and late afternoon. Later the symptoms may be many, but some of the most common somatic complaints are fatigue or exhaustion, headaches, heart palpitations, muscular aching or twitching, prickling or tingling of the skin, excessive sweating, gasping for breath, trembling, dizziness, weak spells, fainting, double or blurred vision, cold hands or feet, craving for sugar, hunger, chronic indigestion and nausea. Psychological symptoms include confusion, absent-mindedness, indecisiveness, loss of memory and/or concentration, irritability, moodiness, restlessness, insomnia, fears, nightmares, paranoia, anxiety and depression.

One symptom which stands out in almost all patients is fatigue, both physical and mental. The FH patient usually feels tired a few hours after meals, notably in the late morning or late afternoon. She may have trouble falling asleep, sleep an abnormally long time (ten to fourteen hours) and then find she cannot get her exhausted, achy body out of bed the next morning.

The patient with FH often tires easily and has little or no physical or mental energy for performing daily tasks. He may even have trouble making it up a single flight of stairs. The manifestations of hypoglycemia are cruel and sometimes they leave the individual unable to perform at a job or in school.

The Body's Sugar Mechanism

"Hypoglycemia" sounds almost like an overly technical name for such a common disorder, but its origins are complicated. At any given time the blood glucose level is the result of many complex factors. Unfortunately, these have not been all sorted out yet, and relatively little is known about the mechanisms of FH. Thus, what follows is speculation, but it is the most logical theory to date.

In simplified terms, we know that in normal people, the sugar hormone insulin is released from the pancreas in response to raised sugar (glucose) in the blood after the intake of food. Insulin *removes* the blood sugar for storage in the liver in the form of glycogen (liver starch). The substances glucagon, growth hormones, glucocorticoids, and adrenalin are antagonists and *raise* the blood sugar. We know, further, that the hormone glucagon and/or these other factors stimulate the conversion of glycogen from the liver back to glucose and its release into the bloodstream to be carried throughout the body for use by cells for fuel. In this way, these two forces work together to maintain the proper blood glucose level at all times.

FH is probably the result of several malfunctions. In some it may be hyperreactivity to the glucose challenge which releases excessive insulin (hyperinsulinism). Insulin secretion by the normal pancreas stops when the blood glucose concentration falls into the hypoglycemic range. A malfunctioning pancreas may continue to secrete insulin. Or, frequently, the release of insulin may be abnormally delayed relative to the glucose load, resulting in a high insulin/glucose level when, a few hours after eating, most of the glucose load has already been absorbed. In other cases, the insulin response may be normal, but the antagonists of insulin (glucagon, glucocorticoids, adrenalin, etc.) may be malfunctioning and not responding sufficiently to the insulin-lowered blood sugar to restore a normal level. Finally, the hypoglycemia may be the result of a combination of excessive insulin *and* deficient glucagon. In all cases, the delicate balance is not maintained between insulin and its antagonists which enables them to work together as a team to regulate blood sugar.

The recently discovered glucose tolerance factor (GTF) is also mobilized from the tissues during the glucose tolerance test (GTTest). The GTF, which contains chromium, nicotinic acid and three amino acids, is essential for the proper functioning of insulin and may be the underlying requisite for proper carbohydrate metabolism, without which diabetes or hypoglycemia develops.

The brain waves (EEG) of an FH patient differ from those of a normal person and, with effective treatment, return to normal. All the body's cells must have the right amount of glucose as fuel for energy to perform their functions. Since the brain cells' sole source of nourishment is glucose, the lowered blood sugar leaves the brain and nervous system in a state of sugar starvation and decreased energy. This deprivation results in depressed, worn-out people and can produce many of the psychiatric symptoms associated with FH.

No one is absolutely certain of the cause of the malfunctions resulting in FH. In some cases it may be due to inborn errors of metabolism. The predisposition towards developing FH later in life also seems to be related to heredity. However, FH is frequently triggered (in genetically predisposed people) by diet or stress.

The major cause is thought to be the tremendous amounts of sugar (sucrose) and other refined carbohydrates and stimulants (caffeine, nicotine, etc.) ingested, especially in the United States. The average American consumes over 100 pounds of sugar a year; the actual estimates are between 115 and 150 pounds per capita per year. This is contrasted with the 5 to 10 pounds per person eaten per year just 100 to 150 years ago. The body's biochemical processes cannot handle this tremendously increased load. It initially seems ironic that *excess* sugar consumption can cause *low* blood sugar, but this is precisely what may happen.

We know that the enormous consumption of sugar-loaded foods, plus refined carbohydrate and starchy foods, constantly overstimulates the pancreas, from childhood on, into excessive production of insulin. This continuous overstimulation of the pancreas may "sensitize" it, resulting in consistent overresponse (with too much insulin) to the intake of sugar and in lowering the blood sugar level below the amount needed to nourish the cells. In addition, hypoglycemia can lead to diabetes; this is believed to come about (after years of overresponding with insulin) from an exhausted pancreas, resulting in less insulin secretion. However, there is probably some more basic cause for the whole mechanism, for decreased insulin is now known to be merely a symptom of diabetes.

All carbohydrates stimulate insulin release; the more refined they are, the more dramatic is the release. Sugar (sucrose) is the most dramatic. This is because the bond in sucrose (consisting of a molecule of glucose and a molecule of fructose, two simple sugars) is very easily broken. Sucrose is rapidly absorbed by the body, releasing a surge of glucose into the bloodstream, which then stimulates the release of insulin to lower the blood sugar again. This is what lies behind the advertising pitch of "quick energy." Most college students have learned that a candy bar before an exam gives them a quick pick-up (a swift rise in their blood sugar), only to be followed a few hours later with the 'fatigue symptoms of lowered blood sugar.

The hypoglycemic response can be triggered by many factors, one of the most important of which is stress. One explanatory theory is that when subjected to sustained stress, the body reacts by lowering the blood sugar level. With a raised sugar level in the blood, the pancreas overreacts and the overabundant insulin lowers the blood sugar.

In addition, the patient's increasing adrenalin (as a result of prolonged stress) may lead to defects in the stress responses, hyperactivity and psychotic behavior (hallucination, delusion, illusions, etc.). The efficiency of the adrenal cortex, which produces the adrenalin, may eventually be reduced, owing to its continual excitation from prolonged stress, and thus sufficient adrenalin may not be produced to raise the blood sugar when needed. The net result of all this is a defective stress mechanism coupled with hypoglycemia. In support of stress causing low blood sugar, Rennie and Howard have observed flattening of the GTTest curves in normal patients during period of emotional stress, with return to normal configuration upon recovery.

Stress, emotional or physical, can result from poor diet, infection, pain, overexertion, pregnancy, lactation, physical injury, chronic worries, drugs or alcohol. An abrupt change or shock can precipitate an otherwise dormant FH. The stress of pregnancy and childbirth often precipitates FH in those women susceptible by constitution and dietary history, resulting in a long-lasting period of postpartum difficulties.

Other causes of hypoglycemia are excessive use of tobacco and alcohol (believed to inhibit the mobilization of reserve glucose from the liver and to depress the demand for more sugar by the hypothalamus in the brain), stimulants (caffeine in coffee, colas and tea, etc.), the birth control pill or high doses of estrogen, some psychotranquilizer drugs (because they may depress adrenalin release) and diuretics. These all may disturb the controlled blood sugar level and contribute to or aggravate hypoglycemia. Also, the liver, essential in maintaining the glucose level, can be damaged by excessive alcohol use, infections

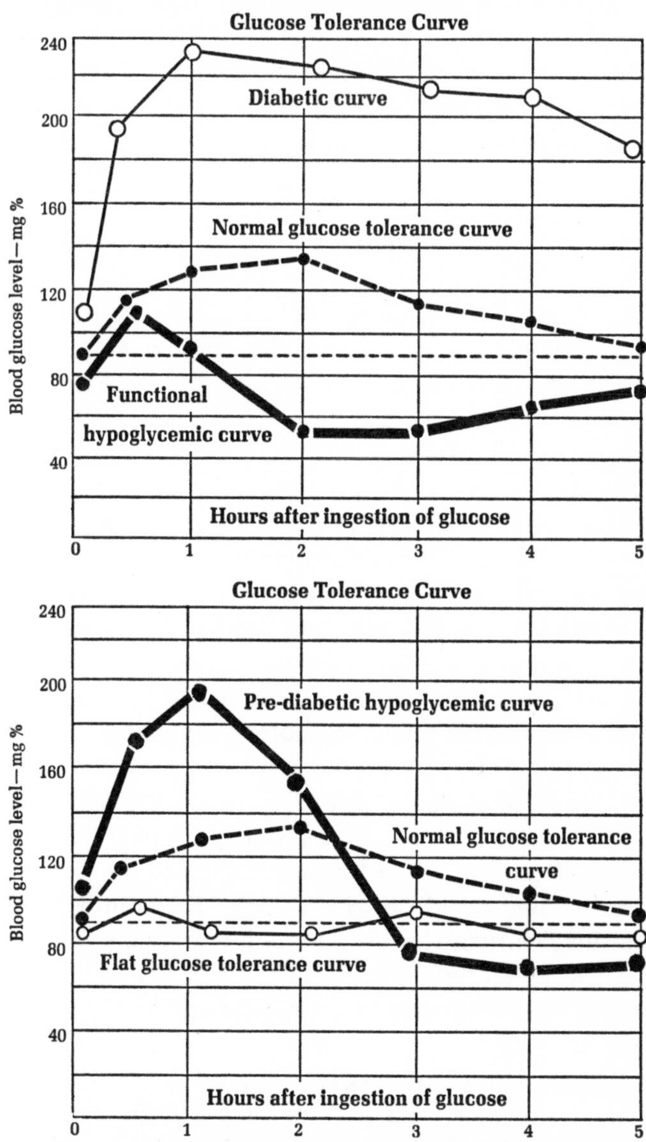

Types of glucose tolerance curves encountered clinically. The typical curve in the hypoglycemic patient has a drop of 20 mg percent or more below the initial value. The prediabetic curve goes much higher and drops 60 mg percent or more in the third and fourth hour. The flat type of curve still indicates hypoglycemia. Other factors to be seriously considered are the occurrence of typical symptoms during the test such as sweating, disperceptions, nausea and tremor. Relief of symptoms with a diet low in starch and sugar also indicates functional hypoglycemia. These patients have a return of their initial symptoms when they eat appreciable amounts of sugar.

and toxic substances. Furthermore, the B-complex vitamins and trace elements are essential for carbohydrate metabolism, and deficiency or poor assimilation of these required nutrients may contribute to FH. Almost any disease is made worse by poor nutrition, including FH.

Diagnosis and Treatment

Unfortunately, too few doctors are knowledgeable about the signs, symptoms and diagnosis of the hypoglycemias. Hypoglycemic patients are often told that their problems are "in their heads" or "just nerves." Even the more serious kinds of hypoglycemia which produce stupor, blackouts, comas, seizures and psychoses may not be diagnosed correctly.

Once organic causes (pancreatic tumors, etc.) of the low blood sugar (which would indicate fasting hypoglycemia) have been ruled out, FH can be confirmed by a five- or six-hour glucose tolerance test. The GTTest monitors the glucose-regulating mechanism following a challenge (oral ingestion of 100 gm of glucose after a fasting period of twelve to fourteen hours.) Blood sugar levels are determined before ingestion (fasting level) and at thirty minutes, one hour and every subsequent hour following. (See Figures 39.1 and 39.2.) The normal configuration of the GTTest has a hyperglycemic (up) and hypoglycemic (down) phase. A peak of 150 to 220 mg/100 ml of the blood sugar is normally reached within thirty to forty-five minutes, and the blood sugar level returns to the fasting level in one and one-half to three hours. In diabetes, the glucose level remains high. In the hypoglycemias, diagnosis is closely related to the rate of fall of the glucose level.

While the patient with organic hypoglycemia shows a low fasting blood sugar level which drops lower with time, the patient with FH usually has a normal fasting blood sugar level. As can be seen from the graph, the latter patient's GTT usually follows the same configuration as normal, but with values declining to the lower limit of the normal range (60 to 120 mg/100 ml) or less and a delayed return to the fasting level. In reading the GTT, the patient's own fasting level is the base or standard from which the other readings are judged. If any subsequent glucose level (usually between the second and fifth hours) drops 20 mg percent (mg per 100 ml of blood) or more below the fasting level, a diagnosis of FH is indicated. A drop of 10 to 20 mg percent below the fasting level is considered borderline. Some consider a drop below 60 mg/100 ml to be FH regardless of the fasting level. Buehler accepted two additional configurations as indicative of FH: one with a moderate peak at one hour without declining below the starting level; the other the so-called flat or low-profile curve. Reading the GTT can be complex since many doctors don't know enough about the subtleties of the GTT involved, such as correlation of glucose levels with symptoms during the test. These can often be more significant than the final low reading. The contraceptive pill or estrogen therapy can alter one's GTT, a fact of which some doctors are not aware.

At present, some further interesting leads in diagnosis are available. The Brain Bio Center has found that hypoglycemics have a significantly lower level of blood spermine. (Refer to Table 39.2.) Spermine level is now used by this group as an indication of hypoglycemia. This is a simple chemical which can be assayed and some knowledge is available on how to elevate blood spermine.

In the body, glucose is rapidly made from refined carbohydrates, especially sugar. However, glucose for energy can also be synthesized from proteins and fats. In all these cases insulin is released, but the glucose from proteins and fats is released into the bloodstream at a much slower rate which does not throw the regulating mechanism off balance. Low-carbohydrate meals will prevent an extreme postprandial (after-eating) rise in the blood sugar.

The normal individual primarily uses carbohydrates for energy. However, the hypoglycemic cannot, because of a malfunctioning mechanism. So, the hypoglycemic must make use of more protein and fat to maintain high blood sugar. For the hypoglycemic, a high-protein breakfast is mandatory! Frequent high-protein snacks are suggested between low-carbohydrate meals, and another protein snack before bedtime. Liberal amounts of protein foods will prevent hypoglycemia for a period of three

TABLE 39.2

Comparison of spermine and histamine levels in normal, hypoglycemic and schizophrenic patients

	Sex	Number	Whole blood spermine levels mcg/ml=S.D.	Whole blood histamine levels nanogram/ml=S.D.
Normals	**Male**	**19**	**1.48±.34**	**46.3±18**
	Female	**10**	**1.27±.48**	**41.7±14.5**
Functional hypoglycemic	**Male**	**35**	**0.81±.16 t[a]=9.9 p=<.001**	**43.4±25.1**
(FH)b	**Female**	**71**	**0.79±.16 t[a]=6.5 p=<.001**	**49.3±21.1**
Pyroluric	**Male**	**27**	**1.17±0.33**	**52.8±23.8**
	Female	**27**	**1.03±0.31**	**46.1±11.7**
Schizophrenic low histamine	**Male**	**28**	**1.17±0.31**	**20.2±10.4 t[a]=6.3 p=<0.001**
	Female	**29**	**1.08±0.32**	**27.6± 8.1 t[a]=2.3 p=<0.05**
Schizophrenic high histamine	**Male**	**29**	**1.52±0.55**	**110.7±16.5 t[a]=12.8 p=<.001**
	Female	**26**	**1.10±0.23**	**107.3±24.4 t[a]= 7.9 p=<.001**

[a] Compared to normal group.

[b] The FH patients are the only group to have spermine levels below 1.0 mcg/ml. Their blood histamine levels are in the normal range.

to six hours. Sugar, refined carbohydrates, alcohol, caffeine, tobacco and other stimulants are absolute No! No!s, and natural carbohydrates and sugars (in fruits and vegetables) are limited to small amounts throughout the day. A regular schedule of daily exercise is an essential part of the treatment.

The hypoglycemic diet was originally designed by Dr. Seale Harris, who first discovered that the pancreas could overproduce insulin. The diet has undergone adjustments, but still makes use of the original principles. At first sight, the diet may seem a bit severe in its restrictions, but the tremendous difference in health and outlook experienced is well worth the effort. Most patients rapidly lose their sweet tooth and find candy too sugary for their newly educated taste buds.

Some who publicize FH, especially the Hypoglycemia Foundation, have advocated the use of injections of adrenal cortical extract (ACE) in the treatment. They claim that it is safe

TABLE 39.3

Foods for hypoglycemic patients

Foods allowed	*Foods to avoid*
All meats, fish and shellfish (except lunch meats)*	Potatoes, corn, macaroni, spaghetti, rice
Dairy products: eggs, milk, butter and cheese; also, margarines	Pie, cake, pastries, sugar (white & brown), candies, dates and raisins; honey except in limited amounts
Milk between meals, milk, cheese and/ or butter (or margarine) before retiring	Cola and other sweet soft drinks
All vegetables and fruits	Alcohol in all forms
Salted nuts (excellent between meals)	Coffee and strong tea
Dietetic (no sugar) peanut butter	All hot and cold cereals, except oatmeal occasionally
Protein or whole grain bread	
Soybeans and soybean products	
Decaffeinated coffee, weak tea (herb teas) and ice water	
Saccharin, as a substitute for sugar, in limited quantity and frequency	

* Lunch meats have carbohydrate extenders.
Having milk, fruit, or nuts between meals is advisable.

and effective for long-term use. Others profess that this preparation is obsolete; that the effective constituent of ACE is cortisone and that it is found in such a minute quantity in ACE that cortisone alone would be better when the patient needs such treatment. ACE has not proven itself as a helpful adjunct for FH. Dr. Atkins of New York feels it may hasten the development of FH into diabetes. Perhaps the few patients who claim benefit from its use are those with adrenal insufficiency or some malfunctioning in their adrenal cortex. (See Table 39.1.) Although FH can be one symptom of adrenal insufficiency, adrenal insufficiency itself is an uncommon condition and is rarely a cause of FH. For the most part, ACE is unnecessary and a waste of time and money.

Some physicians, after thorough testing, may use phenformin (DB1-50) in the treatment of severe hypoglycemia. This is an oral, synthetic insulin-type drug. Initial reaction to even a small dose may be distressing, but if the patient persists, the more serious symptoms may be lessened.

The hypoglycemic diet (see Table 39.3), combined with vitamin and mineral supplementation to correct faulty metabolism, is found to be extremely effective and sufficient in the treatment of FH; such treatment obviates the need for adrenal cortical hormone. To ensure the intake of all necessary nutrients, food supplements are recommended. These may include a high-potency multivitamin formula; choline for fat metabolism; calcium and a good source of the trace elements zinc, manganese, chromium and magnesium; and yeast and B-complex supplements to assure adequate B vitamins. Many physicians also stress the importance of vitamin C, pantothenic acid, niacin, inositol, vitamin E, pyridoxine (B-6), vitamin B-12 and folic acid.

Dr. G. Watson has described two types of patients in studying the effect of nutritional therapy in functional mental illness. On the basis of differences in blood plasma pH as well as carbon dioxide and carbonic acid levels, these two types were characterized as slow (high plasma pH) or fast (low plasma pH) oxidizers. Drs. Currier and Watson have found that patients with dizziness and hypoglycemia were generally fast oxidizers and responded well to nutrient therapy.

Since unprocessed natural foods are emphasized in the hypoglycemic diet, the diet is most nutritious and has also been found helpful for most schizophrenics, whether or not they are hypoglycemic. In many psychiatric institutions, patients receive a high-carbohydrate diet. This can prevent recovery, especially if the patient is hypoglycemic. Dr. Atkins has estimated that there might be a one-third reduction in the number of institutionalized patients if their diets were corrected in this way. Gay Gaer Luce, in her book *Body Time* mentions reports of abrupt changes in the eating behavior of intermittently psychotic patients. Just prior to their acute psychosis, they became restless and anxious and substituted sweets, starches and other carbohydrates for their normal diets of meat and vegetables. The hypoglycemic diet, coupled with nutrient therapy, has also been found effective in the treatment of some psychotic children and some children with learning disabilities.

As we have seen, FH, a debilitating metabolic disorder, is becoming more widespread in the United States and sometimes precipitates or aggravates other conditions such as mental illness and alcoholism. FH can be controlled simply by diet and nutrient therapy. The hypoglycemic can lead a normal or above-normal healthy life. A total improvement can be maintained, but the patient is seldom cured. He or she must stick to the diet, or eventually and gradually the old symptoms will recur. A further worsening of the hypoglycemia or progression toward diabetes may be indicated in the successive GTTests, each time the hypoglycemic patient falls by the wayside and then starts again on his low-carbohydrate diet. (This is particularly true if alcohol is an offending substance in the diet.) With more research, it may be possible to arrest FH completely.

References

Buehler, M. S. Reactive hypoglycemia. *Lancet* 82:289, 1962.

Crofford, O. B. and Graber, A. L. Symptomatic hypoglycemia in adults. *South Med. J.* 66, 1:74, 1973.

Currier, W. D. Dizziness related to hypoglycemia: the role of adrenal steroids and nutrition. *Laryngoscope* 81, 1:18, 1971.

Currier, W. D. and Watson, G. Intensive vitamin therapy in mental illness. *J. Psychol.* 49:67-81, 1960.

Finestone, A. and Wohl, M. *Med. Clin. N. Amer.* 54:531, 1970.

Hawkins, D. and Pauling, L. eds. *Orthomolecular psychiatry: Treatment of schizophrenia.* San Francisco: W. H. Freeman, 1973.

Heninger, G. R. and Mueller, P. S. Carbohydrate metabolism in mania. *Arch. Gen. Psychiat.* 23:310, 1970.

Luce, G. G. *Body time.* New York: Random House, 1971.

Mueller, P. S., Heninger, G. R., and Macdonald, R. K. Insulin tolerance test in depression. *Arch. Gen. Psychiat.* 21:387, 1969.

Rennie, T. A. and Howard, J. E. Hypoglycemia and tension depression. *Psychosom. Med.* 4:273, 1942.

Trotter, R. Aggression: a way of life for the Qolla. *Science News* 103:76, 1973.

Underwood, D. and Thurston, E. W. *Research Bulletin,* Hollywood, California. Institute of Nutritional Research, May 1971.

Watson, G. Differences in intermediary metabolism in mental illness. *Psychol. Rep.* 17:563, 1965.

CHAPTER 40

The Schizophrenias—At Least Three Types

Schizophrenia (better called the schizophrenias), a term which in the past evoked a kaleidoscope of terrifying images ranging from Eve's multifaceted distortion of reality to the demonic "schizoid" character of the Boston Strangler, denotes a complex of thought, perceptual and experiential disorders whose origins long mystified the medical sciences. Since the illnesses prey on that most elusive but vital phenomenon, the "mind," and are therefore subjective or personal maladies with no clear or reliable external manifestations, objective criteria for establishing a cause-effect relationship have seemed to be lacking. Without a clue to the origin of the illnesses, effective treatments could hardly be determined or implemented, and hence many afflicted with the schizophrenias retained the unfortunate status of "wastebasket" or hopeless cases. One young clinical psychologist reported to parents that their son John showed tests "positive for schizophrenia" and warned that the patient should never be told and that they should plan for a lifelong institutionalization of John!

A major breakthrough in the understanding of the schizophrenias resulted from the discovery of the causes of many syndromes which mimic schizophrenia exactly. Included in this group of "facsimile schizophrenias" are dementia paralytica (brain syphilis), porphyria (an abnormal form of chemical blood pigment), homocysteinuria (a metabolic disorder wherein the body secretes an abnormal amino acid, homocysteine), thyroid deficiency, pellagra (niacin deficiency), amphetamine psychosis, vitamin B-12-folic acid avitaminosis and wheat gluten sensitivity. All eight syndromes are chemically-induced metabolic disorders, which suggested the strong possibility that the "true" schizophrenias left in the "wastebasket" might also be due to biochemical abnormalities.

Evidence for this possibility came in 1966 when Pfeiffer and Iliev of the Brain Bio Center showed the possible role of histamine, an amine found in all organic matter and, most notably, in the brain. Having devised a method for accurately assaying tissue histamine content, they discovered that the blood (and therefore presumably the brain) of the schizophrenic patient contained abnormal levels of histamine. On the basis of their research they established two major categories of schizophrenia, thus classifying approximately two-thirds of those afflicted with the illness.

TABLE 40.1

Comparison of blood histamine levels in normal and hypoglycemic patients with means ± standard deviation in three types of schizophrenic patients

	Sex	*Number*	*Blood histamine nanogram/ml ± S.D.*		
Normal	**Male**	**19**	**46.3±18**		
	Female	**10**	**41.7±14.5**		
Hypoglycemic	**Male**	**35**	**43.4±25.1**		
	Female	**71**	**49.3±21.1**		
Pyroluric	**Male**	**27**	**52.8±23.8**		
	Female	**27**	**46.1±11.7**		
Low histamine	**Male**	**28**	**20.2±10.4**	**t*=6.3**	**p=< 0.001**
	Female	**29**	**27.6±8.1**	**t*=2.3**	**p=< 0.05**
High histamine	**Male**	**29**	**110.7±16.5**	**t*=12.8**	**p=< 0.001**
	Female	**26**	**107.3±24.4**	**t*=7.9**	**p=< 0.001**

*Compared to normal group.

The means of normal, hypoglycemic and pyroluric patients are similar and not significantly different.

Histapenic Patients

Normal levels of blood histamine range between 40 and 70 mg per ml. Patients with abnormally low blood (and brain) histamine (50 percent of schizophrenics) are classified as "histapenic," while those with abnormally high levels of blood histamine (20 percent of the total) are termed "histadelic."

Histapenic patients are usually overstimulated, with thoughts hurdling and somersaulting so rapidly through their distraught minds that ideation and speech processes become distorted and bizarre. Severe disperceptions in many spheres, such as sensory, time, body, self and perception of others, cause confusion and render them fearful of themselves, their neighbors and the world around them. Hallucinations plague them, and they frequently report audiences with disembodied voices or contend that their lives are tyrannized by evil spirits. Often these patients turn night into day, and their insomnia becomes another source of torment to them. Histapenic children are hyperactive, unusually healthy and have a very high threshold for pain.

Serum copper levels in histapenic patients are abnormally high. The normal level of serum copper is about 100 mcg percent; the serum copper of the histapenic patient may attain levels as high as 200 mcg percent. Since copper is a brain stimulant and destroys histamine, the elevated serum (and presumably brain) copper level in the histapenic patient probably accounts for many symptoms, including the histapenia.

Hope for the distressed histapenic patient derives from the administration of vitamin C, niacin, B-12 and folic acid. Folic acid in conjunction with weekly B-12 injections raises the blood histamine while lowering the degree of psychopathology, as evidenced by more normal scores on psychiatric rating tests following treatment with these nutrients. Niacin raises the blood histamine and has the added effect of increasing the potency of tranquilizers such as Mellaril and Benadryl, which the patient may receive at bedtime for his insomnia. However, since niacin interferes with the excretion of uric acid by the kidney and may precipitate an attack of gout (a rapid rise in serum uric acid which causes nausea and vomiting), niacin should be increased gradually. In severe cases of histapenia, antipsychotic medication and lithium may be necessary.

For the hyperactive, histapenic child, adequate doses of rutin or Deaner, mild stimulants without the potential hazards of Ritalin and the amphetamines, given in addition to the vitamin C, niacin, folic acid and B-12, effectively reduce the child's hyperactivity and allow learning to proceed.

Histadelic Patients

Histadelia, the biochemical antithesis of histapenia, produces suicidal depression and compulsive or obsessive rumination. Unlike their histapenic counterparts, histadelic patients seldom suffer hallucinations or paranoia, but they do have disperceptions and often lose contact with reality. Frequently histadelic patients experience a state of "blank mindedness" and may sit for hours looking at a book with an uncomprehending mind. Severe headache may also occur with this type of schizophrenia.

Effective treatment for such patients obviously requires chemical factors which will lower their blood and tissue histamine content. Since a high tissue folate level may accompany a high tissue histamine level (hence the use of folic acid to *raise* histamine in histapenic patients), diphenylhydantoin (Dilantin), which produces an antifolate effect, gradually brings about a decrease in histamine. Calcium and the potent analgesics (such as codeine) are histamine-releasing chemicals which will pass to the brain, thereby lowering brain-tissue histamine. Calcium also aids in the relief of the constant or frequent headaches characteristic of histadelia. Methionine, an amino acid, serves as yet another agent in decreasing histamine since it methylates and thus detoxifies histamine. Used in combination, Dilantin, calcium lactate, and methionine plus the trace-metal supplements zinc and manganese (since histadelic patients are usually deficient in these nutrients) provide a powerful and successful therapy for the high-histamine patients. Antidepressants such as thyroid, Deaner, and Elavil and sleep medications including Benadryl, Mellaril, and Trilafon may also help to alleviate the suicidal depression of histadelia. In most cases lithi-

FIGURE 40.1

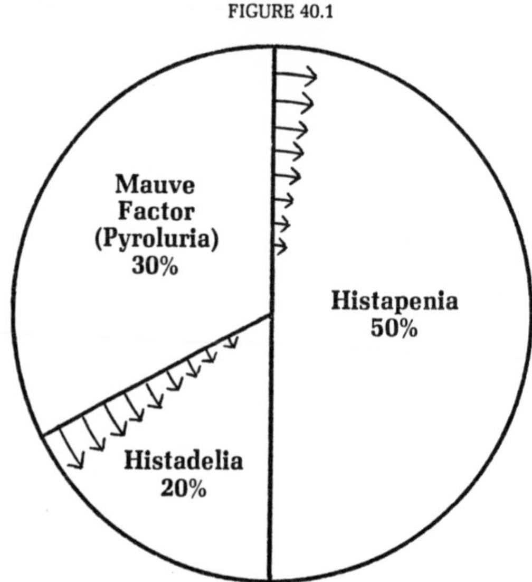

Figure 40.1 **Symptoms: three types of schizophrenia**

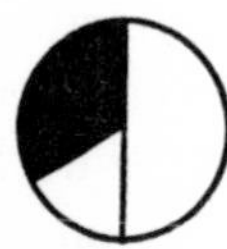
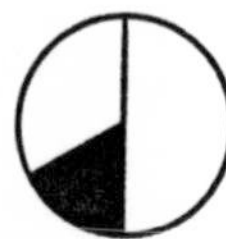
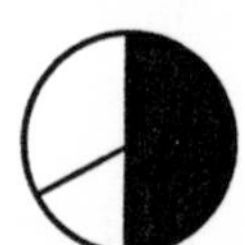

Mauve Factor (Pyroluria)	Histadelia	Histapenia
Stress-induced psychosis	Thought disorder	Thought disorder
Neurological symptoms	Overarousal	Overarousal
Abdominal pain	Compulsions	Grandiosity
White marks—nails	Obsessions	Paranoia
Stretch marks—skin	Suicidal depression	Ideas of reference
Inability to remember dreams		Hallucinations
Iron-resistant anemia		Hypomania
Better affect		Mania

Patients may have two recognizable biochemical imbalances. The most common is pyroluria and histapenia. The second most common is pyroluria and histadelia. Patients who do not respond to therapy for either of these double biochemical imbalances may have a food allergy which is usually characterized by a rapid pulse rate, i.e. 90-120 rather than the usual 60-70 beats per minute.

FIGURE 40.2

The schizophrenias '75: American dietary

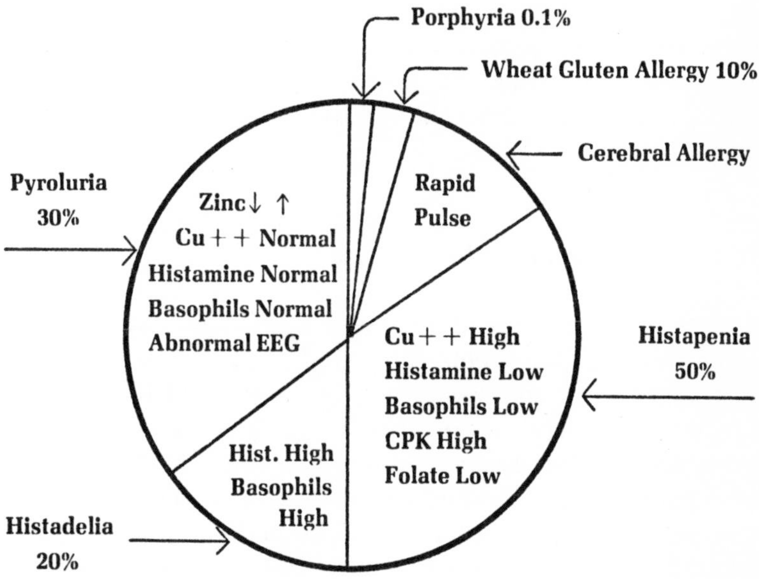

The schizophrenias may have many biochemical facets, since in the past, eight biochemical entities have been separated. We now suggest that 3 major subdivisions may be considered for more intensive research. These are diagramed above. Porphyria, is very rare but should be tested if symptoms warrant. The patients sensitive to wheat gluten are low in blood histamine and represent a special group of the histapenic patients. The few histapenic patients tested are low in serum folic acid but high in creatine phosphokinase (CPK). These paranoid and hallucinatory patients do respond to vitamin B-12, folate and niacin therapy. The histapenic group is low in mean energy content of the alpha waves in their EEG and high in serum copper and ceruloplasm. Ceruloplasm has histaminase activity, and all diaminoxidases contain copper. The high blood histamine group have suicidal depression and high energy content in the alpha waves of their EEG. The blood histamine is contained in the basophils, so they frequently have basophil counts above 1%. Serum copper is low or normal circa 100 mcg%. The pyrolurias are normal in histamine and normal in trace metals except for those who are low or high in serum zinc. The high serum zinc is caused by a marked vitamin B-6 deficiency. The mauve factor (kryptopyrrole) in the patients' urines depletes them of both zinc and pyridoxine. This may result in abnormal EEG's with occasional slow waves and isolated high voltage spikes. These patients may have single convulsions when first placed on neuroleptic medication. They respond best to large doses of pyridoxine A.M. and P.M. and an added dietary source of zinc. Pyroluric patients may have any of the classical symptoms of schizophrenia, but their insight and affect are usually much better than other schizophrenic types.

um treatment may also be necessary.

With the discovery that their schizophrenias result neither from some mysterious and sinister influence on the mind nor from some indeterminable environmental factor such as "lack of mother love," but rather from very real biochemical defects which can be corrected with appropriate chemical treatment, thousands of schizophrenic patients have been spared the misery and hopelessness of a living death and are now able to lead productive lives.

Mauve-factor Patients

More recently, another biochemical syndrome, pyroluria or the "mauve factor," has been separated from the schizophrenias and accounts for the remaining one-third (30-40 percent) of schizophrenics who are normal in their histamine and trace metals, except for those who are high or low in serum zinc. These patients may have single convulsions when first placed on antischizophrenic medication. The mauve factor (kryptopyrrole) in their urine depletes them of both zinc and vitamin B-6, which may result in abnormal EEGs (occasional slow waves and isolated high voltage spikes).

Adequate doses of pyridoxine (B-6), up to 1 gm, administered each morning and evening, provides the best response in pyroluric patients. Because the pyrrole combines with pyridoxal and then combines with zinc to produce a combined deficiency, dietary supplements of zinc must be given with the pyridoxine. Pyroluric patients have many of the classical symptoms of "schizophrenia," but their insight and affect are much better than other "schizophrenic" types. We coined the word "pyroluria" because this describes the condition as we now know it —namely, pyrroles in the urine. When this can be measured in the blood, the condition can be called "pyrolemia."

History of the Mauve Factor In 1963 Drs. Abram Hoffer and Humphry Osmond of Saskatchewan coined the name "malvaria" for those schizophrenic patients who had a mauve factor in their urine. The original observation that an abnormal factor is excreted in greater frequency in the urine of schizophrenics was made by Donald Irvine of the Saskatchewan Laboratory in 1961. Several researchers have since confirmed that this abnormal product of metabolism does, indeed, occur with greater frequency in schizophrenics than in normals.

Ellman et al. erroneously labelled this a drug artifact found only in those taking major tranquilizers. Recently, however, Donald Irvine et al. and subsequently Arthur Sohler of the Brain Bio Center have succeeded in isolating and identifying the mauve factor as 2, 4-dimethyl -3 ethylpyrrole. Neither Irvine nor Sohler could find any relationship between kryptopyrrole excretion and the intake of major tranquilizers. Furthermore, at least 5 percent of so-called "normals," who are not on any major tranquilizers are found to excrete the mauve factor.

Clinical Signs and Symptoms Clinical observation has revealed the following signs and symptoms as being characteristic of pyroluric patients: classical schizophrenic symptoms but better affect, white spots in the fingernails, loss of dreaming or inability to remember dreams, sweetish breath odor, and occasional abdominal pain in the left upper quadrant. Also, constipation, cutaneous striae (stretch marks), inability to tan, sensitivity to sunlight, and possible tremors, spasms and amnesia. They may also be sexually impotent and intolerant of barbiturates, and they may have menstrual irregularities and an anemia which does not respond to iron but will respond to vitamin B-6. Eosinophilia (up to 20 percent) may be present. The individual symptoms vary, but anyone demonstrating a majority of these symptoms is probably mauve positive and should respond well to pyridoxine (B-6) and zinc. The lack of dream recall in pyroluric patients provides a useful yardstick for measuring their degree of B-6 deficiency. When *enough* B-6 is given, then normal dream recall returns. This phenomenon also occurs in "normal" people who do not recall their dreams. According to this criterion, many "normals" may require 25 to 50 mg of B-6 per day rather than the recommended daily allowance of 2.5 mg.

We at the Brain Bio Center, where the treatment for pyroluria was discovered, have now seen more than four hundred cases of this disorder. The treatment with adequate vitamin B-6 and zinc has been 95 percent successful. Patients do extremely well when maintained with minimal or no tranquilizers. Since the patients have good insight with normal affect, they respond to the zinc and B-6 with complete social rehabilitation. Some are witty and even laugh at the horrors of their past mental state. We have therefore wondered as to the stress-induced illnesses that afflicted notables in history. Much has been written about the illness of Charles Darwin and also that of Emily Dickinson. We think they had pyroluria.

Emily Dickinson and Charles Darwin: Partners In Pyroluria? The meaning of life and death: these were the two major influences in the life works of Emily Dickinson and Charles Darwin. Their literary and scientific contributions have been praised for over a century, but only recently has science begun to peek behind the closed doors of their secluded lives and gather the pertinent data that encourages us to suggest that Emily Dickinson and Charles Darwin may have suffered biochemical abnormalities which produced the physical and psychiatric symptoms of pyroluria.

Dickinson and Darwin possessed inner emotional volcanos that erupted and flowed into their work. Because of this intensity, they feared and avoided any outside stress that might upset their delicate balance of emotion and ideas. Any change in routine or involvement with people outside the family group provoked undue stress which could manifest itself as tremor, palpitations, insomnia and (for Darwin), nausea and vomiting as well. As Darwin and Dickinson approached age thirty, they purposely chose voluntary exile. Emily was succinctly subjective when she wrote, "The soul selects her own society then shuts the door."

An amalgam of pyroluric symptoms manifested themselves during the course of their isolated lives. They shared bouts of melancholy, blinding headaches, nervous exhaustion, a change of handwriting and a familial dependence. Darwin endured, usually without complaint, a crippling fatigue and loss of appetite and underwent such extreme depression that it pained him to look at a printed page. Emily became hypersensitive to normal daylight and suffered such extreme eye pains that she, too, could not read.

Many authorities claim emotional, psychological, or simple physical reasons for the reclusiveness of Dickinson and Darwin. For them, seclusion may have been a means by which they could combat the distressing symptoms of pyroluria. A cloistered life provided them with the regulated daily routine and diet, adequate rest and, most important, the avoidance of stressful situations and experiences that enabled them to continue their brilliant studies and productive writing.

Emily Dickinson gave her personal explanation when she wrote, "Insanity for the sane seems so unreasonable."

It is worth mentioning that Dickinson may have had other symptoms than those marked positive; because of her strict seclusion, medical information has been almost impossible to

TABLE 40.2

Comparative symptoms of pyroluria in Emily Dickinson and Charles Darwin

Pyroluria symptoms	*Dickinson*	*Darwin*
Nausea	?	+
Inability to eat breakfast	?	?
Abdominal pains	?	+
Headaches (usually severe)	+	+
Nervous exhaustion	+	+
Emotional response, from flat to hysteria	+	+
Rapid pulse (palpitations)	+	+
Severe inner tension	+	+
Depression (deep)	+	+
Fear of people	+	**Avoidance**
China-doll complexion	+	?
Insomnia	?	+
Unusual time awareness	+	+
Familial dependence	+	+
Coarse eyebrows	?	+
Weight loss	**Thin?**	**Thin?**
Sensitivity to cold weather (frequent chills and fever)	?	+
Personality change	?	?
Inherited illness/characteristics	+	+

obtain. We do know that Emily only wore the color white. Both Darwin and Dickinson worshipped their stern and protective fathers, and were severely affected by their fathers' deaths. As they slipped deeper into seclusion, their handwriting changed and became less legible. Both Dickinson and Darwin enjoyed the company of friends, parties, etc., when young. However, as they grew older, they became retiring and avoided even the closest friends, except through correspondence.

Our First Case 1/29/71 Sara was fifteen, pretty, intelligent and scared. She was wracked with seizures, drained by chronic insomnia and persecuted by bouts of amnesia and vomiting. Through her pleading eyes, Sara viewed her Hadean world in fear. Her past a painful memory, her future a dreaded uncertainty, Sara wanted to die.

Sara's was a perplexing case to the three hospitals through which she ambulance-hopped without relief. Her usual psychiatric and standard blood tests were normal. Her urinalysis profiles were normal, but her seizures, her attempted suicide and her complex miseries were obvious indications of illness. After hospitalization, psychotherapy and tranquilizing medication offered no help, Sara came to the research clinic seeking her sanity. Our laboratory yielded scores that revealed a pattern of biochemical imbalances. Her urine showed a strong mauve factor and a high coproporphyrin excretion, and a psychiatric rating test, the Experiential World Inventory (EWI), showed considerable perceptive disorder.

We administered large doses of pyridoxine (B-6), up to 1 gm per day, supplementary zinc amounting to 160 mg, and 8 mg of manganese. Sara responded to the trace mineral therapy and steadily improved; the antipsychotic and anticonvulsive medications were later dropped. This vitamin B-6 and zinc deficiency syndrome was termed the "Sara syndrome." Today, twenty-year-old Sara has completed the schooling she had missed and is well into premedical training. She continues a maintenance dosage of the vitamin and mineral supplements to prevent relapse. Sara is now a healthy, sane young lady.

Other Cases After finding a practical antidote to Sara's illness, the same principles of treatment were applied successfully to hundreds of mauve-positive patients. One sixteen-year-old boy, who experienced life as a bizarre nightmare, was found to excrete kryptopyrrole at a level of 285 mcg percent (normal is 0 to 20 mcg percent). An EWI test score of 118 (normal is 10 to 20) confirmed his severe psychiatric difficulties. His physical symptoms of pallor, chronic constipation and abdominal pain in the upper left quadrant, together with his high mauve factor, clearly indicated that he was suffering from "Sara's syndrome." His response to large doses of vitamin B-6, plus an extra dietary source of zinc and manganese, was rapid and dramatic. Within one week, his KP urinary excretion had fallen to 90 mcg percent and he could no longer tolerate the large doses of antipsychotic drugs he had been receiving routinely. Further improvement was marked by a steady decrease in KP urinary excretion, which eventually reached the normal range, and by more normal scores on subsequent EWI evaluations.

Freedom from psychiatric difficulties and better health have freed this young man from his hellish existence, allowing him to cope successfully with everyday realities and to pursue his education and hobbies creatively. Continued treatment with vitamin B-6 plus supplementary zinc and manganese will enable him to maintain this condition. Cases such as these indicate that many more pyroluric patients as yet undiagnosed can benefit from vitamin B-6 and zinc therapy.

KP Combines with Zinc and Vitamin B-6 Undoubtedly, the mauve-positive syndrome would have been discovered earlier if the essential relationship between zinc and B-6 had been known. Further testing has indicated that victims of this syndrome excrete, via the urine, significantly more zinc and corporphyrin than do other "schizophrenics." Even in "normals," an oral dose of 50 mg of B-6 results in the reduction of urinary zinc excretion. This dose of B-6 reduces excretion of zinc while increasing copper excretion in both groups, although decreased zinc excretion after B-6 is more pronounced in schizophrenics.

The dose of B-6 needed by the KP-positive patient may be as high as 3 gm per day to prevent psychopathology and to keep the urine free of KP. The present quantitative test for KP measures the total assayable KP.

Although the etiology of the syndrome as a double deficiency syndrome has not been firmly established, we do know that substitution of placebo capsules for the B-6 and zinc therapy may result in rapid return of the previous symptoms or catatonia, muscle weakness, or chills with fever. If such tests are contemplated, slow withdrawal is recommended.

Biochemical advances have thus far identified three syndromes indicative of faulty biochemistry which cause mental illness. Nutrient supplements have relieved these patients of their psychoses, but awareness of dietary intake might have prevented their illnesses from occurring. More research is needed to discover deficiencies or dependencies; but until their discovery, adequate nutrition for prevention is the best medicine.

Childhood Behavioral Disorders

Parents want normal, happy, healthy children who respond favorably to their playful prodding and who become part of an entourage of playmates sharing fun-filled days. Unfortunately, there are many children whose lackadaisical or hyperactive mannerisms prevent them from responding appropriately to the world in which they live. These childhood disorders are manifest in sundry symptomatological categories and may be caused by nutritional deficiencies or dependencies, neurological dysfunctions, or perhaps by environmental events experienced prenatally or postnatally. Many times the "problem child" is ignored or turned away as a "lost cause," and the physician may not explore all the clinical possibilities. A better understanding of the symptoms, possible causes and beneficial treatments is important.

Diagnosis The cause of a child's deviant behavior or learning problems may be difficult to diagnose and treat. The family physician should exercise a high index of suspicion and an awareness that a behavioral problem may be due to a physical disorder. A thorough history that probes into genetics, diet and attitudes, and a battery of tests including eye, ear and natural sidedness examinations is vital if mislabeling and improper treatment are to be avoided.

Minimal brain dysfunction (MBD), hyperactivity, autism, childhood schizophrenia and dyslexia are the major labeled categories. Over fifty terms are used to describe these syndromes, but few of them have much current meaning. There is a very real danger of mislabeling, which often results in ineffective treatment and unnecessary hospitalization.

Minimal brain dysfunction is not a diagnosis but a widely abused label that encompasses a broad spectrum of problems, including retardation, brain lesions, hyperactivity and dyslexia. One cannot expect to treat the causes of the disease if they are not correctly identified. The term "MBD" is as effective in treating a problem child as the term "inoperative" is in repairing a stalled automobile.

Early infantile autism, first described by Kanner in 1943, develops within the first six months of life and is characterized by a total absence of social contact and an obsessive insistence on sameness. These children are well formed, and too intelligent and agile to be considered retarded. The autistic child lives in a private world. He often speaks of himself in the third person, if he speaks at all. He does not relate to people and tends to be interested in mechanical objects more than in people. The classic case is a boy named Joey who believed he was a machine and could not eat or perform daily tasks without first plugging himself in to a wall for power! Bernard Rimland, Director of the Institute for Behavior Research in California, estimates that only one child in three thousand suffers from autism. He believes autism results from an inability to give meaning to incoming stimuli due to an incapacity to relate such stimuli to relevant stored information.

Childhood schizophrenia is a catch-all label used to collect an amalgam of symptoms: hyperactivity, thought disorder, stereotyped and repetitive behavior or thoughts, silly grimacing, inability to distinguish people from objects, severe speech impairment and, rarely, catatonia or waxlike rigidity. Schizophrenia is difficult to diagnose under age ten because the personality has not yet stabilized. A change in personality is a major indicator of the schizophrenias. However, the mauve factor test on the urine, electroencephalographic (EEG) studies, and behavior reports from parents and teachers are valuable adjuncts to the diagnosis. Childhood is the period of life when schizophrenia can do the most harm. Early diagnosis and treatment can prevent later speech and behavior problems.

Hyperactivity strikes 3 to 10 percent of the school children in the United States. The hyperactive syndrome is a disorder of inhibitory mechanisms in the central nervous system which is characterized by fidgeting, inability to sit still, short attention span and impulsiveness. The external stimuli are not filtered by the hyperactive child as by normal children, and therefore the hyperactive child is at the mercy of all the external stimuli in his environment. Hyperactivity is a symptom of some underlying imbalance—not a diagnosis. Furthermore, overactivity can be a manifestation of many things besides "hyperactivity," such as anxiety, boredom or feelings of insecurity.

Dyslexia is a term that identifies difficulty in reading or writing. It is estimated that 30 percent of the school children in the United States are dyslexic. Although this is a high percentage, it should be noted that any child who reads below his grade level due to poor teachers, emotional disturbances, retardation, crossed dominance or any related cause is called dyslexic. Primary developmental dyslexia, which strikes approximately 2 percent of intelligent school children, has no known cause, but nutritional deficiencies and heredity are clearly indicated.

The bright, healthy child who is overactive or who has learning difficulties may be cross-dominant. Cross-dominance is the use of the writing hand opposite the sighting eye. The resulting neural tension can produce hyperactivity and illegible, erratic handwriting. A simple test for natural sidedness during the first grade could eliminate later mislabeling and frustration.

One can readily observe how these categories overlap in their symptomatology; all categories can produce severe learning disabilities and behavioral problems. Nutritional deficiencies manifest themselves in many varying symptoms. The physician must consider each possibility so that the child's real problem can be treated.

What Are the Causes? Controversy rages concerning the etiology (causes) of psychic illness. Until recently, followers of the Bettelheim school of thought believed that autism, deviant behavior and learning difficulties were produced by a faulty environment, such as a poor parent-child relationship. At present, another group of authorities argues that mental illness stems from organic causes, such as brain anatomical disorder. Currently, however, research clearly indicates that many of the schizophrenias, autism, abnormal behavior and subsequent learning difficulties are caused by a biochemical imbalance within the body (too much copper or too much lead). Rather than employ talking therapy or behavior therapy, or remove the child from the "hostile environment," many authorities, like Drs. Allan Cott of New York and Bernard Rimland, approach these abnormalities with nutrient therapy. (Even Freud was of the opinion that schizophrenia had a biochemical basis.) As opposed to the amphetamines or Ritalin, which only mask the illness, nutrients build up a healthy cellular foundation, thereby helping to correct the disorder. Proper counseling and therapy can be effective in alleviating the emotional disturbances brought on by the illness, but a stable chemical balance within the body must first be reached.

Hyperactivity, perceptual changes involving any or all of the five senses, dyslexia, insomnia and irritability—symptoms usually attributed to childhood schizophrenia—are manifestations of nutritional imbalances. Subclinical pellagra, the hidden disease caused by a deficiency of niacin (vitamin B-3), produces symptoms similar to those of hypoglycemia (low blood sugar) and the niacin-dependent schizophrenias (there is a block between the substrate vitamin B-3 and the synthesis into NAD so that extra niacin is needed). Dr. Abram Hoffer, President of the Huxley Foundation, believes that pellagra and some schizophrenias are identical orthomolecular diseases. The resulting symptoms, which include visual distortions (seeing words and numbers move or reverse), auditory dysperceptions (hearing noises or his name called) and excess fatigue will obviously create reading and writing difficulties or dyslexia and should be investigated with blood tests and a nutritional review of the patient's diet to prevent future impaired mental functions.

The importance of the daily diet should not be underestimated. Carbohydrates, especially of the refined variety, play a major role in exacerbating the above syndromes. Studies by Dr. Ben F. Feingold of the Kaiser-Permanente Medical Center, have revealed that the processed foods that children like to eat in abundance (i.e., hot dogs, ice cream, cola, bakery goods, etc.) can produce hyperactivity. During the acute stages of marked perceptual dysfunction, particularly of the senses, nutrients (especially B-3, B-6 and zinc) have proven to be effective treatments.

The family history affords the doctor an insight into the etiology of the illness. Incidences of alcoholism, obesity, and/or "nerves" in any member of the family may be significant.

Sound nutritional practices can be preventive of childhood problems. According to the World Health Organization, over one-half of the one hundred and sixteen million babies born annually are undernourished during the first three years of life. These statistics are frightening when one realizes that severe mental impairment can result from malnutrition. Hypoglycemia and lack of protein during the critical periods of growth—intrauterine life, early infancy, and childhood—can result in severe brain damage, childhood hyperactivity or learning disabilities.

Therapy of Behavioral Disorders The nutrient therapy provides what Linus Pauling calls "optimum concentrations of substances normally present in the body." Vitamins B-1, B-2, B-3 (niacin), pantothenic acid, folic acid, deanol and glutamic acid are used in treatment. The minerals zinc, magnesium and manganese also play major roles. Vitamin and mineral therapy has successfully treated the underlying causes of hypoglycemia, hyperactivity, many of the schizophrenias and autism in many children. Because the nutrients work to correct the imbalance rather than to disguise it, the response to the program is slow. Three to six months is the minimum time for maximal changes to become manifest. Most parents report that the first noticeable change is a slowing of the hyperactivity and a willingness to learn. Unfortunately, the delay in response discourages parents and often causes them to give up the program.

The quick metabolic response in children to stimulant drugs has created a large market for the amphetamines, Ritalin and also for sedatives. Many parents and physicians are relieved to have the child's unruly behavior under control. The use of stimulant drugs has the paradoxical effect of sedating the child and enabling him to concentrate in school. Yet such drugs do not treat the underlying cause of the hyperactivity; they provide temporary control. Furthermore, these drugs can produce adverse side-effects such as insomnia, loss of appetite and weight, tactile hallucinations, tics, nausea and irritability. Evidence suggests that cardiovascular disturbances, possible Hodgkin's disease, and brain damage, as well as drug dependence, may result from continued use of these drugs. All side-effects, regardless of how trivial they may seem, should be reported to the physician. Considerable controversy exists over the mislabeling and subsequent abuse of stimulant drugs in the treatment of young children in the United States today.

Deanol is a natural compound that was introduced in 1957 by Pfeiffer et al. as a biochemical stimulant. The effects of deanol are similar to those of the stimulant drugs, but deanol does not produce adverse side-effects nor the dependency that the stimulant drugs can produce.

The wise physician will first investigate all possible physical disorders, treat primary nutritional imbalances such as copper excess and zinc deficiency and then, if necessary, carefully add metabolic stimulants such as deanol and perhaps thyroid, depending on the patient's symptoms.

The aim in treatment is to eliminate the child's perceptual dysfunctions. Dr. Cott reports that the administration of adequate vitamin B-3 and vitamin C each day provides the optimal treatment. Besides subclinical pellagra, which is caused by a diet deficient in niacin, many of the schizophrenias are believed to be niacin dependent. With large doses of niacin the dependency is fulfilled.

Dr. Rimland has devised a questionnaire useful in differential diagnosis and has recently reported data on the effect of many drugs administered to the autistic child (see Table 40.3). From these reports we can see that, for the total group of children, certain drugs (i.e., phenobarbitol and other sedatives)

TABLE 40.3

Drug- and vitamin-induced changes in the behavior of autistic, schizophrenic and hyperactive children, by percent

	Number of patients	Improved (%)	Unaffected (%)	worse (%)
All drugs	**1591**	**49**	**24**	**27**
Best drug (Mellaril)	**277**	**58**	**22**	**20**
Vitamins	**191**	**86**	**10**	**4**

Note that drugs can make these children worse, whereas the vitamins have the least-worsening effect and the best score for possible improvement.

Calculated from data of Bernard Rimland.

TABLE 40.4

Parent evaluation of drug effects in young patients*

Drug	Number of patients	Improved (%)	Unaffected (%)	Made worse (%)
Mellaril	**277**	**58**	**22**	**20**
Deanol	**73**	**59**	**27**	**14**
Stellazine	**120**	**56**	**34**	**10**
Dilantin	**204**	**46**	**44**	**10**
Benadryl	**151**	**44**	**46**	**10**
Valium	**106**	**44**	**27**	**29**
Thorazine	**225**	**48**	**22**	**30**
Ritalin	**66**	**48**	**25**	**27**
Dexedrine	**172**	**36**	**18**	**46**
Phenobarbital	**52**	**38**	**22**	**40**

*Calculated percentage changes in behavior of autistic, schizophrenic and hyperkinetic children from data of Dr. Bernard Rimland (1972). The drugs are listed in order of merit according to Dr. Rimland and the parents. Potent drugs such as Valium, Thorazine, Ritalin, Dexedrine and phenobarbital are almost as apt to make the patient worse as better. This indicates the multifaceted causes of these disorders. Note also that all drugs have the potential for worsening behavior in these children.

seem to be more harmful than beneficial, while other drugs (i.e. Mellaril and deanol) have a better rating by parents. Although drugs only serve to suppress, not eliminate, the behavior, it is suggested that small doses of the more effective drugs be used as needed. Careful trial of several drugs in turn may be needed before the most effective one is found.

Dr. Rimland has also studied the effect of large doses of certain vitamins and trace elements on autistic behavior and has found positive results. The biochemical treatment is a novel approach which postulates abnormalities (treatable with vitamin and trace element supplements) as the origin of many childhood behavioral difficulties. Vitamins B-1, B-2, B-3, pantothenic acid, deanol and glutamic acid are all used in treatment. Helpful minerals are magnesium, zinc, manganese and sulfur (as in the yolks of eggs). Mellaril has also been found to be effective in small doses. Advocates of nutrient treatment contend that a common misconception exists that anyone who eats a "normal" diet will not require extra vitamins and minerals. Proper nutritional knowledge and adequate supplements can prevent such illness from occurring.

The childhood behavioral disorders have various precipitating factors and have been seen to manifest themselves in diverse symptoms. Diagnostic categories may overlap, and treatment may be tenuous because of the inability of the child to describe his symptoms accurately. Any behavioral abnormality may be a sign of emotional disturbance, possibly precipitated by physical malfunction and malnutrition. Awareness of the optimal dietary intake of vitamins and trace elements may help prevent the onset of mental disturbance; once it is present, nutrient therapy may provide the best relief and may prevent the child from being institutionalized as a mental retardate. Perhaps if doctors would treat these children as being only "mentally dormant," their prognoses for recovery would be greatly improved.

Cerebral Allergy

Medical workers have long known that the obviously allergic

child can have an allergy-tension-fatigue syndrome which results in disinterest in learning and thus decreases learning ability. When they are tested and the offending allergen is removed, these young patients improve remarkably in respect of all of their symptoms, which can range from hyperactivity to somnolence, with headaches and bellyaches in between. The foods that may most commonly precipitate symptoms are milk, wheat, beef, bananas, chocolate and sugar.

The symptoms shown by the child may be those that would previously have produced a diagnosis of minimal brain dysfunction, namely:

1. Specific learning disability: Not reading at his age level, poor spelling, difficulty with arithmetic or abstractions, poor visual-motor coordination, mentally dormant.
2. Perceptual-motor deficits: Poor painting, writing or drawing; poor copying of simple designs.
3. General coordination deficits: Clumsiness or awkwardness.
4. Hyperkinesis: Constantly active, flitting from one object or activity to another, restless and fidgety, voluble uninhibited speech, disorganized thinking.
5. Impulsivity: Unrestrained in touching objects, especially in a new environment, unrestrained speech (even to being insulting), antisocial behavior and nonconformity with school, family, society.
6. Emotional lability: Irritable and aggressive with rapid swings from temper displays to passivity, easily panicked by minimal stress.
7. Short attention span on any one object or subject, and ease of distraction, especially from a subject that does not arouse great interest.
8. "Equivocal" neurological signs: Transient eye muscle paralysis, poor finger coordination, mixed and confused laterality, slow speech development or speech defect.
9. Abnormal electroencephalogram (brain waves).

Fortunately each child does not show all these symptoms or findings, but any one finding may be allergic in origin. Since the allergen may be either of the inhalant or food type, considerable testing may be necessary before the culpable agent is found. If the child is allergic to all things tested, as is frequently the case, then adequate nutrition with trace elements and vitamins may be helpful.

This same syndrome may also occur in adults and has been termed "cerebral allergy" by D. T. G. Randolph and others in this field. Problem schizophrenics who have gone the rounds from clinic to hospital may be markedly benefited when an allergen is removed. Dohan finds that 4 percent of hospitalized schizophrenics are sensitive to wheat gluten. Perhaps 10 percent of outpatient schizophrenics have this sensitivity. The Princeton group finds that 50 percent of schizophrenics have very-low-to-zero levels of blood histamine—a finding that can occur if the patient is allergic to food or inhalants and is constantly depleting his blood and tissue histamine. Doctors who specialize in the treatment of allergies claim that each schizophrenic referred to them has an average of ten allergies and that 92 percent of patients are allergic! (Somewhere between 10 and 92 percent must be the reasonable expectation.)

Randolph has termed slow and adverse reactions "masked food allergy." Allergic-like reactions have been so characterized because of the fact that immediate and/or relatively immediate reactions occur on exposure. Food addiction has been characterized by an initial relief or partial relief on exposure and the emergence of delayed reactions which can again be relieved by eating the offending food. Food addiction has the same characteristics of relief on exposure and emergence of delayed reactions as addiction to tobacco, narcotics or alcohol. Addiction can be converted to allergic reactions by a four-day fast, after which symptoms are immediately evoked with the offending food. This conversion from addiction to allergy is also clearly demonstrable in tobacco addiction, but not so clearly observable in alcohol and narcotic addiction due to the greater symptom-relieving values of alcohol and narcotics. Randolph is probably correct in observing a continuum between allergy and addiction.

The most effective procedure in testing for cerebral allergy is the four-to-six-day fast. The patient continues his essential medication, vitamin and trace element supplements.

Whenever hungry, he drinks water. Sleeping medication may be useful the first two nights. After two days of fasting, the usual hunger pains disappear and the mind becomes clearer and free of disperceptions and anxiety. This clearing of the mind may indicate either food allergies or the cessation of absorption of abnormal toxins or vitamins which are synthesized by the bacteria of the gastrointestinal tract.

The patient is then tested by the insertion under the tongue of various food extracts. One to two hours are allowed to elapse between each test. If the patient reacts to everything, a placebo of saline solution is used to determine the validity of the test. The pulse rate will usually rise with a true allergen, although anxiety and excitement will also elevate the pulse.

Dr. James C. Breneman supervised the testing under blind test conditions of various food extracts in 32 patients who were known to be allergic to foods. In 342 tests, only 31 percent of the patients responded as positive to the sublingual testing. This is probably better than skin testing, but the batting average is still far less than the rotation of foods after a period of fasting.

In older patients dizziness and deafness (frequently diagnosed as Meniere's syndrome) may be caused by food allergies. The elimination diet or testing of foods after a suitable period of fasting may disclose the food allergen.

The stored blood histamine should fall with a substance to which the patient is allergic. As a research project, one might propose to determine the possible allergies of various patients and then, in retesting, confirm this by the response of the blood histamine to the specific allergen.

Patients found to be truly sensitive to foods or other substances have a regimen suggested for the avoidance of the allergens. If, as with the child, the adult is sensitive to all foods tested, then again large doses of vitamin B-6 plus zinc may help to cover the allergic reaction.

Maybe the Pulse Can Guide You Patients who are schizophrenic, headachy or hypoglycemic may have an elevated pulse rate for no apparent reason. This may indicate food allergy. Normal is 70 beats per minute. Smokers have a pulse rate of 80, well-trained runners 50 and nervous people 80 to 110. The pulse rate rises with the daily rise in body temperature, 7 beats for each degree of the rise. The fevered pulse thus will be high. Thyrotoxic patients will have a pulse rate of over 100. Pulse rate rises with exercise but returns to normal within minutes. It does not rise after a meal of food to which the patient is not allergic. A rise in pulse rate after eating may indicate food allergy. The counting of the pulse before and after each meal might therefore be the first step in determining possible food allergy. Some hospitals use this simple test.

A final word of caution on the starvation test: one should note that fasting stops the food supply to the flora of our gastrointestinal tract. Thus, the starving patient also starves and even changes the flora of the intestines. These microorganisms have long been suspected of producing amines which might intoxicate the brain. In earlier times the colon was removed in order to get rid of these presumed toxic amines. We have seen at least four of Dr. Cott's patients who got well during the starvation period. All of these patients had a strong mauve factor (kryptopyrrole) in their urine. This decreases with starvation, so the possibility exists that the intestines may be the source of kryptopyrrole or that the patient may have abnormal vitamins such as biotin antagonists produced by the flora of the intestines. The impact of this on allergen testing is obvious, since the fasting period may be the only symptom-free period and the patient would respond to all foods as allergens.

References

Pfeiffer, C. C. et al. *The schizophrenias, yours and mine.* New York: Pyramid Publications, 1970.

——— A study of zinc deficiency and copper excess in the schizophrenias, *Int. Rev. Neurobiol.* Suppl. 1, 1972.

——— Observations on the therapy of the schizophrenias. Unpublished data. 1973.

Pyroluria and Kryptopyrrole (Mauve Factor)

Pfeiffer, C. C. et al. Pyroluria and the mauve factor. *Journal of Applied Nutrition.* Winter, 1974.

____________ The pyroluric schizophrenic. *Journal of Orthomolecular Psychiatry.*

Pfeiffer, C. C. and Jenny, E. H. Fingernail white spots: possible zinc deficiency. *JAMA* vol. 228, 8 April 1974.

The mauve factor in schizophrenia. *Medical World News,* 14 December 1973.

Childhood Behavioral Disorders

Alvarez, W. C. Why that's our Jimmy. *Mod. Medicine,* March 1968.

Arnold, L. E. Is this label necessary? *J. Health,* October 1973.

Aug, R. and Aldes, B. A clinical guide to childhood psychosis. *Pediatrics* 47, 2:327, 1971.

Bender, L. The brain and child behavior. *Arch. Gen. Psychiat.* 4 June 1961.

Cammer, L. Schizophrenic children of manic depressive parents. Presented at the annual meeting of the Society of Biological Psychiatry, Florida, May 1969.

Cott, A. A hyperactive child needs nutrients, not drugs. *Prevention* 169, April 1971.

Critchley, M. Developmental dyslexia. *Ped. Clin. Pediat.* January 1968.

Does baffling reading disorder stem from inner ear lesion? *Med. World News,* April 1974.

Faigel, H. C. When children can't read. *Clin. Pediat.* January 1969.

Fields, E. M. The effects of deanol in children. *N.Y. State J. Med.* 61:6, March 1961.

Goldfarb, W. An investigation of childhood schizophrenia. *Arch. Gen. Psych.* 11, December 1964.

Green, R. A child's dilemma. *Can. Schiz. Found.* 10:2, 1971.

Hawkins, D. and Pauling, L. eds. *Orthomolecular psychiatry: treatment of schizophrenia.* San Francisco: W. H. Freeman, 1973.

Kysar, J. E. Two camps in child psychiatry. *Amer. J. Psychiat.* 125:1, July 1968.

Loomis, E. Nutrition and the exceptional child. *J. Amer. Inst. Homeopathy for Phys. and Surgeons* 1, September 1972.

Mendelson, W., Johnson, N. and Stewart, M. Hyperactive children as teenagers. *J. Nervous and Mental Dis.* 153:4, 1973.

Ornitz, E. M. and Ritvo, E. R. Perceptual inconsistency in early infantile autism. *Arch. Gen. Psychiat.* 18, January 1968.

Pfeiffer, C. C. Deanol, a precursor of choline. Unpublished data.

Reaser, G. Child health and human development. *Research Progress* (971) HEW 72-39:1.

Rimland, B. Analysis of the diagnostic check list for behavior in disturbed children. Institute for Child Behavior Research, March 1968.

________ *Infantile autism.* Des Moines, Iowa: Meredith Publishing, 1964.

Sleator, E. K., von Neumann, A. and Sprague, R. L. Hyperactive children. *JAMA* 229, 1974.

Stone, F. H. The autistic child. *The Practicioner* 205, September 1970.

von Hilsheimer, G. *Doctor, teacher, parent, child.* Academic Therapy Publications, 1971.

Cerebral Allergy

Frazier, C. A. *Parent's guide to allergy in children.* Garden City, New York: Doubleday, 1973.

Green, M. Sublingual provocative testing for foods and FD&C dyes. *Annals of Allergy* 33:5, November 1974.

Kittler, F. J. and Baldwin, D. G. The role of allergic factors in the child with minimal brain dysfunction. *Annals of Allergy* vol. 28, May 1970.

Mandell, M. An introduction to clinical ecology: allergic, ecologic and addictive factors in physical and mental disease. Presented to the International Academy of Metabology, 23 March 1973.

Philpott, W. H., Nielsen, R. and Pearson, V. Four day rotation of foods according to families. December 1973.

Randolph, T. G. The descriptive features of food addiction. *Quarterly Journal of Studies on Alcohol* 17:2, June 1956.

Speer, F. *Allergy of the nervous system.* Springfield, Illinois: Charles C. Thomas, 1970.

Sublingual challenge inadequate for diagnosing allergy to foods. *Internal Med. News* 1 July 1974.

CHAPTER 41

Insomnia: To Sleep, Perchance to Dream

Sleep is a relaxing enigma. No one can explain why we fall asleep or why we awaken sometimes refreshed and sometimes tired and sluggish. Even to define sleep is an arduous task. Historically, behavioral descriptions of sleep were given. Modern science uses the monitoring of the brain's electrical activity to define, study, and subdivide sleep.

A great contribution was made in 1937 when scientists discovered that brain wave patterns during sleep could be categorized into several classes or stages of sleep. Another great leap forward came in 1953 when Drs. Aserinsky and Kleitman identified one of the stages as REM (rapid eye movement) sleep. During this stage of sleep, the brain's electrical activity is more similar to the awake pattern than at any other stage. Also during this period a person is most likely to report dreaming. Biochemical and physiologic activity often reaches a peak during REM sleep. The eyes move back and forth as if watching players on a stage. The muscles are turned off so that a rat or cat sleeping on a moated pedestal will fall into the water and be awakened. Many REM deprivation studies have been made with rats perched on an inverted flower pot placed in a pan of water.

Dr. William C. Dement demonstrated that normal humans

go through a sleep cycle that includes 3 or 4 periods of rapid eye movements. A person moves successively into "deeper" stages of sleep as the alpha rhythm of the wakeful brain waves is replaced by slower, larger waves. In the third and fourth stages (deep stages) the body mobility is at its lowest levels and if the sleeper is then awakened he will require more time to respond effectively than if he had been in stage 1, stage 2 or the REM stage. During deep sleep the smooth muscle of the urinary valves may open and allow bed wetting to occur. Drugs that prevent deep sleep are sometimes effective in preventing bedwetting (enuresis).

In the 1940s, German researchers described another periodic sleep phenomenon—the nocturnal penile erection of males. Drs. Fisher, Gross, and Zuch have confirmed the finding and discovered that erections were concomitant with REM sleep. These full or partial penile erections occur even in infants. Dr. Fisher and his co-workers state that the so-called "morning" or bladder erection that men have on awakening has nothing to do with a full urinary bladder, but is the erection of the final REM period of the night. Studies have shown, however, that the dream content is most often not sexual, and therefore unrelated to the presence of erections.

What Is Normal Sleep?

To date, there is still no scientific definition of normal sleep, nor the needed sleeping hours. People's needs vary. Long-term sleepers find that nine or more hours are needed, while short-term sleepers require less than six hours of sleep. These groups are the exception rather than the rule. The remaining 98 percent of the population sleeps somewhere between six and nine hours. People who sleep only three to four hours nightly will catnap during the day. A picture of normal sleep should take the age and sex of the sleeper into account. Most people appear to reduce the amount of needed sleep (stages three and four) as they age. Females seem more easily aroused from sleep and more vulnerable to sleep problems than their male counterparts. An effective night's sleep is ordinarily restful, restorative, and easily obtained. Continued insomnia can lead to paranoia, rages and hallucinations.

A persistent myth is that one needs one half an hour of sleep for every hour awake. This notion is contradicted by sleep deprivation studies. Volunteers who have been deprived of sleep for several days recover in no more than fourteen hours of sleep, after which they spontaneously awaken. If sleep deprivation is continued for four or five days most subjects become paranoid.

Millions of people have problems with sleep. The superstitions and remedies (both effective and worthless) are probably just as numerous. Benjamin Franklin had two beds so that he could move into the cold one in the middle of the night, believing that he woke prematurely because the bed was too warm. One woman had to lock her son's shiny red bicycle at night in order to prevent him from bike riding while asleep (somnambulistic sleepwalking). The sale and promotion of items to promote sleep, such as eye covers, ear plugs and sedatives, has created a big, multi-million dollar business.

Insomnia

Insomnia means a total loss of sleep, an exceedingly rare condition. However, difficulty in falling asleep or in staying asleep is often termed insomnia. People often state they have insomnia because their slumber is not restful. If you have any of these problems, you have copious company. At least during part or all of their adult lives, one out of three people worry about their ability to sleep, and one out of four feel exhausted when they awaken.

Anxiety, tension, physical pain or discomfort, can all produce insomnia. However, Dr. Anthony Kales of the Sleep Research and Treatment Center of Pennsylvania State University finds that the majority of cases of insomnia are secondary to mental disturbances. Using the Minnesota Multiphasic Personality Inventory to evaluate insomniacs, Dr. Kales found over 85 percent of those tested had one or more major scores in the high pathologic range. The scales most frequently elevated were depression, sociopathy, obsessive-compulsive personality, and schizophrenic trends. Thus for many, insomnia is a symptom rather than a primary disease. Sleeplessness also may accompany hyper- or hypothyroidism (high or low thyroid).

Sleeping Pills

Sleeping pills come in a variety of shapes, colors, and chemical compositions. Dr. Kales and his co-workers reported in the Journal of the American Medical Association that their sleep laboratory studies of patients who had been chronically (months to years) taking drugs for sleep suggest that with use the drugs become ineffective. Despite their long-term inefficiency, Kales and his colleagues postulate that drug-withdrawal insomnia keeps the patients dependent on their particular drug.

Over the counter (non-prescription) sleeping tablets, like "Sominex" and "Nytol" contain anti-histamines as one of their principal sedative substances. If necessary your physician can prescribe stronger anti-histamines such as Benadryl or Phenergan. Some sleeping pills contain aspirin (acetylsalicylic acid). In our work, we have found that two buffered aspirin are as effective in combating anxiety and promoting sleep as meprobamate (Miltown, Equanil).

Sleep Vitamins and Natural Remedies

Vitamin C and Inositol are referred to as the sleep vitamins because of their actions in promoting restorative slumber. Information on these nutrients and their actions is contained in their respective chapters. Hot milk, an old home remedy, may have a scientific basis. Milk will neutralize stomach acid. Also, the milk contains tryptophan, an amino acid that some researchers believe induces sleep. Perhaps the large amount of tryptophan found in turkey is what makes you feel so tired after Thanksgiving dinner.

The piping hot bath has biophysical logic. Muscle, when tense, is in high state of tone. Heat forces the muscle into relaxed submission. Orientals have made use of this principle for centuries. In Japan, it is not uncommon for businessmen to hold meetings in large, hot, communal baths.

Dreams

A dream is the term for the ideas, images, thoughts, and emotions that come to us during sleep. Humans, young and old, even babies, and if we can apply the same brain wave criteria, most mammals dream. Since dreaming is simultaneous with REM sleep the hypothesis has been made that there is a need for dreaming. An extension of that theory was that dream (REM) deprivation would bring increases in irritability, anxiety, difficulty in recall, and even psychosis.

Pharmaceutical firms spent thousands of dollars on sleep studies to determine whether their sleep drugs reduced REM sleep. Psychoanalysts looked to the statement as proof of Freud's theory that dreams are the "guardian" of sleep. Some biologists postulated that the dream phenomenon burnt up hallucinogenic molecules so that dreaming was necessary to prevent psychosis. Subsequent investigations failed to confirm either supposition or the underlying hypothesis. In 1965, Dement himself stated that he no longer felt that REM sleep occurs in order to satisfy a requirement for dreaming. We are left with the dream as a novel random factor in sleep which has no logical answer.

Nightmares and Night Terrors

The "mare" of nightmare is not a horse but supposedly an evil spirit that oppresses people during their sleep. Nightmares and night terrors are similar, the latter being more severe. During a night terror, the heart rate shoots up above 150 beats per minute and the amplitude and frequency of respiration increases. Accompanying these physiologic changes are strong feelings of doom, anxiety, and difficulty in breathing. Often the dreamer screams, moans and gasps. Although night terrors arise during stage four sleep, a waking alpha EEG pattern is present during the one to two minutes of the event. Night terror or *pavor noc-*

turnus is more prevalent among children than adults, and children usually outgrow these terrors.

Nightmares are far more common and their degree of anxiety is markedly less. The ordinary, frightening dream occurs in all ages and usually occurs during normal REM periods. Autonomic changes, if any, are slight although sufficient adrenalin will be released to cause angina and chest pain in the cardiac patient.

Sleep Under Adverse Conditions

Dr. Warren McCullough, the great neurophysiologist and psychiatrist, recounted the true story of the British submariners during World War I. The crew slept in hammocks in the close quarters of the submarine. When the watch was changed the mate blew a bugle to awaken the new shift. An old submariner stuck one leg out of the hammock automatically at the sound of the bugle but this didn't mean he was awake because the mate next paddled the bottom of the hammock to awaken some men and if this failed the mate cut the rope at the foot of the hammock to awaken the sound sleepers. In other words some of the crew were particularly hard to awaken. These same men, however, were the first to awaken when the skipper changed the course of the submarine during their sleeping period. Out of a sound sleep they would awaken and wonder, why is the skipper changing the course of the ship? What gentle stimulus inside the brain was more powerful than the sound of the bugle in close quarters?

Dr. Leonide Goldstein recalls the French retreat from the Maginot Line when the foot soldiers walked day and night. By walking in threes, the middle man was able to walk and sleep as the two outside soldiers supported their napping comrade. The sleeper was rotated at regular intervals. A modern version occurs also in dance marathons or walkathons when the partners alternate sleeping in the slow shuffle position. Brain waves have not been taken in these upright shufflers so we do not know for sure the degree or type of sleep that is obtained. To the individual, ambulatory sleep is better than no sleep!

The No-Sleep Individuals

We have had many patients who state that they never sleep. Some are disperceptive about their sleep because the relatives report snoring and the patient himself reports "dreams without sleep." We have had several patients who slept so lightly all night long that they concluded that sleep did not occur. A brain wave taken with the patient lying on a bed showed frequent twenty to thirty second periods of sleep. Perhaps this micro sleep did suffice. We did not find the exact nature of the patients' lack of sleep. These patients usually sleep with the bedside radio turned on and report their favorite night-time talk show.

Turning Night Into Day

Many over-stimulated, disperceptive teenagers will feel better at night when the sun is behind the Earth. Long distance radio communication is also better when the sun is below the horizon. The geomagnetic forces of the sun which evolve from sun spot activity are known to disrupt daytime radio communication and make psychiatric patients worse. More psychiatric hospital admissions occur at the time of greater sun spot activity, and the decibelosity as measured by noise recorders in the psychiatric ward is higher. The patients who turn night into day have learned by experience that they do better at nighttime jobs. One of our patients became a short order cook in an all night restaurant. He took his tranquilizer at dawn to sleep through the difficult time of the twenty-four hours, namely the daytime.

Hypnagogic Hallucinations

Predominantly visual hallucinations may occur in normal individuals as they become drowsy prior to sleep. This dream-like state is sometimes reported to the doctor as actual hallucinations. These are normal visions that may take geometric forms such as colored lines or bright points and they resemble the phosphorus which can be produced by pressing on the eyeball or the "stars" that occur when the head is hit. Faces, figures, landscapes and abstract shapes may be seen in hypnagogic hallucinations. How do such visions arise? The retina of the eye is spontaneously active and has an important role in maintaining the level of activity of the reticular formation during darkness. Visual sensations can emanate from the retina without any visual stimulus, and some theorists explain these visions as false perceptions based on this activity. Against this theory there is the apparent fact that visual and auditory hypnagogic images are like other "mental" images, responses which need not depend on sense-organ stimulation at all.

Driving in a snowstorm at night can give rise to feelings of severe unreality because of the auto headlights on the snow flakes. This again is a normal retinal phenomenon. These hypnagogic effects whether produced by input overload, total darkness or total silence are normal factors coincidental to settling down to sleep.

Narcolepsy

Narcolepsy (attacks of irresistible sleep) is sometimes accompanied by cataplexy (loss of muscle tone) and less frequently, by hallucinations while falling asleep, and sleep paralysis. Patients with severe cases of narcolepsy can fall asleep under extraordinary conditions: while dancing, driving, and even during coitus. Narcolepsy, the irresistible sleep, differs from hypersomnia, the condition when normal sleep is of unusually long duration, even up to several days. Hypersomnia is not irresistible.

Sleep studies have shown that during nocturnal sleep, as well as during sleep attacks, the narcoleptic goes directly into REM sleep, whereas the normal sleeper will pass through the usual stages of sleep, namely one through four.

The disease appears to be transmitted genetically. It can

occur during adolescence or early adulthood. Attacks are more frequent during monotonous situations, in the later part of the day, and after meals. Drs. Evans and Oswald report that narcoleptics seem abnormally sensitive to L-tryptophane, an amino acid. Unlike normals, narcoleptics experience increases in the duration of the initial REM periods and increases in the frequency of nightmares in that period as a result of oral tryptophane.

Treatment usually consists in giving the stimulant drugs (amphetamines and Ritalin). Their effectiveness may be due to the suppression of REM sleep or the stimulant effect. Natural stimulants, such as deanol (Deaner) have also been used successfully. Research needs to be done on the possible effectiveness of other natural stimulants, such as rutin. Imipramine (Tofranil) is useful in decreasing any accompanying depression, but offers little relief from the sleep attacks.

Why Don't I Dream?

Dr. Kleitman, the famous sleep researcher, has remarked that Hamlet's line, "to sleep, perchance to dream" should be revised to, "perchance to recall *some* dreams." All humans dream, but some do not remember their dreams.

Goodenough and his co-workers revealed that the EEG and EOG (electro-oculogram—a recording of eye movements) showed that the so-called non-dreamers awakened during REM dreams. Schizophrenic patients more than others are more likely not to recall their dreams. Vitamin B-6 (pyridoxine) has been shown in our work to facilitate dream recall. When given sufficient pyridoxine, persons who have never remembered dreaming, start to recall their dreams. Too much vitamin B-6 will result in such vivid dreams that sleep will be fitful.

Various and sundry theories exist as to the purpose of dreaming, but none has been proven. Popular misconceptions of the role of dreams in our lives include the review or recapitulation of a significant event in one's life, or that dreams are valuable tools to discover one's hidden personality or to predict the future (according to the bible, David, son of Abraham, rose to wealth and power because of his ability to interpret the pharaoh's dreams). A dream analyst may gain profit by interpreting dreams, but mental disease will not be relieved.

We do know that dreams, even unpleasant ones, offer relief for the mate of a snorer, because snoring almost never occurs during dreaming. We need to dream during sleep, but the reason remains a mystery.

References

Dement, W. The effect of dream deprivation. *Science* 131:3415, June 1960.

Evans, J. I. and Oswald, I. Some experiments in the chemistry of narcoleptic sleep. *British J. Psychiat.* 112, 1966.

Fisher, C., Gross, J. and Zuch, J. Cycle of penile erections synchronous with dreaming (REM) sleep. *Arch. Genl. Psych.* 12 January 1965.

Fisher, C.; Kahn, E.; Edwards, A.; Davis, D. M. and Fine, J. A psychophysiological study of nightmares and night terrors. *J. Nervous and Mental Dis.* 150:3, 1974.

Hartmann, E. Science and sleep research you can use. *Med. Opinion.* November 1973.

________ The D-state, a review and discussion. *New England Med.* 290:487-449, February 1974.

Rakstis, T. J. New help for nonsleepers. *Today's Health.* September 1971.

Sega, J. Treating sleep disorders. *Med. Opinion,* November 1973.

Sweet, J. To sleep (perchance to dream). *Hyde Parker* September 1973.

The anatomy of sleep. Nutley, New Jersey: Roche Laboratories, 1966.

CHAPTER 42

Headache

Headache is, believe it or not, the most common complaint of the personnel isolated in the dark winter of Antarctica. Headache is probably man's Number One malady. Very likely its incidence exceeds by far that of the common cold. Can headaches be caused by too much sun, sex, drinking, food, wrong food, sweets, hunger, rain, stress, caffeine, letdown, fever, carbon monoxide, reading or even too much work?

Headaches have been with us for a long time. Migraine-type headaches probably afflicted Alexander Pope, Lewis Carroll, Heinrich Heine, Edgar Allan Poe, Guy de Maupassant, Leo Tolstoi, Frederic Chopin, Peter Ilich Tchaikovsky, Julius Caesar, Madame Pompadour, Karl Marx, Alfred Nobel, Charles Darwin, Mary Todd Lincoln, Thomas Jefferson, Ulysses S. Grant, Sigmund Freud and the philosophers Nietzsche and Schopenhauer. The headache altered the lives of these famous people and entered their works and letters. Many a sufferer is mute about her headache and carries on with aspirin and an occasional whiff of ergotamine tartrate. Between headaches the migrainous individual is usually perfectionistic, productive and unusually healthy. These individuals may actually live longer than others because of having a "safety valve" which creates a headache when too much stress occurs.

The Common and Other Headaches

If you are among the two-thirds of mankind that is subject to headache, you can tell the world that a single head can have several types of headache, but usually not at the same time. A lucky one-third of mankind never has a headache of the kind that occasionally lays the rest of the world low. Excluding neuralgias and (back-of-the-head) muscle tension, one can state flatly that headaches are due to a varying heart and blood-volume output in relation to the local or peripheral resistance to blood flow. Various agents have been used to produce experimental headaches in order to study the biochemical and physiological changes.

Experimental Headaches

Nitrite Headache If 15 mg of nitroglycerine is rubbed on the skin or 1 to 2 mg is given under the tongue, a headache that may last twenty-four hours will be produced in certain individuals. Tolerance is quickly established to this headache. The acute headache occurs after the blood pressure has recovered from the marked drop produced by the nitrites. This was first discovered by dynamite factory workers who had headaches every Monday unless they put nitroglycerine in their hatbands to continue their nitrite exposure over Sunday. Amyl nitrite inhalation is used by some to enhance the orgasmic pleasure of sex. Both amyl nitrite and sex can initiate headache in the susceptible individual. With orgasm or ejaculation histamine is probably released, and histamine can cause headache.

Histamine Headache If a trivial dose of histamine is injected intravenously into *any* individual, a severe throbbing headache will occur in about two to three minutes and will last about five minutes. The headache does not occur during the drop in blood pressure accompanying the initial histamine shock. *The pain can definitely be correlated with a rise in blood pressure above the initial level. If this is counteracted by continuous histamine infusion, the headache is prevented tem-*

porarily. Many physiological procedures, such as jugular vein compression, which affect the cranial blood supply and raise the cerebrospinal fluid pressure will relieve the headache. In the case of cluster headache (described by Dr. Horton of the Mayo Clinic in 1932), a subcutaneous injection of histamine produces the headache. The cluster headache may have its origin in the local release of histamine since on the afflicted side the eye waters, the skin sweats, the nose runs and the area of pain is frequently inflamed. Although the pain is intense, the headache does respond to oxygen therapy and is shorter in duration than a migraine headache.

Caffeine-withdrawal Headache Many individuals will develop a headache if they do not obtain their morning cup of coffee. Making use of this observation, experimental headaches may be produced by giving subjects increasing doses of caffeine. Placebo capsules are then substituted on the fifth to seventh day of caffeine administration. The subject will feel sleepy in the morning, and in the early afternoon a headache starts which reaches a maximum about 4 to 6 P.M. Nausea and vomiting may, as with other headaches, also occur with this type of headache. It is possible to induce this headache in 60 to 70 percent of normal individuals.

Migrainous subjects in the caffeine-withdrawal studies did not have a migraine headache. Instead, the headache was central, full and bursting. At the peak, two of the migrainous subjects had vomiting, which was the only symptom in common with their migraine headache. We postulate that this headache is owing to an increase in arterial blood volume, whereas migraines may be initiated by a decrease in effective arterial blood volume.

Caffeine intake should be carefully regulated by all who are susceptible to periodic headaches. Beverages which contain caffeine are coffee, tea, and cola drinks including some low-calorie ones. A food containing caffeine is coffee ice cream. Liquors with caffeine are creme de cocao, Kaluá, and possibly Benedictine. Many headache remedies contain caffeine. The usual content is 30 mg per tablet, which is one-half that of a cup of coffee and roughly twice that of a cola drink. However, headache tablets are usually taken two at a time, so that the caffeine intake over a twenty-four hour period may be enough to produce a caffeine-withdrawal headache on the day after a migraine headache. Careful label reading will allow the headachy individual to use caffeine wisely.

Relaxation Headache With subjects who are susceptible to this type of headache, one can reproduce it consistently by having them follow a daily cycle of increased activity and decreasing sleep. The headache is then precipitated by having them sleep late. This may be the characteristic weekend headache of the business executive, or the postexamination headache of the student, the Monday headache of the clergy or the day-off headache of the nurse. As one nurse said, "I'm glad it occurs on my day off because I can sleep late." When advised that sleeping late actually precipitated the headache, she was able to avoid the headache by rising on signal from the alarm clock each day of the week. She then caught up on her sleep by napping after working hours.

One can suggest to the migrainous patient that the *worst thing* he can do is work hard all week, sleep late on Saturday, then go fishing in the hot sun in a flat-bottomed boat with a can of beer to assuage the thirst. Headachy persons are knowledgeable enough about their physiology to shudder at this suggestion.

Hypertensive Headache Patients with labile blood pressure, as at the beginning of high blood pressure, will be plagued by headaches. When the blood pressure is stabilized at a high level or, with therapy, regulated to a normal level, the headaches do not occur. This headache can be duplicated in normal individuals by elevation of blood pressure with a simple pressor amine such as ephedrine or Neosynephrine. Tyramine is such a pressor amine which occurs in aged cheese, pickled herring and other aged, protein foods. These foods can cause headache which may be particularly severe if the tyramine food is combined with glutamic acid (as in MSG) foods such as are provided in a Chinese restaurant. Soy sauce is not only loaded with glutamic acid but also with salt. One physiologist didn't urinate for a day after a heavy Chinese banquet. During this twenty-four hour period he was extremely thirsty and, of course, salt- and water-logged. Patients on antidepressant drugs designed to prolong the action of pressor amines may not only have headache with tyramine-containing food but may also have stroke because of the great rise in blood pressure. The MAO inhibitors are the worst offenders, and patients on these drugs are warned to avoid cheeses and pickled herring. An oral dose of 100 mg of tyramine will produce a migraine headache in a susceptible subject.

Fever Headache The onset of fever may cause a headache and since artificial fever has, in the past, been used to treat patients, this type of headache has had considerable study. It has been found that in fever therapy the headache is accompanied by an increased excursion of the visible blood vessels of the head. Many febrile diseases may have severe frontal headache as their initial symptom; of these, the typhus group (rickettsial type) is the most prominent. Patients with undiagnosed malaria may have a periodic headache produced by slight fever, with the periodic headache as the main symptom. Aspirin reduces fever and increases the blood volume. Both actions will help to alleviate fever headache.

Carbon Monoxide Headache The mechanism of this headache has been studied extensively by Swedish scientists and others. A rise in cerebrospinal fluid pressure has characteristically accompanied the headache when produced in volunteer subjects. The headache is central, generalized and bursting, and may be accompanied by nausea and vomiting. The similarity to a caffeine-withdrawal headache is striking. Poorly ventilated tunnels or garages and faulty exhaust systems on autos can produce carbon monoxide intoxication, with the characteristic headache presenting as one of the first warning symptoms.

Definite Types of Clinical Headache

(Not in the order of frequency or importance.)

1. *Eyestrain headache* frequently affects the back of the head or neck. It is usually relieved by prescription lenses or change of occupation.

2. *Pus in a nasal sinus* usually follows a cold and requires X-rays of sinus to prove. The popular expression "sinus headache" usually refers to a one-sided migraine-type headache or cluster headache, either of which may be accompanied by a watery but not purulent nasal discharge.

3. *Brain-tumor headache* is usually a morning frontal or generalized headache which is aggravated by elevating the head or any change of posture. For instance, sitting up in bed may cause severe headache with projectile vomiting. The age groups most susceptible to brain tumor are childhood up to puberty and forty to fifty years in both sexes. Severe blows to the head can cause subdural bleeding which can in later months give all of the symptoms of a brain tumor.

4. *Post spinal puncture headache* may occur for several days after a spinal tap. Rest in bed provides the best treatment. Such a headache is thought to be due to continued leakage of the cerebral spinal fluid.

5. *Early hypertensive headache* may be of two types: (a) dull headache as the blood pressure rises during the busy day, or (b) severe headache on awakening because the blood pressure during the night has fallen to a lower level. For the patient who usually awakens with a headache, elevation of the head of the bed (two bricks under the head end) may serve to prevent its onset. Control of the elevated blood pressure also provides relief.

6. *Relaxation headache.* See the section on this under the heading, *Experimental Headaches.*

7. *Caffeine-withdrawal headache.* See the section on this under the heading, *Experimental Headaches.*

8. *Toxic headache* may be produced by carbon monoxide, lead poisoning, tissue copper excess, paint fumes, shellac fumes (methanol), insecticides, nicotine (smoking) and nitrites. Alcohol in excess greatly upsets the fluid balance of the body and liberates adrenalin from the adrenal glands. The total impact may be hangover-headache, and even seizures (rum fits) in the susceptible individual. For those who have over-indulged, the best treatment is prophylactic—namely, an antihistamine such as Benadryl or Phenergan plus two to three

buffered aspirin (Bufferin) before going to bed. The headachy individual usually learns early in life that alcohol is not an ideal sedative.

9. *Hunger headache* may be produced by going too long without food. The hypoglycemic patient is particularly susceptible. The snack food to prevent this may be a hard-boiled egg, a piece of cheese, or meats, all of which may be wrapped up and carried in the pocket or purse. The incidence of functional hypoglycemia is twice as frequent in the female as in the male. The careful choice of food for high trace mineral content and the avoidance of sweets will prevent hunger headache.

10. *Food-allergy headache* is most commonly precipitated by garlic, onions, green peppers, chocolate, watermelon, cabbage, cucumbers, parsley and radishes. Most of these contain sulfur or other compounds which lower blood pressure. Classes of protein foods to which the patient may have a real allergy are wheat and dairy products. Cooked wheat gluten is the usual offender in bread. Milk protein is the offender in dairy products. Tyramine in food produces headache.

11. *Cluster (Horton's) headache* is usually on one side of the face and head, is sudden in onset, is severe, and may be due to the local release in the tissues of histamine or serotonin. The duration is only several hours, compared to twenty-four hours for the usual migraine. Sweating and tearing occur on the side of the headache. The only therapy is the inhalation of pure oxygen. The patients are usually loaded with copper, so relief may be obtained in several months' time if the tissue copper level is lowered by zinc therapy.

12. *Unphysiological or psychic headache*. The patient will complain of such symptoms as a tight band around the head or headache on top of the head or head pain on swallowing. Since these symptoms do not follow any regular nerve distribution, the patient's senses may be playing tricks on him. In other words a disperception occurs.

13. *Migraine headache* starts at puberty, may have eye signs such as photophobia or dancing bright dots before the eyes or a defect in the visual field. The very first sign of the headache may, however, be a copious flow of water-white urine as the kidney arterioles relax. Migraine is twice as frequent in the female, is usually one sided at onset and has a familial history. The headache stops with pregnancy (increased blood volume),

with the menopause or at age forty-five when some mild degree of elevated blood pressure may be present. The headache afflicts 10 percent of the population, but among nonagenarians 20 percent had a previous history of migraine, so that migraine patients are endowed with longevity—perhaps because of the headache-enforced rest periods. These patients are perfectionists and make excellent club secretaries, etc.

Mechanism of Migraine

The famous physiologist, Lauter Brunton, suggested near the close of the nineteenth century that the cerebral blood vessels must be involved in migraine headache, inasmuch as he was able to obtain relief of his unilateral headache by pressure on his carotid artery. Ray, Graham and Wolff in 1937 demonstrated adequately that the migraine headache is associated with an increased excursion of the temporal blood vessels. The excursion of the vessel returns to normal with ergotamine injection.

Theoretically, an increased excursion of the temporal blood vessels could result from an increased arterial blood volume, decreased blood volume, increased blood pressure, decreased blood pressure, increased cerebrospinal fluid pressure or decreased cerebrospinal fluid pressure. Most unlikely is the possibility that a local hormone is released to dilate a major blood vessel such as an artery and cause the headache. Most migraine headaches are perhaps accompanied by a decreased blood volume with a relaxed peripheral vascular tone. Therapy should, hence, be directed at increasing the peripheral vascular tone (ergotamine tartrate) or increasing the blood volume (salt mixtures or mineral solutions). We have found that most migrainous patients are high in copper and that the incidence and severity of their headaches is decreased when a zinc dietary supplement is given.

Therapy of Acute Migraine

The ascribed etiology and resultant therapy of migraine and most recurrent headaches depend on the kind of specialist consulted. The endocrinologist is likely to ascribe much of migraine to endocrine deficiency; the allergist claims a high percentage of these cases when he diagnoses the condition; the psychiatrist is likely to apply psychotherapy for headache. In most cases the interested general practitioner or neurologist can determine the cause of the migraine syndrome, so that the patient obtains the proper therapy for his particular case.

Ergotamine Tartrate or Gynergen

Either 0.3 cc intravenously, or 0.5 cc to 1.0 cc of 1-2000 Gynergen intramuscularly, given at the onset of an attack, will result in relief in one to two hours in 90 percent of patients. For nausea and vomiting produced by Gynergen, 0.5 mg atropine may help, and 10 cc of 10 percent calcium gluconate may relieve the muscle cramps produced by Gynergen.

Most effective, at present, is the use of inhaled ergotamine. This comes as a Medihaler Ergotamine marketed by Riker Laboratories. The inhaler contains twenty-five doses, and one to three inhalations will usually suffice to stop a migraine headache if the inhaler is used early in the course of the headache.

For prevention of headache all migraine patients should take at bedtime two Bufferin and one diphenhydramine (Benadryl). This produces better sleep, and the aspirin in the Bufferin will keep the blood more liquid (prevent clots). Niacin (100 mg) should be taken morning and night and 500 mg calcium gluconate should be taken each morning. Occasionally extra potassium may also be needed. A source of zinc should be taken morning and night. This is available with magnesium in the preparation called Vicon C of Meyer Laboratories. If the patient's blood pressure is abnormally low, Vicon Plus should be used. This is similar to Vicon C but provides 4 mg of manganese chloride.

In treating menstrual migraine the patient should have available a "water pill," usually in the form of Diuril or Hydrodiuril to be taken each morning at the time of the menstrual period. Digoxin in a small dose of 0.25 mg may stabilize heart output and prevent chronic headache.

Inderal (propanolol) is a blocking compound for adrenalin

and may help the tense headachy patient. Since the duration of action is short, frequently three to four doses are needed each day. Valium may also be helpful in tense individuals. Phenobarbital is disliked by most migrainous patients because they cannot, under phenobarbital, organize their day exactly as it should be.

The migrainous patient must learn to regulate: 1. her perfectionistic capabilities, productivity and mental stimulation; 2. her daily routine of activity, sleep, meals, etc.; 3. her caffeine intake; 4. her salt and water intake; and 5. her hours of sleep.

This is not an impossible life prescription and, if followed carefully, will usually be more rewarding in terms of freedom from headache than any number of doctors' prescriptions for drugs.

References

Anthony, M. Histamine and serotonin in cluster headache. *Arch. Neurol.* 25:225-231, 11 September 1971.

Berde, B. Recent progress in the elucidation of the mechanism of action of ergot compounds used in migraine therapy. *Med. J. Aust. Special Supp.* 2:15-26, 1972.

Clark, D., Hough, H., and Wolff, H. G. Experimental studies on headache: observations on histamine headache. *The Proceedings of the Association for Research in Nervous and Mental Disease.* vol. 15, December 1934.

Dreisbach, R. H. and Pfeiffer, C. Caffeine-withdrawal headache. *Journal of Laboratory and Clinical Medicine* vol. 28, no. 10, pp. 1212-1219, July 1943.

Duvoisin, R. C. The cluster headache. *JAMA* 222:11, 11 December 1972.

Edmeads, J. Management of the acute attack of migraine. *Headache* pp. 1-9, October 1973.

Friedman, A. P., and Frazier, Jr. S. H., with Dodi Schultz *The Headache Book.* New York: Dodd, Mead, 1973.

Friedman, A. P. The headache in history, literature, and legend. *Bull. N.Y. Acad. Med.*, vol. 48, no. 4, May 1972.

Malvea, B. P., Gwon, N. and Graham, J. R. Propranolol prophylaxis of migraine. *Headache* vol. 12, no. 4, January 1973.

Moser, M., Wish, H., and Friedman, A. P. Headache and hypertension. *JAMA* 28 April 1962.

Pfeiffer, C.; Dreisbach, R. H.; Roby, C. C., and Glass, H. G. The etiology of the migraine syndrome—a physiologic approach. *Journal of Laboratory and Clinical Medicine* vol. 28, no. 10, pp. 1219-1225, July 1943.

Pfeiffer, C.; Dreisbach, R. H., and Roby, C. C. Therapy of migraine by electrolytes affecting the blood volume. *Journal of Laboratory and Clinical Medicine* vol. 29, no. 7, pp. 709-714, July 1944.

Rothlin, E. Historical development of the ergot therapy of migraine. *Int. Arch. Allergy* vol. 7, 4-6, 1955.

Ryan, R. E. Histaminic cephalalgia differentiated from acute nasal sinusitis. *Eye, Ear, Nose and Throat Monthly* vol. 49, May 1970.

Sandok, B. A. Temporal arteritis. *JAMA* vol. 222, no. 11, 11 December 1972.

Shapiro, R. S. and Eisenberg, B. C. Allergic headache. *Annals of Allergy* vol. 23, pp. 123-126, March 1965.

Smith, I., et al. Dietary migraine and tyramine metabolism. *Nature* 230:246-248, 26 March 1971.

Stowell, A. Physiologic mechanisms and treatment of histaminic or petrosal neuralgia. *Headache* vol. 9, no. 4, January 1970.

von Storch, T. J. C. Relation of experimental histamine headache to migraine and non-migraine headache. *Archives of Neurology and Psychiatry* vol. 44, pp. 316-322, August 1940.

Weber, R. B. and Reinmuth, O. M. The treatment of migraine with propranolol. *Neurology* vol. 22, no. 4, April 1972.

Widerøe, Tor-Erik, Tor Vigander. Propranolol in the treatment of migraine. *British Medical Journal* 29 June 1974.

Wolff, H. G. Headache mechanisms. *Int. Arch. Allergy* vol. 7, no. 4-6, 1955.

CHAPTER 43

Aging and Senility

Our biological timeclock starts ticking from the moment of birth, not stopping until the moment of death. Although aging is a natural biological process, improper diet, bad habits or infections in early life may predispose an individual to premature aging or death. The very inevitability of death has not prevented scientists from continuing to study the causes of aging, in the hope of eventually discovering methods of prolonging life. Diseases of the aged are numerous, among them atherosclerosis, chronic infection, diabetes, arthritis, emphysema, osteoporosis, presenile and senile dementia and various cerebrovascular and cancerous diseases. Treatment is often difficult, but contemporary scientific breakthroughs have isolated possible causes, and many potentially useful treatments are now being discovered.

Cardiovascular diseases rank high among hospitalized geriatric patients—hypertension and atherosclerosis being the predominant ones. Atherosclerosis is a metabolic disturbance in which cholesterol and its derivatives are deposited in the walls of arteries (hardening of the arteries), causing slower bloodflow. Popular theory designates high serum cholesterol as the prime causative factor in heart disease—cholesterol being a white, odorless, tasteless and ubiquitous fatty alcohol found in eggs, meat, butterfat and shellfish.

Although it is widely known that animals fed a diet high in cholesterol and saturated fats will develop atherosclerosis, the same is not true for human beings if adequate amounts of other nutrients, such as zinc and chromium and vitamin C, are also ingested. Nonetheless, some evidence seems to support the present theory. In a two-year study in which one group of men was fed a low-fat diet and another group was given a normal diet, the men on the low-fat diet showed a 10 percent drop in serum cholesterol. Another study in which the high-cholesterol patients were given the cholesterol-reducing drug clofibrate or a placebo resulted in a significantly lower incidence of heart attacks in the patients on the drug. J. Rinse has reported successful treatment of atherosclerosis with lecithin, wheat germ, brewer's yeast and vitamins C and E. Lecithin binds with the cholesterol and thus may prevent extra cholesterol from depositing in the arteries. No study has yielded conclusive evidence, but implications are that a steady blood serum level of cholesterol above 300 mg percent will result in ischemic heart disease (angina).

High serum cholesterol is among many possible causative agents designated "high-risk factors." Others include diabetes, high blood pressure. EKG abnormalities and cigarette smoking—heavy smokers are three times more likely to die from heart disease than nonsmokers. Also, men are more likely to die from heart disease than women. Recently, considerable statistical evidence has led some doctors to suggest that *excesses* of cadmium or copper or *deficiencies* of zinc, vanadium or chromium (trace metals) might be critical factors in causing death from heart attacks. The controversy centers on the trace element content in hard and soft water, with the underlying hypothesis being that the concentration and interrelationships of calcium, magnesium and sodium are fundamentally related to the association of cardiovascular disease with drinking water. Other harmful elements, particularly the metal contaminants from pipes, may also predispose individuals to cardiovascular death.

Dr. Henry Schroeder pioneered in this field of research by initially studying the toxic cadmium in rats. His studies revealed that a high cadmium content in the rats' drinking water precipitated hardening of the arteries, high blood pressure, heart enlargement and a shortened life span. Retrospective studies on people dying from hypertension revealed a higher cadmium level in their kidneys than in those of people dying from accidents or other diseases. Other evidence has also confirmed that hypertension is highly correlated with high cadmium levels, which would seem to indicate that cadmium is a factor in human high blood pressure and its corresponding death rate. This is supported by the fact that soft well water tends to be acidic and acid water corrodes pipes, releasing the cadmium contained in galvanized pipes, which is then ingested by its users. Copper plumbing contributes excess copper, and lead from the joints, when acid well water is used!

Findings by Schroeder, Crawford and others have indicated that the absorption by the body of trace elements such as lead and cadmium is inversely related to the concentration of calcium in the medium, so that lead absorption and possible toxicity is more likely to be a problem in soft-water areas where the calcium content is low. Calcium may act by inhibiting the absorption of toxic elements from pipes and soil. Stitt and Crawford have found that high blood pressure, plasma cholesterol and heart disease were higher in soft-water towns and have indicated that hypertension and "sudden death" are more prevalent in these towns. The geographical diversity of the many studies testing the hypothesis that the harder the water, the less the degree of cardiovascular disease, and the mortality data, would seem to validate this claim. This evidence gives a strong indication that contamination of man's drinking water by excessive amounts of some of the trace elements such as copper, which are known to be essential in smaller quantities to man's existence, may result in metal intoxication which manifests itself as cardiovascular disease in later life. More research is needed to facilitate treatment and prevent this possible intoxication.

Premature Senility

Two important mental disorders that have their origin in later life are presenile and senile dementia. Senility accounts for 10 to 15 percent of the cases in mental hospitals; its onset is insidious, with the mean age of presenile patients being fifty-six. (Presenile dementia, by definition, is senile dementia before the age of sixty.) Memory loss for recent events is the first symptom, accompanied by disorientation, repetition of phrases, inability to perform fine muscular movements and, finally, psychotic behavior. The EEG of the senile individual will often demonstrate theta or delta waves in a symmetrical pattern, and this is the most useful method of distinguishing organic dementia from functional depression.

The etiology of senile dementia has often been associated with atherosclerosis, but at autopsy this has been found in only one-third of those afflicted. Other conditions that have been associated on a theoretical level with the etiology of these diseases are gradual cellular or nerve degeneration, growth of plaques, and low spermine levels in the blood and presumably the brain.

Lysosomes, small organelles inside the cells, are concerned with cellular digestion, protein turnover, tissue remodeling and autolysis of dead cells. They may take part in the cellular aging process by causing damage to the cell, by damaging extracellular structures through enzyme activity, or by an inability to perform their digestive function. DeDuve and Watteaux propose that an inability of most cells to eliminate engorged lysosomes may disrupt cellular organization. Free radical lysosomal DNA-ases penetrate lysosomal membranes to destroy the DNA. Allison has reported that carcinogenic agents release lysosomal enzymes, among them DNA-ases, which penetrate cell nuclei to cause genetic changes and cancer.

Beginning with childhood, some of our brain cells are lost each day; the suspected killers are faulty genetic material, autoimmunity (the body's natural defenses attack themselves), toxins and poor nutrition. Dr. F. Straub feels that the loss of normal cellular activity is caused by changes in the cellular environment and the accumulation of the altered enzymes which eventually produces death in tissue culture. Normal cells divide fifty times and stop, but in some children afflicted with the disease progeria, the cells only divide a few times before stopping. In these children, the life cycle is so accelerated that they may begin aging at two and will have reached old age by eight. Another condition, Werner's disease, is similar but aging begins after adolescence. If cell deterioration causes senile dementia, then accelerated cellular aging may generate dementia or the previously mentioned childhood diseases.

There are various disorders associated with presenile or senile dementia that display the nerve degeneration postulated to cause these disorders. The two lesions associated with dementia are senile plaques and the tangle of nerve fibers found in patients with Alzheimer's disease. The concentration of these lesions is strongly correlated with the loss of recent memory and behavioral deterioration in the aged; the lesions seem to be localized in the hippocampus, temporal or frontal regions. Dr. Robert Terry has described these two types of lesions: the neurofibrillary tangle of Alzheimer's is most concentrated in the hippocampal gyrus. This involves emotions and personality. Senile plaques occur most often in the frontal or temporal areas and are composed of clustered enlarged or abnormal synaptic endings, altered axons and dendrites filled with degenerating cell organelles and loaded with aluminum.

In 1964, Dr. Terry discovered that senile plaques are abnormally high in a protein, amyloid, that is also known to accumulate in the body with aging. His theory is that the senile plaques originate with the degeneration of the nerve cell or axon. As the cell begins to die, it initiates the secondary deposition of amyloid through blood capillaries. When he investigated the neurofibrillary tangles, he found them to be composed of the neurofibril bundles occupying neuronal cytoplasm and displacing other organelles. It may be that increased amyloid accumulation precipitates senile plaques, which then cause memory deterioration and the perceptual and motor disturbances associated with the dementias.

Alzheimer's disease, as previously mentioned, is a presenile dementia characterized by cerebral atrophy, senile plaques and neurofibrillary degeneration. Aluminum, which can be used to induce neurofibrillary formation in the brains of higher animals, has been found in significant concentrations in some regions of the brain of Alzheimer's patients.

Creutzfeld-Jakob's disease, another of the very rare presenile dementias, has a worldwide distribution. It is caused by a transmissible viral agent, although the symptoms are not characteristic of infection. There is premature mental deterioration with lesions occurring in the gray area of the brain. Both these diseases have the characteristics of senile dementia, but with much earlier onset.

We at the Brain Bio Center in Princeton have found a correlation between low spermine levels in the blood and the recent memory loss displayed by presenile and senile dementia patients. Spermine, a simple polyamine containing four amino nitrogens, is known to occur in large quantities in semen, blood tissues and brain. When measured in the blood, it has been found in high concentration in patients and normals with adequate memory for recent events, and low in patients with presenile and senile dementia. Patients on estrogen therapy, pa-

TABLE 43.1

Presenile and senile dementia—spermine levels*

Sex	*Age*	*Diagnosis*	*Spermine (mcg%)*
Patients			
F	50	Presenile dementia	0.39
F	75	Senile dementia	0.63
M	71	Senile dementia	0.38
M	85	Senile dementia	0.58
Controls			
F	91	Normal	0.81
M	80	Normal	0.94
M	75	Normal	1.00

* Those individuals labeled as having presenile or senile dementia have significantly lower spermine levels than do normal controls.

tients with hypoglycemia, and patients with normal aging are found to have low blood spermine levels. (See Table 43.1.) The level is lower in senility than in hypoglycemia.

Forgetfulness of recent events is a hallmark of senility; notebooks and frenzied jottings are used in attempts to compensate. One current theory holds that recent memory depends on the brain's ability to synthesize ribonucleic acid (RNA). The continual synthesis of RNA depends on RNA polymerase, which is activated by spermine. The four aminonitrogen groups of spermine neutralize the acidic phosphate groups of the nucleic acids in RNA and allow the synthesis of more RNA. The recent memory is encoded in the RNA, so that without adequate spermine the recent memory may be faulty. Almost all of the presenile and senile dementia patients seen at the Brain Bio Center show exceedingly low blood spermine levels when compared with controls.

Since spermine levels in the blood decrease with age, young patients with Tourette's syndrome (swearing and motor tics) are also particularly low in spermine for their ages. Spermine can be elevated by trace element supplementation of the diet; of the trace elements, manganese appears to be the most important. The combination of zinc with manganese is most effective in mobilizing copper from the tissues. Copper is high in many neoplastic diseases. This element may be a factor in reversing the usual spermine to spermidine ratio to less than 1. Normal is Sp. 1.50/Spd. 0.90—i.e., about 1.70.

Although little is known about the many possible functions of spermine in the body, the consistently low levels of spermine found in patients suffering from senility warrants further investigation. Trace element and vitamin supplementation are beneficial and should be used to relieve the patient of his mental confusion and memory loss. Some confused geriatric patients become rational when Theragran-M is stopped and a source of zinc and manganese started.

Preventive Nutrition

Biochemical research has not yet discovered a way to prevent aging. To the best of our knowledge, preventive nutrition is the best medicine for the aging body and mind. It has been shown that cholesterol deposition in the arteries may cause heart disease. Thus, as one advances in age, there should be a reduction in saturated fat intake to prevent unnecessary arterial cholesterol deposits. Refined sugars and carbohydrates have been shown to be consumed in varying amounts by all ages; the elderly would do better to rely on the natural sugar content found in fresh fruits and vegetables.

Alcohol has also been proven harmful when taken in large quantities; liver damage, diabetes and hypoglycemia are only a few diseases possibly precipitated by prolonged alcohol use. An occasional drink or two will not unduly damage our vital organs, but the aging individual should acquaint himself with the bodily deterioration accompanying excessive alcohol intake.

We cannot prevent aging, but with good nutrition and moderate exercise, we can enjoy our lives longer. The older patient should avoid strong alcoholic drinks and be content with beer or wine, both of which are loaded with nutrients and free of the quinine present in gin and tonic. If hard liquor is used by the elderly, the adrenalin released may produce a poor night's sleep. Aging is still a major medical problem, whether it be how to prevent aging or how to relieve the various degenerative symptoms that occur.

Although genetic diseases are usually associated with childhood, some do manifest themselves in later life. Adult polycystic kidney is caused by an autosomal dominant gene with high penetrance (a single mutant gene will cause the disease). Familial polyposia and Huntington's chorea are other late-developing genetic disorders. These, in addition to cancer, osteoporosis, atherosclerosis, and presenile and senile dementia, constitute the major diseases afflicting the aged. The human code may be designed to deteriorate with age, but proper care, nutritional guidance and avoidance of toxins and infection may retard or relieve the unwanted symptoms of cellular and bodily degeneration that make inevitable aging uncomfortable.

References

Altman, L. *The New York Times* 22 October 1973.

Aronson, S. and Perl, D. *Dis. Nerv. Sys.* 76:286, 1974.

Bowen, D., Smith, C. and Davison, A. *Brain* 96:849, 1973.

Coblentz, J. et al. *Arch. Neurol.* 29:299, 1973.

Crawford, M. and Stitt, F. *Medical World News* 76B, 1972.

DeDuve, C. and Watteaux, R. *Ann. Rev. Physiol.* 28:435, 1966.

Fister, W. P. et al. The treatment of hepatolenticular degeneration with penicillamine with report of two cases. *Can. Med. Assoc. J.* 78:99, 1958.

Hochschild, R. *Exp. Geront.* 6:153, 1971.

Horwitt, M. K. et al. *Arch. Neurol. Psychiat.* 78:317, 1957.

Jarvic, L. *Geriatrics* 7:13, 1973.

Rinse, J. Atherosclerosis, chemistry and nutrition: some observations, experiences and an hypothesis. *American Laboratory* July 1973.

Schroeder, H. *Proc. Sixth Ann. Water Qual. Symp.* 1972.

Terry, R. D. The fine structure of neurofibrillary tangles in Alzheimer's disease. *J. Neuropath. Exp. Neurol.* 22:629-642, 1963.

——— Ultrastructural studies in Alzheimer's presenile dementia. *Amer. J. Pathol.* 44:269-281, 1964.

Wilkins, R. and Brosy, I. *Arch. Neurol.* 21:109, 1969.

CHAPTER 44

Arthritis and Joint Disorders

Rheumatoid arthritis (RA) is a persistent, serious disorder; its exact cause is unknown. Psychiatric theory claims RA as one of the stress-induced (or even psychically induced) disorders. Poor nutrition, repeated bacterial infection and a host of other causes are more apt to be the real cause of RA.

Drugs and hormones give symptomatic, anti-inflammatory relief which can usually be measured in hours rather than days. Hydrocortisone and other synthetic steroids give relief for days, but they are scarcely the answer because of cumulative side-effects. With this in mind, the prudent physician uses steroids only in an emergency and on a decreasing dosage schedule.

Gold therapy, the injection of soluble salts of the precious metal, is sometimes effective when other therapy fails. This may result in weeks and even months of complete remission. But gold has serious side-effects such as severe skin rashes and depression of the formation of red and white blood cells. The gold level can be monitored along with the blood cell counts. When this is done, and the side actions are explained to the patient, then such therapy is useable. However, gold therapy is empirical. The mechanism of action is unknown. Do gold molecules interfere with other trace elements which may be in excess in the tissues of the joints? Does gold act to alter the immune response?

Large doses of nicotinic acid (niacin) will increase joint mobility, decrease stiffness and relieve joint deformity and pain associated with rheumatoid arthritis. According to Dr. William Kaufman, who pioneered this treatment in 1941, no adverse side-effects result from niacin therapy.

Niacin should be administered with equal or greater amounts of vitamin C. Niacin causes a red flush around the blush area in many patients which can be mildly uncomfortable, but this is harmless and usually passes in less than an hour. The arthritic may benefit from 100 mg of niacin (with meals) and 500 mg vitamin C three times a day. This is a considerably smaller dose than that recommended by Dr. Kaufman, but it has the advantage of being tolerated by almost all patients.

The typical rheumatoid arthritic patient has a serum copper level twice normal and the iron level is one-half of normal. The patient has plenty of iron, however, in the joints, lymph nodes and other tissues. Perhaps the excess iron in the joints may give rise to the painful inflammatory response.

Case Histories

We have seen RA occur in a vigorous man of 72 who used modern cutting blades to cut through a 100-year-old brick wall in his New Jersey home. This wall was painted with lead-containing paint on either side and the dust engendered by the saw was dense. He wore only a gauze mask and had black dust in his throat and lungs. Five days after completing the job he was afflicted with generalized RA in all his joints.

Hospitalization disclosed all of the clinical signs of RA. Since steroids and anti-RA remedies gave little relief, he tried, in addition to his aspirin schedule, large doses of vitamin C, a vitamin which mobilizes lead. This was the turning point; he again could walk; he was no longer bedridden. With an adequate nutritional program, his recovery continues.

C. T., aged twenty-four, came to us with a ten-year history of RA and pitifully deformed hands and feet. She had not responded to steroid or gold therapy and, in spite of a full aspirin schedule, each movement was like walking on her eyeballs. Her serum copper (she was never on the birth-control pill) was 238 mcg percent (normal 110), and her zinc was 78 mcg percent (normal 100). One year later her weight has risen from 100 to 115 and her copper is a normal 114 mcg percent. Her zinc and iron are still low, but her active disease process is arrested.

A patient who spends her summers in the copper-mining region of Upper Michigan, states that their well water is so metallic-tasting that she won't drink it straight but only as tea or with orange juice concentrate. Each summer in Upper Michigan she is plagued with aching and swollen joints and frequent migraine headaches. All of her relatives who live the year round in that area are afflicted with arthritis.

Some claim that a copper bracelet, worn by the arthritic patient, will relieve joint pains. Maybe the copper bracelet is a solid clue and will be more effective against arthritis when it is made from the actual excess copper taken out of the patient's blood and tissues.

Since copper in the serum rises because of a lack of zinc and manganese in the diet and blood, we usually find these two essential elements to be low. The high copper may also be the result of lack of elemental sulfur in the diet. These patients usually do not have eggs for breakfast, and the egg yolk is almost the only food that has enough sulfur to turn a silver spoon black (silver sulfide).

RA patients should have zinc, manganese, niacin and vitamin C with two eggs per day. If they cannot eat eggs, then elemental sulfur can be supplied at the level of 200 mg per day. This was available as sulfur water at the spas and as sulfur and molasses from grandmother each springtime.

The eggs need not be eaten at breakfast. They can be eaten hard boiled later in the day. Some patients will not eat eggs unless they are deviled or put in eggnog. The yolk is the sulfur-containing portion and this can be mixed with milk by simply stirring. This may be necessary to increase the appetite. The patient should in addition have a carefully balanced diet high in B vitamins. Ten brewer's yeast tablets twice a day are needed.

Nutrition and Arthritis

Dr. Williams notes in his book, *Nutrition Against Disease*, the important link between poor nutrition and arthritis. Specific foods which have been reported to help are cod liver oil and royal jelly (which is rich in pantothenic acid). Dr. Williams contends that many arthritics are deficient in niacin, pantothenic acid, folic acid and vitamin B-6. Supplemental doses of these nutrients as well as the trace metals zinc and manganese may help. Ziman, a zinc and manganese dietary supplement, causes iron to be displaced from the tissues and the serum iron usually rises. The blood iron level should then be maintained. Therapy in the form of Mol-Iron might be indicated if the serum iron falls to 0.3 ppm or 30 mcg percent. The high copper level goes to normal in about six to twelve months' time and joint symptoms subside.

The use of the chelating agent D-penicillamine has proven useful in several controlled studies. D-penicillamine (P) under the name Cuprimine removes large amounts of copper and some zinc from the body via the urinary pathway. One of the side-effects of the P therapy is loss of taste, which is a sign of zinc deficiency. In 1964, Fister et al. suggested that P should always be used in conjunction with a trace metal supplement excluding copper. This prevents zinc and other trace element deficiencies. The success of P therapy in RA may point to copper or other heavy metal excess as a factor in the inflamed joints.

Experimental Findings on Copper and Iron in Joint Disease

The first direct study of copper and iron in the synovial fluid of joints was made by Dr. W. Niedermeier in 1965. The copper level of joint fluid was three times as high as in normal joints. This was confirmed by Niedermeier and Griggs in 1971 when again copper was 27.5 for postmortem normals and 84.8 mcg percent for RA patients. Iron is also doubled, but Bennett et al. in 1973 ascribed the high iron to frequent bleeding into the joint.

Zinc is also greatly increased, which we would ascribe to vitamin B-6 deficiency. Bonebrake et al. in 1972 ascribed the high zinc levels in the synovial fluid to the presence of white blood cells as part of the inflammatory process.

The trace elements that are greatly decreased in RA are molybdenum, chromium, tin and aluminum. When blood serum was compared, the RA patient was very low in zinc and iron and high in copper, manganese and molybdenum. Thus, copper was the only element found to be significantly high in both joint fluid and blood serum. Other types of arthritis do not show this high zinc level in the joint fluid.

Angevine and Jacox pointed out in 1974 that patients with hemachromatosis or siderosis show joint changes similar to those of RA patients. In the former, large deposits of iron are found in the joints. Brighton et al. in 1970 injected baby rabbits with iron and produced an arthritis similar to that of RA patients. In mature rabbits only the joint lining was affected, but the baby rabbit also had changes in the cartilage of the joints. The same authors called attention to the study of the Japanese worker Hiyeda in 1939 who was able to produce arthritis in rabbits with large doses of iron salts in the rabbit chow. In eastern Russia, where iron content of the drinking water is high, many children have degenerative joint disease which responds to a change of their drinking water.

Gordon et al. found in 1974 that degenerative changes in the hip joints of older patients is frequently due to an iron overload as shown by high blood serum, liver and synovial iron levels. Muirden of Victoria, Australia in 1970 found high levels of iron in the synovial membrane of the joints of RA patients. Thus, while iron serum levels may be low in RA, the tissue storage is high.

Niedermeier in 1971 reported that gold therapy in RA patients lowers the serum levels of molybdenum and manganese but not copper. The low levels of serum zinc and iron were not raised by the gold therapy. Copper in serum was actually raised by gold therapy from 111 mcg percent to 152 mcg percent. This type of change we see when zinc and manganese mobilize copper from tissues. Finally, RA patients improve when given either histidine or D-penicillamine, both of which chelate and remove copper and lead from the body via the urinary pathway.

These data suggest, in toto, that RA may be caused by an excess of either copper or iron and that therapy should be directed toward an active program of heavy metal chelation (copper, iron and lead) with a good supportive nutrient program.

References

Andrews, F. M.; Golding, D. N.; Freeman, A. M.; Golding, J. R.; Day, A. T.; Hill, A. G. S.; Camp, A. V.; Lewis-Fanning, E. and Lyle, W. H. Controlled trial of D(—) penicillamine in severe rheumatoid arthritis. *Lancet,* 275-280, 10 February 1973.

Angevine, C. D. and Jacox, R. F. Unusual connective tissue manifestations of hemochromatosis. *Arthritis & Rheumatism* 17:477-485, 1974.

Boddy, K. and Will, G. Iron absorption in rheumatoid arthritis. *Ann. Rheumatic Dis.* 28:537-540, 1969.

Bonebreak, R. A.; McCall, J. T.; Hunder, G. G. and Polley, H. F. Zinc accumulation in synovial fluid. *Mayo Clin. Proc.* 47:746-750, 1972.

Brighton, C. T., Bigley, E. C. and Smolenski, B. I. Iron-induced arthritis in immature rabbits. *Arthritis & Rheumatism* 13:849-857, 1970.

Gerami, S.; Payan, H. M.; Easley, G. W. and Zimmerman, B. Arteriosclerosis and iron metabolism. *J. Surg. Res.* 10:105-110, 1970.

Gordon, D. A., Clarke, P. V. and Ogryzlo, M. A. The chondrocalcific arthropathy of iron overload. *Arch. Intern. Med.* 134:21-28, 1974.

Gordon, M. H. and Ehrlich, G. E. Penicillamine for treatment of rheumatoid arthritis. *JAMA* 229:1342-1343, 1974.

Hiyeda, K. The cause of Kaschin-Beck's disease. *Jap. Med. Sci.* 4:91-106, 1939.

Muirden, K. D. Lymph node iron in rheumatoid arthritis. *Ann. Rheum. Dis.* 29:81-88, 1970.

———The anemia of rheumatoid arthritis: the significance of iron deposits in the synovial membrane. *Aust. Ann. Med.* 2:97, 1970.

Neidermeier, W., Prillaman, W. W. and Griggs, J. R. The effect of chrysotherapy on trace metals in patients with rheumatoid arthritis. *Arthritis & Rheumatism* 14:533-538, 1971.

Niedermeier, W. and Griggs, J. H. Trace metal composition of synovial fluid and blood serum of patients with rheumatoid arthritis. *J. Chron. Dis.* 23:527-536, 1971.

Rheumatoid arthritis patients improve when given histidine. *JAMA* 215:551-556, 1971.

Trethewie, E. R. Gold, histamine and rheumatoid arthritis. *Med. J. Australia* 2:1136-1137, 1970.

CHAPTER 45

Skin Problems in Patients of All Ages

Almost every teen-ager at some point has to face up to the annoying problem of acne. Although American teen-agers spend approximately forty million dollars a year on over-the-counter acne lotions and creams, these remedies are not very effective and the pimples remain, often causing embarrassment and social withdrawal. Let's look at the problem more closely: What is acne? How is it caused? How is it best treated?

What Is Acne?

Acne is characterized by blackheads, whiteheads and pimples, and occurs primarily on the face, neck, back and chest and rarely on the arms and legs. It appears most frequently during adolescence, when the hormones of growth and development, testosterone and progesterone, are at a high level of activity. Also, during this time of life, the oil glands are secreting profusely.

Testosterone, known as the "male hormone" but also produced in females, though in lesser quantities, causes an increased output of the sebaceous (fat, keratin) glands. When this happens, a keratinous plug may fill the sebaceous gland duct and later extend into the common duct. Inflammation of the superficial skin layer near the ducts occurs and pustules may develop. The pustules extend into the wall of the sebaceous gland duct, which may disintegrate, thus becoming continuous with the inflamed skin. At this point cystic lesions (lesions of the sacs filled with fluid) may evolve and leave permanent scars after healing. The last two steps in this process occur only in very severe cases of acne; permanent scarring is not a common result of acne, or *acne vulgaris,* as it is called medically.

Therapy for Acne

Now what can be done about acne? During Chaucer's time little could be done; and in his famous *General Prologue* to the *Canterbury Tales* he describes the Summoner's terrible case of acne and lists all the cures he has tried without success.

> A Summoner there was in that place
> That had a fire-red cherubim's face.
> There was neither quicksilver nor lytarge [lead] nor brimstone,
> Borac, ceruce [white lead] nor oil of tartar none
> Nor ointment that would cleanse and bite
> That him might help of his whelkes [pimples] white
> Nor of the knobs sitting on his cheecks.

Today, however, we are fortunate in having several remedies, some more effective than others. Fresh air, sunlight, exercise and adequate rest—to start with the simplest—are known to be helpful.

We have seen Navy trainees (nineteen years of age) who have never before had acne come into the services from an active, outdoor life such as cowboy or forester and after boot-camp training come down with disabling acne of the entire face and back. Part of the cause is dietary, since all institutions serve too many refined starches and sugars; part is decreased exercise (desk jobs); but the most important cause is the lack of the ultraviolet light of the sun which sterilized the skin daily with actinic rays. This leads to one simple treatment, the daily exposure of the face to sunlight. Since this is frequently impossible, the purchase of a sunlamp, with a timer, allows the acne patient to apply a strong dose of ultraviolet light to the face and back three times each week. The U-V light subdues bacterial infection and prevents the large boil-like bumps. The timer can prevent serious overexposure.

Many authorities believe that excessive use of carbohydrates, especially candy and sugared soft drinks, and fatty foods such as chocolate, fried foods and nuts, produce or aggravate acne and should therefore be avoided. This contention, however, has been disputed. In an experiment in 1969 at the University of Pennsylvania Medical School, forty teen-age girls with acne were given, in addition to their regular diet, a chocolate bar to eat each day for four weeks. All of the subjects had moderate cases of acne at the beginning. At the end of the four-week period, none of them experienced a worsening of their condition. Perhaps one chocolate bar was not a sufficient test.

Iodized salt has also been linked to the aggravation of acne in teen-age girls. Scientific tests are not available, but the other halogen, bromide, greatly increases fat gland secretion and produces skin pustules.

One corrective measure that is universally approved is careful cleansing of the skin, and especially the affected areas, each day. The purpose of this is to remove any dirt and oil—or waxy sebum—which, as we have seen, clogs the pores and causes blackheads. The cleansing process can be a soap-and-water one such as a daily shower in which hair shampoo is used on both the hair and face in the case of males and perhaps only on the face in the case of females. The hot water on the face is beneficial. Bactericidal soaps may not help much and may do harm because of passage through the skin of the germicide.

There are several nutritional cures. Folklore has it that garlic, which contains sulfur, works, but the greater amount of sulfur in an egg yolk is probably more effective. Vitamin A taken internally helps to maintain clear, healthy skin. The daily dose should be 10,000 to 25,000 units. Riboflavin and vitamin B-6 help reduce facial oiliness and blackhead formation. Vitamin C may aid in preventing acne infection, and vitamin E may be helpful in preventing acne scars. The daily facial redness produced by 50 to 100 mg of niacin (vitamin B-3) will increase the blood supply to the infected area. Finally, 15 mg of zinc as the gluconate should be taken morning and night since many skin disorders respond to zinc and teen-agers are usually zinc deficient.

Topical agents (those applied directly to the skin) include sulfur-resorcinol and vitamin A acid. The first of these is a water-soluble powder which is antiseptic and antifungal and is used in many skin diseases. A 0.05 percent solution of vitamin A acid will take about six weeks to clear the skin. It generally causes redness and irritation at the beginning of the treatment and therefore should be used only under medical supervision.

Conjugated estrogens (1.25 mg) taken ten days before the onset of menstruation may prevent premenstrual flare-ups of acne, although there has been some debate as to the effectiveness of the hormone and the possibility of secondary complications such as delayed menstruation.

A more drastic treatment, and one that should be reserved for acute cases only and used only under medical supervision, is the administration of 250 mg of the antibiotic tetracycline A.M. and P.M. While the tetracyclines are sometimes curative, there is a danger since the drug inhibits protein synthesis in the mammalian cells and stains the teeth of growing individuals.

An even more stringent measure is the use of peeling agents which cause the top layers of the skin to shed. Used twice a week for six weeks, these prevent follicular plugging or help to discharge follicles already blocked. Since peeling agents cause severe inflammation, they should be carefully supervised by a physician or dermatologist. The sunlamp can be used safely for this purpose as long as a timer is properly utilized.

A warning to those who suffer from acne: pimples around the nose and upper lip should not be squeezed since this can lead to spreading infection and meningitis. Acne is still not fully understood. We do not know all the biochemical changes involved or why only some adolescents are afflicted while others are immune.

Psoriasis

Psoriasis (ps) is a skin disease in which lesions develop at pressure points such as elbows, knees, bra line, and belt buckle, and large amounts of the epidermis become scaly and are continually shed. Psoriasis is unusual in children but can occur at any time after puberty. Psoriasis affects five million people in the United States. With sunlight exposure it disappears but may return each winter. A sunlamp used during the winter will prevent this occurrence when only a mild degree of ps is present.

Severe ps may be accompanied by arthritic changes in the joints which lead us and others to suspect that excess copper and deficient zinc and sulfur may be one metabolic factor. Ps patients require more than the usual amount of zinc to restore their serum levels to a normal of 100 mcg percent. We use as much as 220 mg of zinc sulfate morning and night along with sufficient vitamin B-6 to produce normal dream recall.

Treatment includes vitamin A cream or retinol. Further clinical research is needed to understand more fully the effect of vitamin A cream; we do know that the vitamin is necessary for the normal functioning of all epithelial tissues. Although the cream helps, the skin lesions frequently reappear one to three months after the initial treatment.

Psoriasis is certainly not treatable by over-the-counter drugs, and all such advertised lotions and preparations should be avoided. Like other serious collagen diseases, ps responds to glucocorticoids, but the side-effects of this therapy relegate steroids to next-to-the-last resort.

The last resort—and the most dangerous therapy—is methotrexate, an anticancer drug which can produce dramatic relief for a short period of time. However, because the methotrexate decreases the formation of all rapidly growing cells in the body, the red and white blood cell formation may become seriously low. At this point the cure is worse than the disease.

As early as 1956 Braun-Falco and Rathjens found that zinc was markedly decreased in the outer layers of the skin of patients with psoriasis. This was confirmed in 1966 by Ponomareva, who found high levels of zinc in the scales. Plasma zinc levels were low in psoriasis according to a 1967 report by Greaves and Boyde, and this was confirmed by Vorhees et al. in 1969. In 1962, Lipkin et al, found serum copper levels to be increased while ceruloplasmin was not proportionately increased and red-cell copper might be decreased.

Molokhia and Portnoy in 1970 again found significantly higher serum copper levels in psoriasis but no significant deviation in zinc levels. Again Zackheim and Wolf in 1972 found much the same—an elevated serum copper. Finally, in 1973, Zlatkov et al. found elevated serum copper which decreased with effective therapy—in this case, ultraviolet tanning of the skin.

Sunburn

A new, and apparently most effective, treatment for sunburn is indomethacin, a nonsteroidal, anti-inflammatory agent resembling aspirin. It decreases the redness and pain within a few hours. Sunburn develops when sunlight strikes the skin and arachidonic acid is released. This can be converted to prostaglandin, the fatty acid which mediates inflammation. If the enzyme action which occurs in this conversion process is stopped by indomethacin, then the inflammation causing sunburn could also be prevented. Although no harmful side-effects of indomethacin have as yet been noted, it is not known what might result from the administration of large quantities of the drug.

Adequate vitamin B-6 will promote tanning of the skin, and sun screen lotions contain p-amino benzoic acid (PABA) or its derivatives. The best "cure" for sunburn is adequate protection in the form of skin lotion and limited exposure. The sun contributes to wrinkling and premature aging of the unprotected skin.

Aging Skin

Winter itch, or just dry skin, is probably the commonest skin complaint of old age. This should not be surprising, since the aging process results in a change in keratinization with a thinner more friable skin plus a diminished number of oil and sweat glands and less active ones. Add overbathing to this and intense itching results. Winter itch is one condition in which the patient can cure himself by less frequent bathing and a good afterbath skin oil.

Any discussion of itching in the elderly must include senile pruritus. It is one of the most distressing of diseases, and it does not respond to the regimen outlined for winter itch. Furthermore, drugs commonly used to allay itching, such as cyproheptadine (Periactin, Merck) or trimeprazine (Temaril, SK&F) are relatively ineffective, as is topical antipruritic therapy, although both approaches should be tried. It is imperative that patients with senile pruritus be given a thorough physical examination to rule out such underlying diseases as diabetes, blood disorders, lymphoma, liver and kidney disease, and internal malignancies. Some patients have senile pruritis of neurogenic origin, but it is dangerous to assume that this is the cause. The origin should be determined by elimination. Neither female sex hormones in creams nor added vitamins (such as E or A) have proved beneficial.

In taking blood specimens we note that some patients at eighty have thick elastic skin but that others at forty-five may have wrinkled, sagging transparent skin wherein the veins appear as raised as boundaries on a relief map.

Many factors cause loss of elasticity, drooping and transparency of the skin. Of these, poor nutrition and undue exposure to the sun predominate as causes of early skin failure. The drooping can be corrected surgically but the transparency (like stretch marks and scars) can only be arrested or slowed. The skin of the elderly must be constantly examined for senile moles, warts, plaques and keratoses which should be carefully removed to prevent skin cancer.

Cellulite (pronounced sell u leet)

A checkered, quilted appearance to excess layers of fat in the skin of the thighs and hips gives a waffle-like appearance to the skin of many inactive females. We have not seen this in males.

With adequate nutritional changes, including exercise and weight reduction, the fat is redistributed and the condition is corrected. Massage, mineral baths and deep breathing are probably ineffective.

Striae or Stretch Marks

These may occur in the skin of the abdomen in pregnant women who are deficient in zinc. These should not occur in the skin of teen-agers, yet teen-age girls frequently have stretch marks on the breasts, belly, hips and thighs so severe that they are embarrassed to appear in a two-piece swimsuit, let alone a string bikini. These striae also occur in young males, usually on the thighs, but also on the shoulder girdle in some who engage in weight lifting. One teen-ager who had pyroluria which robbed him of his zinc and vitamin B-6 reported that in a weight-lifting class he could feel his skin breaking as he lifted the weights. Out of twenty-five students in his class who increased their muscle size, he alone developed stretch marks. His serum zinc level was 60 mcg percent when he presented himself for treatment of his disperceptive mental disorder.

Excessive Hair Loss

When hair starts to clog the comb, most women run to their hairdressers. Hair stylists have ideas, but often these are commercially oriented toward the sale of shampoos and tonics. Hair is not grass and seldom can be fertilized from above. Because the hair must be fertilized from below the hair root via the blood and lymph, most excessive hair loss is either a nutritional or hormonal problem.

In times past, severe fevers frequently resulted in loss of head hair. For instance, typhoid fever was frequently followed by hair loss. We find that excess copper will result in hair loss in women, and this may be caused by the birth control pill or by the last trimester of pregnancy—in both instances the serum copper has been doubled. It can also be caused by excess copper in the drinking water or lack of zinc in the diet. Heavy metal intoxication other than copper, such as mercury, lead and cadmium will also cause excessive loss of hair.

Dietary factors which may be deficient in hair-loss patients are vitamin B-6, zinc and sulfur. The first two may be lost because of pyroluria, while sulfur may be low in the diet because of failure to eat sulfur-containing nutrients such as the yolk of the egg. Some of the best results in hair strength and restoration have occurred when patients got adequate zinc, vitamin B-6 and egg yolks. Of course, patients on the birth-control pill must discontinue this at the first sign of excessive hair loss. The hair loss during the last months of pregnancy will return within three months after delivery of the baby.

Male hair loss and a receding hair line usually follow genetic or familial traits. At present the best and only therapy is the transplant of hair from the neck to the balding parts of the head.

References

Beveridge, G. W. and Powell, E. W. The problem of acne. *The Practicioner* 204:635, May 1970.

Braun-Falco, O. and Rathjens, B. Histochemische darstellung von zink in normaler menschlicher haut. *Arch. Klin. Exp. Derm.* 203:130.

Greaves, M. and Boyde, T. R. C. Plasma zinc concentrations in patients with psoriasis, other dermatoses and venous leg ulceration. *Lancet* II:1019, *1967.*

Griffiths, W. A. D. Diffuse hair loss and oral contraceptives. *Brit. J. of Derm.* 88:31, 1973.

Guthrie, M. B. Treating acne in teenage girls. *The Consultant* p. 87, February 1972.

Hair changes in human malnutrition. *Nutrition Reviews* pp. 143-145, June 1971.

Kuschonann, J. D., director, Nutrition Search, *Nutrition Almanac,* U.S.A. Minneapolis, Minnesota, 1973.

Look out America, the "cellulite" problem has arrived. *Medical World News,* 25 January 1974.

Molin, L. and Wester, P. O. Cobalt, copper and zinc in normal and psoriatic epidermis. *Acta Dermatovener* 53:477-480, 1973.

Molokhia, M. M. and Portnoy, B. Neutron activation analysis of trace elements in skin v. copper and zinc in psoriasis. *Br. J. Derm.* 83:376, 1970.

Sternberg, T. S. and Reisner, R. M. The aging skin. *Geriatrics* 14:50, 1971.

Stoughton, R. The heartbreak of psoriasis. *JAMA* 229:3, 15 July 1974.

Voorhees, J. J.; Chakrabarti, S. G.; Botero, F.; Miedler, L. and Harrell, E. R. Zinc therapy and distribution in psoriasis. *Archs. Derm.* 100:669.

Zackheim, H. S. and Wolf, P. Serum copper in psoriasis and other dermatoses. *J. of Investigative Dermatology*, Vol. 58, 1:28-32.

Zlatkov, N. B., Bozhkov, R. and Genov, D. Serum copper and ceruloplasmin in patients with psoriasis after helio- and thalassotherapy. *Arch. Derm. Forsch.* 247:289-294, 1973.

CHAPTER 46

Nutrients for a Better Sex Life

Male patients on Mellaril may complain that with masturbation a climax comes with a throbbing of the glans penis but no ejaculate. With larger doses of the drug (or greater susceptibility of the patient to the drug) the penile erection cannot be attained, the male is impotent and his sexual partner is disappointed. Impotency can also occur in the pyroluric patient who is deficient in zinc and vitamin B-6. This is the most common cause of impotency in the young male and amenorrhea in the female. With adequate dosage of vitamin B-6 and zinc, the sexual ability of the male should return in one to two months' time.

Histapenic Males

The low-histamine male cannot attain ejaculation, although erection is no problem. Similarly, the low-histamine female may go through life and marriage without orgasm—although as a child before puberty she, as a young girl, may have had occasional orgasm when climbing a pole or riding a bike. We would conclude that somehow at puberty her tissue histamine level decreased since the ability to attain orgasm or ejaculation with sex or masturbation is directly correlated with the level of blood histamine and perhaps with the level of tissue histamine.

The failure of the histapenic male to ejaculate is corrected when his blood histamine is brought to normal by adequate therapy. At the other end of the scale, a male patient with a blood histamine higher than normal may have ejaculation when he reads a pornographic paragraph or gets hugged by a girl. This, again, is corrected by therapy which lowers his blood (and presumably his tissue) histamine.

Microscopic examination of the penis from autopsy specimens discloses mast cells containing histamine concentrated in the glans but not in the skin of the shaft or the foreskin of the penis. A collection of objective reports from twenty-eight male schizophrenic patients shows that the quickness of ejaculation is significantly correlated with the blood histamine level.

This indicates that ejaculation may be a local reflex which is activated by the disruption of mast cells and liberation of histamine. Without adequate histamine levels in the mast cells, ejaculation may be difficult or absent. With excess histamine, the clinical phenomenon known as "premature ejaculation" may occur. A literature survey does not disclose any information on this subject, although a high histamine content occurs in the accessory male sex organs that have been examined.

Other Aspects of Histamines

Low-histamine females, without orgasm, would be labeled frigid. We know, however, that the high-histamine female may have repeated orgasm with sex, or a sustained orgasm.

Also, one should note that in discussing the physiology of sexual intercourse Masters and Johnson describe a sex flush in both male and female which is characterized by a reddening of the skin of the entire trunk at the time of ejaculation or orgasm. This they have confirmed by use of color photography. Many of the reports and queries in the *American Medical Journal* and *Human Sexuality* deal with "peculiar" reactions at the time of orgasm. These may be cutaneous hives, flow of saliva, repeated sneezing, asthma attacks, migraine headaches, pain in the clitoris or glans penis, or even a shaking chill. All of these could be due to histamine release with orgasm and ejaculation. None of the answers by sexologists or psychiatrists have suggested histamine as a factor although, to us, dealing daily with histamine levels, this would seem the obvious answer.

Role of Zinc

Finally, one should note that in the nineteenth century many patients, both male and female, were hospitalized with a diagnosis of masturbation insanity. The doctors probably mistook a common symptom for cause. The male does lose zinc with each ejaculate, but if masturbation were repeated in a given day the ejaculate would become smaller and less zinc would be lost. Prostatic secretion appears at the mouth of the erect penis with sex or masturbation, and the male may lose 5 ml of this fluid as well as 5 ml of ejaculate with each sexual effort. This fluid loss of 10 ml would be equal to 1.4 mg of zinc. Perhaps with zinc-deficient males some degree of nervousness and even psychosis might result from excessive masturbation, but since the female loses little by way of secretions with masturbation, the old nineteenth century diagnosis of masturbatory insanity could scarcely be applied accurately to women.

Zinc is important for the formation of active sperm in all mammalian species, including man. The prostate and the prostatic secretions are high in zinc. In the final formation of sperm, zinc is firmly bound within the keratin of the tail of the sperm. This keratin is similar to the keratin layer of the skin, which also contains and needs zinc for perfect formation. The zinc in the tail of the sperm is strongly attached chemically to reduced sulfur in the form of sulfhydril groups. Drs. Calvin and Bleau of Columbia University report that this action in keratin accounts for the need for zinc in normal reproduction. Certainly, patients both male and female whom we have seen for problems of lack of menses, potency and fertility have successfully produced children when their zinc and vitamin B-6 deficiency was corrected. Cadmium, which antagonizes zinc, can, in excess, stop the formation of sperm in the testes.

Content of Semen

The trace metal content of semen is of interest because of the prominence of zinc and sulfur. Calcium is 25 mg percent, zinc 14 mg percent, magnesium 14 mg percent and copper only 0.015 mg percent, while sulfur is 3 percent of the ash. The odor of semen is due to amines such as spermine and spermidine. These odors come from the testes and are greatly diminished by vasectomy. The known vitamin content of semen is vitamin C, 13 mg percent and inositol 53 mg percent. Fructose is the main nutrient energy source at 224 mg percent.

Summary

In summary, the use of folic acid to elevate blood and tissue histamine will provide easier orgasm in the low-histamine female. Pyrolurics may need both zinc and adequate vitamin B-6 for normal sexual function. Zinc is important for the production of normal sperm and ova. Zinc is needed by the normal prostate and testes.

References

Mann, Thaddeus. *The biochemistry of semen and the male reproductive tract.* New York: John Wiley & Son, 1964.

CHAPTER 47

Side Effects of Hormones

Hormones are chemicals produced by an organ, or by certain cells of an organ, and transmitted by body fluids to carry out specific body functions. When there is a deficiency of certain hormones, the deficiency can often be corrected with an effective natural replacement therapy.

A physician may recommend gradually increasing doses of desiccated thyroid to correct signs of thyroid deficiency. This straightforward replacement therapy is highly effective. Other simple replacement therapies such as insulin for lack of insulin and human growth hormone for lack of growth hormone are also highly effective. Other hormones cannot be easily replaced, and attempts to use corticosteroids as drugs result in many unwanted side actions. Here, again, we are pulling on one portion of a giant endocrine spider web, in that overdose can distort the actions of other hormones and even cellular metabolism.

The best female sex hormone (estrogen) comes from the urine of the pregnant mare and is called conjugated estrogens (Premarin). This is a natural product; all others on the market are synthetic, and chemists have made these synthetic estrogens by the hundreds. Most are more potent than the standard conjugated estrogens, and all the synthetics are unknowns in respect of their cancer-causing ability. For example, about fifteen to thirty years ago diethylstilbestrol (DES) was given to some pregnant women to help prevent threatened miscarriage. Because of DES, many girl babies born to these mothers have developed clear cell cancer of the vagina and cervix and all require careful annual examinations of the vagina and cervix as a preventive measure. Young ladies often, of course, do not know what their mothers took during pregnancy, and no great effort is being made by doctors who used DES to warn all of the young patients at risk.

Herbst et al. of Boston have analyzed 170 reported cases of clear cell cancer of the vagina and cervix. These were divided as follows: 100 of the vagina and 70 of the cervix. The age range of the patients was seven to twenty-nine years, and the in utero exposure of the patients to nonnatural estrogens was confirmed. The synthetic estrogen exposure in utero began as early as the seventeenth week of pregnancy and was continued for as short a period as one week and as long as thirty-three weeks—i.e., throughout the rest of the pregnancy. Of the 170 patients found positive, 24 have died of the cancer, and recurrences of cancer have occurred in 37. Only 9 percent of the cancers evolved before the age of twelve years. The occurrence of this type of cancer, in normal life, is almost nil in patients in this age group.

One wonders about *other synthetic* hormones and their possible side-effects, and at the same time we thank our lucky medical stars that some hormones such as thyroxin are so specifically complex that the chemists have only been able to isolate and synthesize the exact molecules used by the body. This specificity protects man from tinkered and more potent thyroids and probably from cancer of the thyroid.

Progesterones Have Side-effects Too

Progesterone and synthetic progestogens have also been given to prevent threatened abortion, and in this instance boy babies have paid the penalty. Among the male babies born of these treated mothers there was a high incidence of hermaphroditism or transsexualism. The testes and the scrotum just failed to develop normally.

Now proposed for human use is Depo-Provera (DMPA), an injectable synthetic progestogen which, in a dose of 150 mg, will act as a birth control pill so that no pregnancy will occur for at least three months and maybe (24 percent incidence) not for a whole year. Some Depo-Provera-injected women will become sterile and never produce babies, and Depo-Provera causes breast cancer in beagle dogs and cervical cancer in women at a rate 9.1 times the national rate of the underdeveloped countries in which it was tested. Population control groups are still highly optimistic about the continued use of this two-edged sword.

The drug is now available in vial form (as a palliative of uterine cancer) so some doctors will use it for birth control purposes. Make sure that you (or your loved one) are not the one to receive these injections.

Other Risks

In various other ways, women may be exposed to hormones during pregnancy: through the unintentional use of birth control pills after conception has already occurred, and the administration of hormones during certain types of pregnancy tests. The birth control pills are synthetic chemicals which have been inadequately tested for their long-term cancer-producing effect.

In discussing DES, we reported that the female offspring of contaminated mothers are especially susceptible to clear cell cancer of the vagina and cervix. At one time people could also obtain residues of DES from eating meat and poultry products or mixing cattle feed! DES was fed to cattle to increase weight, and to chickens for caponizing. At one time, the USDA suggested that whole chicken heads and necks be used as food for mink. Some caponized chickens, however, retained the implanted pellets of DES in their necks, and the female mink, subsequently became sterile as a result of eating the DES in the contaminated chicken necks! The use of DES as a preventive measure for miscarriages and in animal feed has since been prohibited. However, some hazards remain. This dangerous synthetic continues to be legally recommended in some emergency situations for the "morning after" pill. While such a pill may offer some convenience, we believe that menstrual extraction is preferable when the woman at risk has missed a menstrual period.

The status of DES in cattle and chicken feed is constantly changing, but at the moment of writing, it is prohibited in feed and permitted in implants.

Chorionic Gonadotrophin (CGT) Is Hopelessly Overused

A natural female hormone, chorionic gonadotrophin, is extracted from the urine of pregnant women and sometimes injected daily into obese women for the purpose of weight control. Research is currently in progress to determine the effectiveness of this use, and to uncover possible harmful side-effects. The "Simeons regimen" consists of 125 units daily six days a week until forty injections have been given. A 500-calorie daily diet is recommended, and the daily interview and injection seems to have a very expensive placebo effect as a morale builder.

Drs. Ballin and White of Chicago conclude:

> Since no evidence exists that human chorionic gonadotrophin effects weight reduction, any claims to the contrary are a misrepresentation of the scientific facts. Scientific evidence does not support the claim that HCG causes preferential mobilization of "abnormal" fat. Except as a placebo, there is no rational basis for its use in weight reduction. The "Simeons regime" causes weight loss by means of a required semistarvation diet reinforced by daily visits to a "clinic" and daily injections of a "drug" presented to the patient as an aid to weight reduction. The safety of the "Simeons regimen" is questionable, especially where medical supervision is minimal, because it is unphysiological and can lead to substantial protein loss. Physicians should consider carefully before participating in the Simeons weight "clinics" or using their methods.

Summary

Research is continuing to probe and uncover positive links between hormones and birth defects. In the meantime, however, steps should be taken to protect the mother of the present and her future baby. First, a physician should thoroughly examine and question the patient for possible pregnancy before prescribing birth control pills. Second, safer alternatives should be substituted for pregnancy tests involving the use of hormones. Finally, physicians should be prudent in their use of hormones as supportive therapy. The administration of hormonal treatments to women with problems during a previous pregnancy, but not during the current one, is an unnecessary risk. Through the reckless use of synthetic hormones, doctors can produce cellular alterations which can vary from cancerous changes in cells to endocrine imbalance wherein sex function can be altered. Insulin and thyroid are the two safest hormones.

References

Ballin, John C. and White, Philip L. Fallacy and hazard. *JAMA* 230: 5, 4 November 1974.

Herbst, A. L., et al. Clear-cell adenocarcinoma of vagina and cervix in girls: analysis of 170 registry cases. *Am J. Obstet. Gynecol.* 119:713-724, 1974.

Science Newsletter, 26 October 1974.

Taft, P. D. et al. Cytology of clear cell cancer. *Acta Cytol.* 18:279, 1974.

Zwerdling, R. Depo-Provera. *New Republic*, 9 November 1974.

CHAPTER 48

The Contraceptive Pill: The Mental and Metabolic Havoc It Evokes

The first oral contraceptive pill, a combination of a synthetic estrogen and progestin, was released for the treatment of menstrual disorders in 1957 and as a contraceptive in 1960. Since then dozens of pills containing various combinations and potencies of these female hormones have reached the market. Although sequential medications and a purely progesterone pill are now available, the most widely used pills are of the combination type, and it is these preparations which are most commonly referred to as "the pill."

Nutritionally Related Effects

Since the introduction of oral contraceptives, much research has been done to determine what effect, other than the desired one, these agents have on body composition and functioning. A considerable amount of recent research has been devoted to the nutritionally related effects of "the pill." It is now known that in addition to causing alterations in carbohydrate and lipid metabolism, combination oral contraceptives have a marked effect on the body's need for and use of the trace metals copper, zinc and iron and the vitamins B-2, B-6, B-12 and folic acid.

In both animal and human studies it has repeatedly been shown that the estrogen component of "the pill" causes an increase in serum copper and a decrease in serum zinc. The copper-elevating effect of "the pill" is due to an increased absorption of copper from the intestine and an accelerated synthesis in the liver of ceruloplasmin, a copper-binding protein. Approximately 95 percent of serum copper is bound to this protein.

In a similar manner, "the pill" causes an increase in serum iron and iron-binding capacity. Increased production in the liver of two iron-binding proteins, apoferritin and transferrin, seems to be responsible for an increased absorption of this trace metal and an elevation of its level in the serum.

The Pill and the Schizophrenic

If high serum, and presumably tissue, iron and copper and low serum zinc are involved in the etiology of some of the schizophrenias, "the pill" might be expected to aggravate the symptoms of some schizophrenic women. Clinical observations have, in fact, shown this to be the case. Furthermore, schizophrenic women appear to be particularly susceptible to the copper-elevating effect of "the pill." Their serum copper has been found by Pfeiffer to exceed that of normal women taking combination oral contraceptives and of normal women during the ninth month of pregnancy, a time when endogenous estrogen is high.

The Pill and Copper

"The pill" has also been reported to cause migraine headaches both in women previously susceptible to these headaches and in those who have never experienced them before. Migraine headaches and other pill-related side-effects such as insomnia and depression may be related to excess copper, since individuals with high serum copper have been found to experience these symptoms. A few patients find the excess copper to produce a hypomanic state which is like that produced by amphetamines. Even though their health may be endangered by this overactivity, they will not give up the pill.

There is general agreement that the use of oral contraceptives increases the rise of hypertension or high blood pressure, and of thromboembolism or the occlusion of veins and arteries by blood clots. Although it would be an oversimplification to blame excessive copper for these diseases, it is possible that increased amounts of this trace metal are a contributing factor. Considerable evidence supports this contention. For example, copper is known to be a brain stimulant and could cause a constriction of the blood vessels resulting in increased blood pressure. Furthermore, McKenzie and Kay found in 1973 that hypertensive women excrete more copper than do normotensive women. (In 1967, Rachinski found that individuals with high blood pressure had elevated levels of copper in their blood.)

As for thromboembolism, in a report published by the American Medical Association in 1970 it was noted that "the pill" causes an increase in the number of blood platelets, and possibly in their tendency to clump together, and in blood coagulability. In 1971 Aronson, Magora and Shenker found that this medication causes greater blood viscosity. It has also been reported (by Lages and Stivala in 1973) that the presence of copper ions causes increased clotting. Sacchetti et al. have reported that manganese ions, which are antagonized by copper, ordinarily inhibit platelet aggregation.

It has also been reported that increased serum ceruloplasmin causes the decrease in plasma and platelet ascorbic acid seen in women using "the pill." Ceruloplasmin is known to oxidize vitamin C. This alteration, according to Kalesh et al. in 1971, could cause changes in the electrical activity of the blood and reduce the repulsion of platelets from one another, thereby favoring the formation of clots. Saroja et al. in 1971 pointed out that if, as seems to be true in guinea pigs, the ascorbic acid content of the blood vessel walls is also reduced, there might be a greater attraction between the vessels and the platelets as well.

The Pill and Other Vitamins

The effect of oral contraceptives on vitamins other than ascorbic acid has also been studied, and estrogen-containing pills have been found to lower the serum concentration of vitamin B-12 and the serum and red blood cell concentrations of folic acid. A deficiency of either nutrient can cause anemia, a disease sometimes reported in oral contraceptive users. Reduced serum and red cell folate seem to be the result of a reduction in the absorption of folate polyglutamic phosphate, the form of folic acid most commonly found in food. Both reduced folate and the resulting anemia respond to folic acid and B-6 supplementation.

In addition to increasing the body's need for B-12 and folic acid, "the pill" appears to create a functional vitamin B-6 deficiency. Women using "the pill" have repeatedly been found to excrete increased amounts of xanthurenic acid, a metabolic intermediate in the tryptophan-to-niacin pathway, both spontaneously and after an oral tryptophan load. Increased excretion of xanthurenic acid is generally recognized as symptomatic of a relative B-6 deficiency because many enzymes dependent on B-6 are required for the complete conversion of tryptophan to niacin. The estrogen-induced abnormal tryptophan metabolism and resulting excretion of excessive xanthurenic acid can be corrected with oral doses of B-6.

It was suggested, by Luhby et al. in a 1971 report and by Winston in a 1973 report that the depression and mood and sleep pattern changes sometimes associated with the use of oral contraceptives may be related to abnormal tryptophan metabolism and a relative B-6 deficiency. It is postulated that the control of mood is in some way dependent on the central nervous system concentrations of biogenic amines such as serotonin and that the estrogen component of "the pill" interferes with serotonin production. In animals, estrogen has been shown to divert tryptophan from the serotonin-to-niacin pathway and to compete with pyridoxal phosphate, the metabolically active form of B-6, for binding sites on the enzymes which are necessary for both niacin and serotonin formation. If the same mechanism were operating in oral contraceptive users, it would explain both the increased excretion of xanthurenic acid and the hypothesized reduction in brain serotonin. Whether or not reduced serotonin production is involved in "pill"-related depression and altered sleep patterns, it is significant that these side-effects are frequently alleviated with oral doses of 50 mg of vitamin B-6.

Administration of B-6 has also been shown, by Winston in 1973, to improve the impaired glucose tolerance curve frequently observed in women taking combination oral contraceptives. Many such women show a diabetic-type reaction to a glucose tolerance test. Supplemental B-6 may be effective because it reduces the formation of excess xanthurenic acid. This substance has been shown to combine with circulating insulin to form a complex which reduces the insulin's effect on the blood glucose level.

By increasing the body's need for vitamin B-6, "the pill" also appears to increase the need for vitamin B-2. This nutrient is involved in an enzyme system which converts B-6 into its metabolically active form.

The Pill and Blood Pressure

In 1966, a thirty-three-year-old woman was referred to Dr. John H. Laragh, Professor of Clinical Medicine and Director of the Hypertension Center, Columbia-Presbyterian Medical Center, New York City, for a workup because her blood pressure was 250/150. He did renal arteriography and every other test.

As she was going out the door she said, "Dr. Laragh, I've been on 'the pill' for five years. Do you think that matters?" He said, "I don't know that it matters, but why don't you stop it and see what happens?"

She wasn't keen to, but she did. She came back two months later and her blood pressure was down to 120 over 80. At that point she didn't believe it was "the pill," and she wanted to go back on it again. The doctor switched her to another brand, and in two months the blood pressure was back up to 250. She was convinced that time, and so was he. Dr. Laragh began to look for additional cases, and he found them.

The Pill and Lipids

Finally, combination oral contraceptives may alter lipid metabolism. Small increases in plasma triglycerides are common and increases in plasma cholesterol, phospholipids and lipoproteins have been reported.

Advantages and Disadvantages

Despite the multitude of potential side-effects, oral contraceptives are popular, convenient and effective. In an age of frighteningly rapid population growth, it is unlikely that their use will be abandoned or curtailed. It is therefore important that both physicians and oral contraceptive users be familiar with the mental and metabolic havoc that these agents can evoke.

If the use of an oral contraceptive is contemplated, serious risk factors such as preexisting hypertension, habitual smoking, thromboembolism, atherosclerosis, zinc deficiency, or copper-excess schizophrenia should be considered. If major complications are not foreseen, a pill low in estrogen should be selected, since estrogen seems to be responsible for the nutritionally related adverse side-effects of oral contraceptives. And finally, the body's increased need for zinc, B-2, B-6, B-12, folic acid and C should be met with nutritional supplements.

References

Aronson, H. B., Magora, F. and Shenker, J. G. *Am. J. Obstet. Gyn.* 110:997, 1971.

Kalesh, D. G. Mallikaryuneswara, V. R., and Clemetson, A. B. *C.A.B. Contraception* 4:183, 1971.

Lages, B. and Stivala, S. S. *Biopolymers* 12:961, 1973.

Luhby, A. L.; Brin, M.; Gordon, M.; Davis, P.; Murphy, M. and Spiegel, H. *Am. J. Clin. Nutr.* 24:684, 1971.

McKenzie, J. M. and Kay, D. L. *New Zeal. Med. J.* 79:68, 1973.

McQueen, E. G. *Drugs* 2:138, 1971.

Pfeiffer, C. C. *Unpublished data.*

Rachinski, I. D. *Pat. Fiziol. Eksp. Ter.*·11:74, 1967.

Sacchetti, G.; Gibelli, A.; Bellani, D. and Montanari, C. *Experientia* 30:374, 1974.

Saroja, N., Mallikarjuneswara, V. R. and Clemetson, A. B. C. *A. B. Contraception* 3:269, 1971.

Schenker, J. G.; Hellerstein, S.; Jungreis, E. and Polishuk, W. Z. *Fertil. Steril.* 22:229, 1971.

Tagatz, G. E. and McHugh, R. B. *Clin. Pharmacol.* 50:121, 1971.

Winston, F. *Am. J. Psychiat.* 130:11, 1973.

CHAPTER 49

Hexachlorophene Poisoning

In an age which views cleanliness not only as an insurance against disease but also as a primary social virtue, many of those engaged in the cause for hygiene have become all too willing to exploit every weapon in the crusade against "germ-produced" odors and infections. Often the chemical preparations designed to combat germs are not adequately tested before being sent into action and may prove more hazardous than their tiny adversaries. Hexachlorophene, the well-known antibacterial agent, offers a dramatic case in point.

For more than twenty-five years, hexachlorophene (HCP) enjoyed wide use as the leading skin disinfectant. It served as the "germ-killing" ingredient in countless brands of soap, detergent, shampoo, vaginal spray, mouthwash and infant preparations and as a preservative in sundry cosmetics. Early research with the chemical involved the evaluation of its bacteriostatic action, but only in recent times have studies explored the potential toxic effects of HCP. Results of these crucial investigations have produced evidence linking HCP to brain disturbances in laboratory animals and man.

HCP Is Poison for Rats

Experimental research using rats first determined the brain-damaging properties of hexachlorophene. Rats orally fed HCP in repeated high doses developed anorexia, convulsions, hind-limb weakness and progressive paralysis. It was reported by Kimbrough and Gaines in 1971 that microscopic examination revealed injury to the tissues—namely, holes in the brain stem, an area that controls our vital functions. Curley and Hawk, in the same year, stated that rats fed smaller doses of HCP exhibited no overt toxic symptoms but that microscopically visible damage still appeared. HCP concentrations in the blood of these animals measured an average of 1.2 ppm, suggesting that HCP blood levels might gauge the degree of brain toxicity.

In an experiment with newborn rhesus monkeys reported in 1971, researchers at Winthrop Laboratories further discovered that HCP can enter the bloodstream not only via the digestive tract but through the intact skin. A residue of HCP remains on the skin following topical application and cannot be completely removed by rinsing since the chemical is insoluble in water. While this residue makes HCP a potent skin germicide, it also allows appreciable amounts of the chemical to penetrate the skin and pass into the blood. Monkeys bathed daily for ninety days with a 3 percent HCP solution achieved mean blood concentrations of 1.5 ppm. Although the animals never demonstrated detectable signs of poisoning, on autopsy all had holes in the brain stem resembling those observed in the HCP-fed rats.

HCP Is Poison to Man

Additional discoveries established the relevance of the animal data to man. Newborn infants, medical and dental personnel, wound and burn patients and people with germ phobias were found to be most seriously threatened by the adverse effects of HCP.

The immature skin of the newborn is vulnerable to penetration by HCP. Before the potential hazards of HCP became a major issue, many hospitals routinely used HCP preparations for bathing newborns to protect the infants' delicate skin from harmful bacteria. At one hospital in 1971, blood samples taken from fifty newborns who had received several daily baths with a 3 percent HCP emulsion showed HCP concentrations ranging between .009 ppm and .646 ppm. Although the babies displayed no signs of neurological abnormality, the high level of HCP concentration was near the level associated with brain damage in rats, suggesting the presence of similar damage.

Further studies indicated that cutaneous absorption of HCP occurs more rapidly and completely in premature infants than in full-term newborns, probably because the skin of premature infants is less developed and therefore more permeable than that of full-term babies. Also, the liver, an organ which detoxifies many foreign chemicals that enter the bloodstream, is not as completely formed in the premature infant and might have a limited ability to detoxify HCP once it has been absorbed. Five premature infants bathed daily with a diluted 3 percent HCP solution for twenty-one to fifty-six days had blood HCP levels of 0.21 to 1.1 ppm. Kopelman reported in 1972 that immediately recognizable HCP-induced signs or symptoms of poisoning were not manifested. But what about the motor and learning abilities of these children later on?

To determine whether infants treated with HCP suffered any degree of brain damage despite the absence of any written diagnosis of intoxication, pathologists at the University of Washington Medical School in Seattle in 1972 examined the files of brain stem sections, which had been in storage since 1966, of 250 infants who had died at two Seattle hospitals. Twenty-one of the 250 autopsy specimens reviewed showed characteristic brain stem holes, and all but one of the twenty-one cases had occurred in a hospital where the infants received three or more sponge baths per day with 3 percent HCP. In the one case excepted, the infant had been treated with HCP at one hospital before being transferred elsewhere. The remaining 189 infants in this study who never were treated with HCP had normal brain stem sections by microscopic examination. The failure to diagnose troubles in the first group merely means that "you can't diagnose a disorder unless you think of it."

HCP at 6 Percent in Dry Talcum Powder Is Fatal

An incident in France conclusively demonstrated the clinical and functional significance of the brain lesions found in children treated with HCP. During the spring of 1972, thirty to forty infants in certain areas of France developed an unusual combination of dermatological and neurological miseries. Symptoms peculiar to this condition included a strange diaper rash, lack of appetite, low-grade fever and generalized convulsions which frequently terminated in sudden respiratory arrest and death. Autopsy reports described extensive damage to nerve tissue in the infants' brains. Blood levels of HCP in some of the babies measured as high as 14 ppm. Common to all cases of the illness was exposure to talcum powder accidentally contaminated with 6 percent HCP. An effective remedy for HCP intoxication might have reduced the tragic number of victims.

Suspected Cases of HCP Poisoning

Recently, the Princeton group found vitamin and trace element therapy useful in alleviating some symptoms of HCP poisoning in a child. A three-year-old girl was treated for HCP-induced physiological and neurological impairment. After a premature birth, she was bathed daily for over one year with 3 percent HCP. Three years later, mental retardation was indicated by her short attention span, her frequent lack of response to surrounding people, her lack of toilet training and her speech difficulties. In addition, a biochemical disorder was suggested by her poor appetite, insomnia and intermittent muscle pain. Given substantial daily doses of vitamins plus supplementary zinc and manganese, her condition has slowly improved. Within six months, she became more responsive, was learning to speak, and was no longer plagued by poor appetite and insomnia.

While infants are most likely to suffer the full adverse effects of HCP, adults are by no means immune to the hazards of the chemical. In 1973 Butcher et al. found that surgeons, dentists and other professionals who had used this disinfectant routinely had blood concentrations seven times greater than those measured in nonmedical personnel.

A fifty-six-year-old orthodontist conscientiously washed his hands between treating patients—approximately every five to ten minutes—with a 3 percent HCP soap. At home, he washed his entire body with a hexachlorophene soap during regular bathing. He became severely intoxicated. Muscle degeneration, with tongue immobility and inability to swallow, speak or eat marked the onset of a progressive bulbar palsy. His constant exposure to HCP is thought to be a causal factor of his paralysis. Total elimination of HCP from the patient's use slowed the rate of the disease's progress. The symptoms were alleviated when nutrients were administered by the doctors of the Princeton group.

Burns and wounds disrupt the skin and open the underlying tissue to bacterial infections. Larson, in 1968, stated that burn victims treated with a 3 percent HCP solution to prevent such infections have often developed a state of coma and muscle twitching. HCP concentrations in the blood of some of these victims have attained levels as high as 17 ppm indicating that skin rendered especially permeable by burns or other wounds readily absorbs HCP in amounts large enough to cause severe intoxication.

In our opinion, cases such as these clearly reveal that HCP at the 3 percent level should never have been placed on the market.

Why Germ Phobia in Modern Times?

Fears of germs should have diminished with the discoveries of germ-fighting antibiotics, yet germ phobia has increased with the public awareness of body odor. Why?

One of the answers may be the persistent advertising campaigns leading the consumer in a war on germ-caused odors. There are sprays to fight vaginal odors, sprays to stop underarm odors and sprays to disguise fecal, food and tobacco odors. Mouthwashes claim to swish away germs that can cause bad breath, and soaps are promoted as attacking the bacteria that may cause body odor. Germs and bad odors have received the chief focus as the enemy of the cleanliness-conscious citizen, while hexachlorophene remains the hidden villain.

Advertising teaches the consumer that the HCP germ-fighting ingredient is an aid to good personal hygiene and a desirable protector during social interactions. The consumer must also be made aware of the potential dangers. All bacteria are not harmful; some help combat skin disease by creating a fatty acid barrier to fungi which may infect the skin, perianal region and vagina. Antibacterial soaps thus can deplete the body of its own germ fighters. A female patient, after using an HCP preparation soap, developed a fungus infection on an open area of her arm; normal fungus growth areas would be between the fingers and toes, under the breast or in the groin area. Her body's natural protectors, bacteria and the acid cover, had been washed away by the germicidal soap.

Antibacterial soaps and deodorants may not even be necessary to solve the problems of perspiration odor. In the past few years, medical researchers have been discovering the many unusual benefits of zinc supplementation in the diet. Currently being researched is the postulate that zinc supplements can eliminate perspiration odor, regardless of how much sweat is produced. We know that vitamin B-6 and zinc will prevent the odor in the pyroluric patient.

The sale of vaginal sprays containing HCP soared to a multimillion-dollar business after their introduction seven years ago. Countless cases of irritation were reported which were attributed both to HCP and the perfume. HCP is not even claimed to be the ingredient effective in fighting any possible odor!

Are Warnings Adequate?

Clearly, the use of a chemical which disinfects the skin but makes holes in the brain entails more risks than benefits. Several years ago, this consideration compelled FDA officials to place an almost total ban on HCP in drugs and cosmetics sold over the counter. Items containing more than 0.75 percent HCP can now be purchased on prescription only and must be labeled with warnings concerning absorption and potential toxicity.

Warnings must plainly indicate the potential health hazards. pHisoHex, although now only available on prescription, still contains 3 percent hexachlorophene. With repeated doses, this amount could produce holes in the brain stem and mental retardation. The pHisoHex advertisement provides us with an example of a vague and stupid warning: "pHisoHex should be discontinued promptly if signs or symptoms of cerebral irritability occur." I, for one, do not want any brain irritability caused by holes in my brain stem! The brain is not a bone which knits when broken. Cells and nuclei of the brain, when lost, are lost forever.

In summary, then, all products claiming antibacterial power should list their contents for consumer review. Many do not. Experts question the safety and effectiveness of the popular germ-fighting products and urge that the scores of products already on the market and those in the preparation stage should pass new, rigid tests.

For now, advertisers will continue to exploit the germphobia market in its relentless witch-hunt for germ-caused odors. The HCP story has been told in minute detail in order to save consumers from fungus infections, contact dermatitis, germ phobia and needless holes in the brain stem. We don't need germicides. Let the body function normally. When needed, potent antibiotics can do the germ-killing and lifesaving work.

References

Black, J. G.; Sprott, W. E.; Howes, D. and Rutherford, T. Percutaneous absorption of hexachlorophene. *Toxicol.* 2:127, 1974.

Butcher, H. R., et al. Hexachlorophene concentrations in the blood of operating room personnel. *Arch. Surg.* 107:70, 1973.

Curley, A. and Hawk, R. Hexachlorophene I. Presented at the 61st Annual Meeting of the American Chemical Society, Los Angeles, Ca., 1971.

De Jesus, P. V. and Pleasure, D. E. Hexachlorophene neuropathy. *Arch. Neurol.* 29:180, 1973.

Kimbrough, R. D. and Gaines, T. B. Hexachlorophene effects on the rat brain. *Arch. Environ. Health* 23:114, 1971.

Kimbrough, R. D. Review of toxicity of hexachlorophene. *Arch. Environ. Health* 25:119, 1971.

Kopelman, A. E. Cutaneous absorption of HCP in low birth weight infants. *J. Pediat.* 82:972-975, 1973.

Larson, D. L. Studies show hexachlorophene causes burn syndrome. *Hospitals* 42:63, 1968.

Lockhart, J. D. Hexachlorophene and the food and drug administration. *J. Clin. Pharm.* 13:445, 1973.

Powell, H.; Swarner, O.; Gluch, L. and Lampert, P. Hexachlorophene myelinopathy in premature infants. *J. Pediat.* 82:6:976, 1973.

Shuman, R. M., Leexh, R. W. and Alvord, E. C., Jr. Neuropathology in newborn infants bathed with hexachlorophene. *Morbidity and Mortality* 22:93, 1973.

Trout, M. E. Hexachlorophene in perspective. *J. Clin Pharm.* 13:11, 12:451, 1973.

Ulsamer, A. G. and Marzulli, F. N. Hexachlorophene concentrations in blood associated with the use of products containing hexachlorophene. *Toxicol.* 11:625, 1973.

CONCLUSION

The Good Life can be enhanced most effectively by nutrient methods. "Good Food" containing an adequate amount of minerals, trace elements, vitamins and protein serves as the best possible means of keeping the body mechanism in optimum functioning order. When people are starved and malnourished they become weak, depressed and sleepy and may be victimized by an infinite variety of psychiatric disorders.

Certain foods, rich in trace elements, vitamins and protein, act as brain and muscle stimulants; having a more prolonged and therefore better effect than the sugar and caffeine upon which the "dietary dub" relies for his quick, but temporary, energy pick-up. Fractions of these foods can produce an even more stimulant effect than the whole food. Substances which have been separated and identified as stimulant include: 1) thyroid as in some sweetbreads; 2) ornithine, deanol and methionine as in proteins and 3) rutin and biotin and other vitamins such as B-12. Among the trace elements, copper, iron and cobalt can lead to stimulation and insomnia when ingested in excess.

Other foods have a natural anti-anxiety effect. Hot milk neutralizes stomach acid and promotes sleep. Vitamin C in megadoses of one to two grams helps to relax the individual, and the vitamin inositol, one gram at bedtime, provides calm and promotes sleep. Two buffered aspirin tablets have been found to produce the same anti-anxiety effect in man as do two meprobamate tablets and the hazard is less with aspirin. L-tryptophan, an amino acid, is presently under study as a sleep-producing compound.

Street drugs contain almost anything, so the fool who uses these "uppers" or "downers" as stimulants or anti-anxiety agents plays a dangerous game of Russian roulette with a bullet in every chamber. A physician can provide prescriptions for thyroid, deanol or anti-depressants if needed. He can also prescribe sleep-producing antihistamine drugs which are more effective and physiological in their action than commercially sold sedatives such as Sominex and Nytal. Zinc salt dietary supplements relieve tension and insomnia. On a high-zinc low-copper diet, the problems of insomnia will disappear since zinc drives excess iron and copper (both of which are stimulants) from the body. Zinc gluconate is now available at all health food stores.

Above all, tests for biochemical imbalances which may be causing depression or overstimulation and insomnia should be administered. Most doctors do not quiz the patient adequately about his eating habits and may therefore apply inappropriate and ineffective treatment for a misdiagnosed nutrient deficiency syndrome which could be corrected with trace elements and vitamin dietary supplements.

In our continuing search to identify biochemical markers of psychotic disorders, we have determined three major types of schizophrenia, all of which can be treated with appropriate nutrient therapy. About 50 percent of schizophrenics are low in blood histamine and serum folic acid but high in serum copper (histapenia). These paranoid and hallucinatory patients respond to vitamin B-12, folate and niacin therapy. Their biochemical counterparts, the 20 percent of schizophrenics who are high in blood histamine (histadelia) and who suffer suicidal depression, respond to treatment with calcium lactate, zinc, manganese and Deaner. A remaining 30 percent of schizophrenics excrete large amounts of urinary pyrrole (mauve factor). This syndrome, "pyroluria," is characterized by amnesia, muscle spasms, malformation of the knee cartilage, white spots in the fingernails and cutaneous striae, and results from a combined vitamin B-6 and zinc deficiency. Large doses of B-6 and zinc provide effective therapy for these patients.

Victims of these three syndromes as well as those suffering the symptoms of other biochemical disorders such as hypoglycemia would be greatly benefited should more doctors recognize the compelling need for trace element therapy and the value of eating foods rich in the essential nutrients.

Professionals and public alike should be alerted as to the shortcomings of stored, processed and tinkered-with foods. Even under the best storage conditions, vegetables kept too long will lose up to 50 percent of their vitamin C, a natural factor essential for the regulation of blood cholesterol levels, the prevention of atherosclerosis and the detoxification of toxic substances in the liver. Vegetables treated with EDTA lose considerable amounts of zinc and manganese, both of which remove excess copper from the body.

Processing deprives the nutritious wheat kernel of B vitamins, vitamin E and lecithin, all of which are necessary for maintaining healthy tissues and normal metabolism of fats, proteins and carbohydrates, and for building antibodies, regulating blood cholesterol levels and regulating chromium, which is needed to burn sugar.

Manufacturers of "fake foods" wherein synthetic ingredients are used plus a few inexpensive vitamins have, or will, come to grief because of the lack of essential trace elements in their products. Man cannot make an artificial orange juice, lemon juice or egg that is as nutritious as the natural product. People eating "fake foods" will show trace metal deficiencies which may appear as loss of taste, mental disease or widespread degenerative diseases, including premature aging, heart disease, loss of resistance to infection and diabetes.

Tinkered-with foods are those in which the nutrients are removed and then an attempt made to fortify the product with nutrients which are blatantly deficient because of the tinkering. A proposal has been made to add ten nutrients to white flour, which is obviously better than the four additions we have at present. But what about manganese, molybdenum, vanadium, tin, sulfur, selenium, silicon, chromium and the undiscovered vitamins which may be needed by man but not the laboratory rat? Nutritional studies in man are needed which may disclose many more nuances than the ratkeeper ever dreamed of.

Efforts should be made to prevent the use of food dyes in basic staple foods. Egg yolks are nutritious. Yellow dyes are not. Whole-wheat bread should have color provided by the bran and germ of wheat and not by a brown dye. Red dyes should not be used to make fish or soybean protein (or oatmeal!) look like red meat. And, if you think about it, the number of artificial ingredients in ice cream is a disgrace!

Processed and synthetic foods simply cannot replace nutrient-rich natural foods in promoting the Good Life.

General References

Adams, R. and Murray, F. *Minerals: Kill or Cure?* New York: Larchmont Books, 1974.

Furia, T. E. *Handbook of Food Additives.* Cleveland: Chemical Rubber Co. 1973.

Hawkins, D. and Pauling, L., eds. *Orthomolecular Psychiatry: Treatment of Schizophrenics.* San Francisco: W. H. Freeman, 1973.

Hoffer, A. and Osmond, H. *How to Live with Schizophrenia.* New York: University Books, 1966.

Lappé, F. M. *Diet for a Small Planet.* New York: Ballantine Books, 1971.

Pfeiffer, C. C. and Iliev, V. A study of zinc deficiency and copper excess in the schizophrenias. *Intern. Rev. Neurobiol. Suppl.* 1:141-165, 1972.

Robinson, C. H. *Fundamentals of Normal Nutrition.* New York: Macmillan, 1973.

Schroeder, H. A. *The Trace Elements and Man.* Old Greenwich, Connecticut: Devin-Adair, 1973.

Sebrell, W. H. and Harris, R. S. *The Vitamins.* New York: Academic Press, 1973.

Snyder, S. H. *Madness and the Brain.* New York: McGraw Hill, 1974.

Sollman, T. *A Manual of Pharmacology* (8th edition). Philadelphia: W. B. Saunders, 1957.

Trager, G. T. *The Big, Fertile, Rumbling, Cast-iron, Growling, Aching, Unbuttoned Bellybook.* New York: Grossman, 1972.

Underwood, E. J. *Trace Elements in Human and Animal Nutrition.* New York: Academic Press, 1971.

Books for Further Reading

Abrahamson, E. M. and Pezet, A. W. *Body, Mind, and Sugar.* New York: Pyramid Publications, 1971.

Adams, R. and Murray, F. *Megavitamin Therapy.* (on low blood sugar) New York: Larchmont Books, 1973.

Carson, Rachel. *Silent Spring.* New York: Fawcett World Library, 1973.

Cheraskin, Ringsdorf and Clark. *Diet and Disease.* Emmaus, Pa.: Rodale Press, 1968.

Committee on Food Protection. *Chemicals Used in Food Processing,* Washington, D.C.: National Academy of Sciences, 1965.

Cooper, Paulette. *The Medical Detectives.* New York; David McKay, 1973.

Davis, Adelle. *Let's Cook It Right.* New York: New American Library, 1970.

________*Let's Eat Right to Keep Fit.* New York: New American Library, 1970.

———*Let's Get Well,* New York: New American Library, 1972.

Department of Agriculture. *Safe Use of Agricultural and Household Pesticides.* (SDA Handbook, 321).

Dubos, Rene. *So Human an Animal.* (health consciousness) New York: Charles Scribner's Sons, 1968.

———*The Mirage of Health.* (health as an idealized condition) New York: Harper & Row, 1971.

Fredericks, C. *Eating Right For You,* New York: Grosset & Dunlap, 1972.

von Hilsheimer, George. *Understanding Young People in Trouble.* Washington, D.C.: Acropolis Books, 1974.

Himwich, Harold E. *Biochemistry, Schizophrenias, and Affective Illnesses.* Baltimore: Williams & Wilkins, 1971.

Hunter, Beatrice Trum. *Consumer Beware! Your Food and What's Been Done to It.* New York: Bantam Books, 1972.

Jacobson, Michael. *Eater's Digest.* (factbook of food additives) Garden City, N.Y.: Doubleday, 1972.

Longgood, William. *The Poisons in Your Food.* New York: Pyramid Publications, 1969.

Pauling, Linus. *Vitamin C and the Common Cold.* New York: Bantam Books, 1971.

Porter, J. W. G. and Rolls, B. A., eds. *Proteins in Human Nutrition.* New York: Academic Press, 1973.

Rodale, J. I. and staff. *The Health Finder.* Emmaus, Pa.: Rodale Books, 1954.

Spain, David M. and Kole, J. *Post Mortem.* Garden City, N.Y.: Doubleday, 1974.

Turner, James. *Chemical Feast.* New York: Grossman, 1970.

Watson, George. *Nutrition and Your Mind.* New York: Harper & Row, 1972. 1972.

Williams, Roger J. *Nutrition in a Nutshell.* Garden City, N.Y.: Doubleday, 1962.

Yudkin, John. *Sweet and Dangerous.* New York: Peter H. Wyden, 1972.

Canadian Schizophrenia Foundation Publications: Regina, Saskatchewan.

Cott, A. *Orthomolecular Approach to the Treatment of Learning Disabilities.*

———*Orthomolecular Treatment: A Biochemical Approach to Treatment of Schizophrenia.*

Galton, Lawrence. *Why Young Adults Crack Up.*

Green, R. *Sub Clinical Pellagra, the Hidden Disease.*

Hawkins, David. *The Development of an Integrated Community System for the Treatment of Schizophrenia.*

Hoffer, A. *Megavitamin B-3 Therapy for Schizophrenia.*

Hoffer, Cott, Ward, Hawkins, Green and Kowalson. *Doctors Speak on the Orthomolecular Approach.*

Kahan, F. H. *How to Judge a Mental Hospital.*

________*In Search of Therapy, a Program for Public Action.*

________*What to Do If You Have a Troubled Child.*

________*Which Treatment Should a Schizophrenic Seek?*

Newbold, H. *How One Psychiatrist Began Using Niacin.*

Osmond, H. *The Medical Model in Psychiatry.*

Pauling, Linus. *Orthomolecular Psychiatry.*

Rimland, B. *Freud Is Dead.*

Report on the C.S.F. International Conference. *Research and Troubled Children.*

Saskatoon Branch, D.S.F. *Favorite Recipes for Hypoglycemics and High Protein Diets.*

Index

Name Index

A

B

C

D

E

F

G

H

M

N

O

T

U

V

Subject Index

B

C

I

N

O

P

Q

R

S

T

U

V

W

X

Y

Z